FOCUS Psychiatry Review

Volume 2, DSM-5® Revised Edition

FOCUS Editors

Deborah J. Hales, M.D.
Mark Hyman Rapaport, M.D.

Contributing to *FOCUS Psychiatry Review* Volume 2, DSM-5® Revised Edition

Robert J. Boland, M.D.
J. Michael Bostwick, M.D.
John H. Coverdale, M.D.
Arden D. Dingle, M.D.
Laura Fochtmann, M.D.
Suzanne Garfinkle, M.D.
James W. Jefferson, M.D.
Martin H. Leamon, M.D.
Vishal Madaan, M.D.
Annette M. Matthews, M.D.
David W. Preven, M.D.
Rima Styra, M.D.
Lowell D. Tong, M.D.
Marcia L. Verduin, M.D.
Eric R. Williams, M.D.
Isaac K. Wood, M.D.
Joel Yager, M.D.

AMERICAN PSYCHIATRIC ASSOCIATION

FOCUS Psychiatry Review

Volume 2, DSM-5® Revised Edition

A workbook with questions covering the
ABPN outline of topics for recertification:

Anxiety Disorders
Child and Adolescent Psychiatry
Disorders of Sleep, Eating, and Sex
Ethics and Professionalism
Genetics and Genomics
Geriatric Psychiatry
Mood Disorders
Obsessive-Compulsive Disorder
Personality and Temperament
Posttraumatic Stress Disorder and Disaster Psychiatry
Psychopharmacology
Psychosomatic Medicine
Psychotherapy
Schizophrenia
Substance Use Disorders

Editors

Deborah J. Hales, M.D.

Mark Hyman Rapaport, M.D.

AMERICAN
PSYCHIATRIC
ASSOCIATION

Note: The authors have worked to ensure that all information in this book concerning drug dosages, schedules, and routes of administration is accurate as of the time of publication and consistent with standards set by the U.S. Food and Drug Administration and the general medical community. As medical research and practice advance, however, therapeutic standards may change. For this reason and because human and mechanical errors sometimes occur, we recommend that readers follow the advice of a physician who is directly involved in their care or the care of a member of their family.

Manufactured in the United States of America on acid-free paper

American Psychiatric Association

1000 Wilson Boulevard Arlington, VA 22209-3901 www.psych.org

ISBN 978-0-89042-462-9

Contents

Introduction

In today's world it is hard to keep up with the explosive growth in knowledge. Psychiatric practice is rapidly improving thanks to developments in evidence-based practice and advances in neuroscience research. The editors of *FOCUS* developed the *FOCUS Psychiatry Review* as an aid for psychiatrists in lifelong learning in the field. This workbook contains 400 board-type multiple-choice questions developed from *FOCUS*'s annual assessments that can help psychiatrists prepare for examinations and identify areas for further study. The questions, developed by the *FOCUS* Board, are consistent in form and process with the questions used by high-stakes examinations. They cover important clinical areas of psychiatric practice and closely follow the American Board of Psychiatry and Neurology (ABPN) outline of topics for the recertification examination in psychiatry. This version of *FOCUS Psychiatry Review*, Volume 2, DSM-5 Revised Edition, was updated in January 2014 for consistency with DSM-5.

The *FOCUS Psychiatry Review* is designed to test current knowledge and its clinical application. The workbook is flexible in format, allowing readers to use the educational approach that works best for them. Readers can review resource materials prior to answering questions, or they can use the workbook to review the references listed in the critiques after scoring test sections. A minimum performance of 70% is required. This material is self-scored.

The workbook will be useful for anyone committed to lifelong learning in the field—psychiatric residents, practicing psychiatrists, and psychiatrists preparing for examinations.

- The *FOCUS Psychiatry Review* contains 400 clinical questions that can be used to study or identify areas of strength and weakness.
- It provides up-to-date critiques and current references to facilitate further study.
- It is a complementary component to a larger overall program of lifelong learning for the psychiatrist who wants to keep current in the field.

This volume covers the following topics:

Anxiety Disorders
Child and Adolescent Psychiatry
Disorders of Sleep, Eating, and Sex
Ethics and Professionalism
Genetics and Genomics
Geriatric Psychiatry
Mood Disorders
Obsessive-Compulsive Disorder
Personality and Temperament
Posttraumatic Stress Disorder and Disaster Psychiatry
Psychopharmacology
Psychosomatic Medicine
Psychotherapy
Schizophrenia
Substance Use Disorders

The *FOCUS Psychiatry Review* provides up to 50 hours of Continuing Medical Education Credit.

American Psychiatric Association (APA) is accredited by ACCME to provide continuing medical education for physicians. APA designates this enduring material for a maximum of 50 AMA PRA Category 1 Credits.™ Physicians should claim only the credit commensurate with the extent of their participation in the activity.

Educational Objectives

At the completion of the activity, participants will

1) have an increased understanding of new developments in psychiatric diagnosis and treatment;
2) be aware of resources available for learning more about these developments; and
3) recognize areas of strength and areas where more study is needed.

FOCUS Editors and Editorial Board Contributing to *FOCUS Psychiatry Review* Volume 2, DSM-5® Revised Edition

Disclosure of Financial Interests or Other Affiliations With Commercial Organizations

Deborah J. Hales, M.D.
Director, American Psychiatric Association Division of Education, Arlington, Virginia
No financial affiliations with commercial organizations

Mark Hyman Rapaport, M.D.
Chairman, Department of Psychiatry and Behavioral Sciences, Emory University School of Medicine; Chief of Psychiatric Services at Emory Healthcare in Atlanta, Georgia
No financial affiliations with commercial organizations

Robert J. Boland, M.D.
Associate Professor of Psychiatry and Human Behavior, Division of Biology and Medicine, Brown University, Providence, Rhode Island
No financial affiliations with commercial organizations

J. Michael Bostwick, M.D.
Assistant Professor of Psychiatry, Mayo Medical School Consultant, Department of Psychiatry and Psychology, Mayo Clinic and Foundation, Rochester, Minnesota
No financial affiliations with commercial organizations

John H. Coverdale, M.D.
Associate Professor of Psychiatry and Medical Ethics, Baylor College of Medicine, Houston, Texas
No financial affiliations with commercial organizations

Arden D. Dingle, M.D.
Associate Professor, Department of Psychiatry and Behavioral Sciences, Training Director, Child and Adolescent Psychiatry, Emory University School of Medicine, Atlanta, Georgia
No financial affiliations with commercial organizations

Laura Fochtmann, M.D.
Practice Guidelines Medical Editor, American Psychiatric Association; Professor, Department of Psychiatry and Behavioral Sciences, Department of Pharmacological Sciences, and Department of Emergency Medicine, Stony Brook University, Stony Brook, New York
No financial affiliations with commercial organizations

Suzanne Garfinkle, M.D., M.Sc.
Fellow in Child and Adolescent Psychiatry, Mount Sinai School of Medicine, New York, New York
No financial affiliations with commercial organizations

James W. Jefferson, M.D.
Clinical Professor of Psychiatry, University of Wisconsin Medical School; Distinguished Senior Scientist, Madison Institute of Medicine, Inc.; Director, Healthcare Technology Systems, Inc., Madison, Wisconsin
Grant/Research Support: Bristol-Myers Squibb, GlaxoSmithKline, Lilly, Novartis, Pfizer, Wyeth. Consultant: GlaxoSmithKline. Lecture Honoraria: Bristol-Myers Squibb, GlaxoSmithKline, Lilly, Wyeth Stock Shareholder: Bristol-Myers Squibb, GlaxoSmithKline, SciClone. Principal: Healthcare Technology Systems, Inc.

Martin H. Leamon, M.D.
Associate Professor of Clinical Psychiatry, University of California-Davis, Sacramento
No financial affiliations with commercial organizations

Vishal Madaan, M.D.
Director, Child and Adolescent Psychopharmacology, and Staff Child and Adolescent Psychiatrist, Creighton University Medical Center, Omaha, Nebraska
No financial affiliations with commercial organizations

Annette M. Matthews, M.D.
Psychiatrist, Portland Veterans Affairs Medical Center, Portland, Oregon; Assistant Professor of Psychiatry, Oregon, Health and Science University, Portland, Oregon
No financial affiliations with commercial organizations

David W. Preven, M.D.
Clinical Professor, Department of Behavioral Sciences and Psychiatry, Albert Einstein College of Medicine, Montefiore Medical Center, Bronx, New York
Speaker: Pfizer, Forest

Rima Styra, M.D.
Toronto General Hospital, University Health Network; Associate Professor, Department of Psychiatry, Toronto, Ontario, Canada
No financial affiliations with commercial organizations

Lowell D. Tong, M.D.
Associate Chair of Education, Department of Psychiatry, University of California San Francisco School of Medicine
No financial affiliations with commercial organizations

Marcia L. Verduin, M.D.
Associate Professor of Psychiatry, Assistant Dean for Students, University of Central Florida College of Medicine, Orlando, Florida
Grant/Research Support: Robert Wood Johnson Foundation

Eric R. Williams, M.D.
Assistant Professor of Child and Adolescent Psychiatry, University of South Carolina School of Medicine, Charleston, South Carolina
No financial affiliations with commercial organizations

Isaac K. Wood, M.D.
Associate Professor of Psychiatry and Pediatrics, Associate Dean of Student Activities, Director of Medical Student Education in Psychiatry, Virginia Commonwealth University School of Medicine, Richmond, Virginia
No financial affiliations with commercial organizations

Joel Yager, M.D.
Professor, Department of Psychiatry, School of Medicine, University of Colorado; Emeritus Professor, Department of Psychiatry, University of New Mexico School of Medicine and Department of Psychiatry and Biobehavioral Sciences at the David Geffen School of Medicine at UCLA
No financial affiliations with commercial organizations

Kristen Moeller
Editorial Staff *FOCUS Psychiatry Review*, Director of Continuing Medical Education, American Psychiatric Association, Arlington, Virginia
Reports no competing interests

Disclosure of Unapproved or Investigational Use of a Product

FOCUS examination questions may contain information on off-label uses of particular medications. Off-label use of medications by individual physicians is permitted and common. Decisions about off-label use can be guided by the evidence provided in the scientific literature and by clinical experience.

To obtain Continuing Medical Education Credit, complete and send this page to:

American Psychiatric Association
Department of CME
1000 Wilson Blvd., Suite 1825
Arlington, VA 22209
Fax: 703-907-7849
E-mail: educme@psych.org

Begin date: January 2011
Review and update: January 2014
End date: January 2017

AMERICAN PSYCHIATRIC ASSOCIATION

FOCUS Psychiatry Review: Volume 2, DSM-5® Revised Edition

I have participated for______________ hours (up to 50) in completion of this CME activity.

I have self-scored the material and obtained a passing grade of 70% or better.

Date of completion: ________________________________

Name (please print): ____ Degree _________

Address: ____

Address: ____

City/State/Zip: ____

E-mail: ____ Fax ___________________________

Please send my certificate by: Mail _________ Fax _________ E-mail _________

1. The quality of the *FOCUS Psychiatry Review* workbook was excellent.
   Strongly agree_________Agree_________Disagree_________Strongly disagree_________

2. The *FOCUS Psychiatry Review* workbook was useful to me in preparing for examinations.
   Strongly agree_________Agree_________Disagree_________Strongly disagree_________

3. The workbook was useful in helping me understand my areas of strength and weakness.
   Strongly agree_________Agree_________Disagree_________Strongly disagree_________

4. The workbook will be helpful to me in my clinical practice.
   Strongly agree_________Agree_________Disagree_________Strongly disagree_________

5. The material in the *FOCUS Psychiatry Review* was presented without bias.
   Strongly agree_________Agree_________Disagree_________Strongly disagree_________

6. The questions were: too hard _________, just right _________, too easy _________.

Comments:

____

____

SECTION 1
Multiple-Choice Questions

1 An 18-year-old woman is brought to the emergency department after collapsing at a party. She appears delirious and confused, with a temperature of 104°F. The friends who brought her to the emergency room say that she might have taken some pills. She was talking about feeling blissful and dancing a lot until she collapsed. Which of the following is the most likely drug ingested?

A. Methylenedioxymethamphetamine (MDMA).
B. Ketamine.
C. Flunitrazepam.
D. Gamma-hydroxybutyrate (GHB).

2 Which one of these terms defines the most common form of genetic variation observed in the genome?

A. Short tandem repeat.
B. Single nucleotide polymorphism (SNP).
C. Haplotype.
D. Allele.
E. Variable number of tandem repeat.

3 In adults, which of the following disorders is diagnosed in nearly equal numbers in men and women?

A. Generalized anxiety disorder.
B. Panic disorder.
C. Specific phobia.
D. Obsessive-compulsive disorder (OCD).
E. Agoraphobia.

4 Which of the following selective serotonin reuptake inhibitors (SSRIs) is most likely to be "self-tapering," thereby decreasing the chances of withdrawal effects?

A. Citalopram.
B. Escitalopram.
C. Fluoxetine.
D. Paroxetine.
E. Sertraline.

5 Dialectical behavior therapy (DBT) was developed specifically for the treatment symptoms associated with which one of the following personality disorders?

A. Antisocial.
B. Borderline.
C. Avoidant.
D. Obsessive-compulsive.
E. Histrionic.

6 The most common cause of treatment failure in HIV/AIDS patients on antiretroviral medications is that most patients:

A. Have infections that are resistant to most available medications.
B. Fail to maintain the required adherence to the medication regime.
C. Do not start treatment until the infection is in the terminal stages.
D. Refuse to participate in medical treatment and take medications.
E. Have such severe side effects that medications cannot be used.

---

7 Advanced paternal age is a well-established risk factor for which of the following psychiatric illnesses?

A. Schizophrenia.
B. Substance dependence.
C. Major depressive disorder.
D. Generalized anxiety disorder.

---

8 A 21-year-old woman presents with questions about her risk of developing schizophrenia. She is worried because her 18-year-old brother has recently been diagnosed with schizophrenia and required hospitalization for psychosis. There are no other family members who have a history of schizophrenia. Having a sibling with schizophrenia increases a person's risk of developing schizophrenia by approximately what amount?

A. The sibling is no more likely to develop schizophrenia.
B. The risk of developing schizophrenia for a sibling is 50%.
C. The risk of developing schizophrenia for a sibling is 10-fold.
D. The risk of developing schizophrenia is 30-fold.
E. It is almost certain the sibling will develop schizophrenia.

---

9 An 18-year-old female has high scores on scales of the personality traits of Harm Avoidance and Reward Dependence. On the basis of these personality traits, she is at HIGHEST risk for developing which one of the following disorders?

A. Anorexia nervosa.
B. Major depressive disorder.
C. Obsessive-compulsive disorder.
D. Schizophrenia.
E. Social anxiety disorder.

---

10 A 40-year-old man with a 20-year history of heroin dependence and high tolerance is admitted to the hospital for IV antibiotic treatment of bacterial endocarditis. To prevent opioid withdrawal, considering his opioid tolerance, he is prescribed a moderately high dose of buprenorphine. He is just beginning to experience withdrawal symptoms before the first buprenorphine dose, but shortly thereafter, his anxiety, muscle aches, and rhinorrhea worsen. At this point, the best option would be to:

A. Increase the dose of buprenorphine.
B. Decrease the dose of buprenorphine.
C. Change to methadone.
D. Add a benzodiazepine.
E. Add naltrexone.

---

11 A 35-year-old man with obsessive-compulsive disorder presents for treatment. He would prefer not using medication because of possible side effects. Which of the following psychotherapies would be the treatment of choice for his disorder?

A. Supportive psychotherapy.
B. Exposure with response prevention.
C. Hypnotherapy.
D. Interpersonal therapy.
E. Psychodynamic psychotherapy.

12 An adolescent with mild intellectual disability continues to be significantly depressed despite actively participating in psychotherapy for several months. Which of the following is the best clinical option?

A. Start treatment with an atypical antipsychotic.
B. Start treatment with an SSRI.
C. Change psychotherapeutic approaches.
D. Implement intense behavioral management.

13 Personalities characterized by the traits of persistence, perfectionism, and decreased flexibility in "set shifting" (i.e., the ability to move back and forth between tasks, operations, or mental sets) are associated with which of the following disorders?

A. Alcohol dependence in full-sustained remission.
B. Delusional disorder.
C. Anorexia nervosa.
D. Early Alzheimer's disease.
E. Traumatic brain injury.

14 Which of the following treatments is considered the best approach to managing a patient with panic disorder, unresponsive to initial treatments with an SSRI and a benzodiazepine?

A. Serotonin-norepinephrine reuptake inhibitor (SNRI).
B. Buspirone.
C. Atypical antipsychotic.
D. Another SSRI.
E. Cognitive-behavioral therapy (CBT).

15 A 27-year-old man has borderline personality disorder, primarily manifested by an inability to control his urges to hurt himself. As a result, when frustrated, he will frequently superficially cut his wrists. Which of the following medications has been found to be most helpful in curbing this behavior?

A. Olanzapine.
B. Fluoxetine.
C. Clonazepam.
D. Divalproex.
E. Naloxone.

16 A visibly pregnant 29-year-old woman presents seeking treatment for oxycodone dependence. Because of her pregnancy, she wants to stop using all drugs and does not want to take any medications. She went through untreated opiate withdrawal in the past when she couldn't get any pills, and although it was very uncomfortable, she thinks she could do it again with intensive social support and counseling. At this point, the best treatment recommendation would be to initiate:

A. Methadone maintenance.
B. Methadone-assisted withdrawal.
C. Clonidine-naltrexone-assisted withdrawal.
D. Buprenorphine maintenance.
E. Daily clinic visits to provide support.

17 A 38-year-old female patient with schizophrenia has been treated with haloperidol and risperidone at different times in the past. Currently, she exhibits a nonrhythmical hyperkinetic movement disorder of the lips and jaw. The movement disorder most likely consistent with this finding is:

A. Akathisia (motor restlessness).
B. Parkinsonian's tremor.
C. Tardive dyskinesia.
D. Tardive dystonia.

18 Which one of the following dimensions assessed on the Temperament and Character Inventory (TCI) is MOST likely to increase with age?

A. Cooperativeness.
B. Harm avoidance.
C. Persistence.
D. Reward dependence.
E. Self-transcendence.

19 A 74-year-old man presents with a history of rapidly progressive cognitive decline with ataxia, multifocal myoclonic jerks, and visual field cut. MRI reveals increased T2 and FLAIR signal intensity in the basal ganglia. Which of the following is the most likely diagnosis?

A. Alzheimer's dementia.
B. Huntington's chorea.
C. Creutzfeldt-Jakob disease.
D. Vascular dementia.
E. Lewy body disease.

20 Genome-wide association studies (GWAS) have implicated regions of which chromosome in autism spectrum disorders (ASD)?

A. Chromosome 1.
B. Chromosome 5.
C. Chromosome 8.
D. Chromosome 22.

21 A 16-year-old woman presents with fatigue and dehydration. On physical examination, she is noted to have swollen salivary glands and calluses on her knuckles. She is also hypokalemic. These findings are most consistent with which of the following diagnoses?

A. Chronic fatigue syndrome.
B. Bulimia nervosa.
C. Obsessive-compulsive disorder.
D. Anorexia nervosa.
E. Rumination disorder.

22 A 21-year-old college student is seen in the university counseling center because of relationship problems. He has had one serious relationship with a woman that lasted about 6 months. He terminated the relationship because he discovered that the woman was seeing someone else. Although he wants to engage in a new relationship, he is extremely reluctant, stating: "Women just can't be trusted." Which of the following BEST describes this thinking error?

A. Arbitrary inference.
B. Dichotomous thinking.
C. Magnification.
D. Overgeneralization.
E. Selective abstraction.

23 A 40-year-old patient is diagnosed with Alzheimer's disease (AD). Which of the following genes is associated with this very early form of Alzheimer's disease?

A. Presenilin 1.
B. Presenilin 2.
C. Apo E2.
D. Apo 3.
E. Apo 4.

24 During an interview of a patient with a substance use disorder, the therapist asks the patient about the pros and cons of specific behaviors, explores the patient's goals and associated ambivalence about reaching those goals, and listens reflectively to the patient's response. This treatment approach is most consistent with:

A. Cognitive-behavioral therapy.
B. Contingency management.
C. Interpersonal therapy.
D. Motivational enhancement therapy.
E. Psychodynamic psychotherapy.

25 Which of the following antidepressants has the greatest body of evidence for efficacy in treating major depressive disorder in children and adolescents?

A. Citalopram.
B. Fluoxetine.
C. Fluvoxamine.
D. Sertraline.
E. Paroxetine.

26 A city is attacked by terrorists intermittently over a 3-week period. There is no indication that the attacks will stop. Which of the following interventions is most likely to be effective in lowering the risk of developing posttraumatic stress disorder (PTSD) in the months following exposure?

A. Educating the public about symptoms of PTSD.
B. Evacuating the most vulnerable population.
C. Limiting exposure to media coverage of the attacks.
D. Providing psychological debriefing to survivors.
E. Reestablishing a relative sense of safety.

27 Defining high-risk situations, covert antecedents, and stimulus control techniques are a focus of which of the following therapeutic modalities?

A. Brief psychodynamic psychotherapy.
B. Cognitive-behavioral therapy.
C. Supportive therapy.
D. Interpersonal therapy.
E. Relapse prevention therapy.

28 A 42-year-old patient with schizophrenia presents to the emergency department with confusion and agitation following an overdose of antipsychotic medication. The patient has a temperature of 101.7 degrees Fahrenheit, blood pressure of 140/80 mm Hg, and pulse of 112. Physical examination reveals hot, dry skin, dilated pupils, and decreased bowel sounds. This patient's symptoms are most likely caused by medication effects at which of the following receptors?

A. Muscarinic cholinergic.
B. Nicotinic cholinergic.
C. α_1-adrenergic.
D. Histaminergic.
E. Dopaminergic.

29 Which of the following therapies for borderline personality disorder incorporates psychoeducation about the illness, emotional management skills training, and behavior skills training?

A. Mentalization-based therapy.
B. Schema-focused therapy.
C. Trauma-focused cognitive-behavior therapy.
D. Eye movement desensitization and reprocessing.
E. Systems Training for Emotional Predictability and Problem Solving (STEPPS).

30 When managing a chronically suicidal patient, respecting the patient's preference to remain at home and not be admitted to the psychiatric unit for additional care reflects which of the following ethical principles?

A. Autonomy.
B. Beneficience.
C. Nonmaleficence.
D. Egalitarianism.

31 A 12-year-old boy is hospitalized after a serious suicide attempt. His parents report that they noticed a difference in his behavior about a year ago. He became increasingly withdrawn; he was preoccupied with mythical creatures; his academic performance declined significantly; and he had difficulty sleeping and a decreased appetite. Over the past 2 months, he has seemed progressively worse. He has demonstrated both persecutory and somatic delusions and has reported he hears voices telling him to "beware—they are watching you—you're a naughty little boy." Today he heard a voice telling him that he was "rotting inside," and in response, he attempted to hang himself. On examination, he denies a mood disturbance. His thinking is illogical and nonlinear. What is the most likely diagnosis?

A. Bipolar disorder.
B. Attention-deficit/hyperactivity disorder.
C. Schizophrenia.
D. Major depressive disorder.
E. Autism spectrum disorder.

32 Individuals with two copies of which one of the following genes develop Alzheimer's disease (AD) eight times more frequently than those without it?

A. APOE E1.
B. APOE E2.
C. APOE E3.
D. APOE E4.
E. APOE E5.

33 In the Alternative DSM-5 Model for Personality Disorders (DSM-5 Section III), personality disorder trait domains of psychopathology and their polar opposites are described with a listing of personality facets under each domain. In addition to negative affectivity (vs. emotional stability), detachment (vs. extraversion), disinhibition (vs. conscientiousness), and psychoticism (vs. lucidity), which of the following is included as the trait domain polar opposite of antagonism?

A. Agreeableness.
B. Brightness.
C. Happiness.
D. Humor.
E. Optimism.

34 A 32-year-old man with a history of bipolar I disorder has been off all medication for more than 6 months. He currently presents with symptoms consistent with a moderately severe major depressive episode. Which of the following has the best evidence as a pharmacologic treatment for him?

A. Clonazepam and lithium.
B. Olanzapine and fluoxetine.
C. Lithium and paroxetine.
D. Valproate and fluoxetine.
E. Bupropion alone.

35 Which of the following psychiatric disorders confers the highest genetic relative risk for first-degree relatives?

A. Panic disorder.
B. Alcoholism.
C. Major depression.
D. Bipolar disorder.
E. Schizophrenia.

36 A 35-year-old woman began taking citalopram, 20 mg, daily about 3 months ago when she presented with symptoms consistent with panic disorder. On the current regimen, her symptoms are under control. Until her recent episode of illness, she has had no other history of psychiatric symptoms, and there is no family history of psychiatric illness. How long should she continue this medication?

A. 4 weeks.
B. 3 months.
C. 1 year.
D. 3 years.
E. Indefinitely.

37 On the basis of the results of the National Institute of Mental Health funded multisite Multimodal Treatment Study of Children with Attention Deficit-Hyperactivity Disorder (MTA), which of the following interventions was proven to be the MOST effective in treating the majority of children with ADHD?

A. Medication alone.
B. Medication with an intensive summer treatment program.
C. Medication with community referral.
D. Medication with parent training.
E. Medication with school consultation.

38 Which of the following personality disorders (PDs) is most common in the biological relatives of patients with schizophrenia?

A. Schizoid.
B. Paranoid.
C. Schizotypal.
D. Histrionic.
E. Antisocial.

39 Which of the following symptoms is a diagnostic feature of atypical depression?

A. Insomnia.
B. Weight loss.
C. Suicidal ideation.
D. Mood reactivity.
E. Inappropriate guilt.

40 A 33-year-old man whose bipolar I disorder has been well controlled on medication presents to the emergency department with severe left upper quadrant pain radiating to his back, nausea, and vomiting. Which medication is most likely contributing to these symptoms?

A. Lamotrigine.
B. Lithium.
C. Olanzapine.
D. Valproate.
E. Ziprasidone.

41 A sniper attacks a city hall building, killing 13 individuals and significantly injuring another 12 before he takes his own life. Therapists from the local mental health clinic are dispatched to the scene to provide psychological debriefing to prevent PTSD symptoms. Using an evidence-based framework, what is the most likely impact of this intervention on direct survivors?

A. It will be ineffective or harmful to the direct survivors.
B. It will decrease the probability of developing PTSD symptoms.
C. It will decrease the severity of PTSD symptoms.
D. It will decrease the time period for recovery from PTSD symptoms.
E. It will delay the onset of PTSD symptoms.

42 You are asked to write 22 questions for a board-type examination in less than 4 weeks. Your first thought is, "I will never be able to get all those questions written in such a short time!" You ignore the fact that you seem to have been able to be successful at this several times before. From a cognitive therapy perspective, what is the best description of this type of thinking?

A. Magnification.
B. Minimization.
C. Personalization.
D. Selective abstraction.
E. Catastrophic thinking.

43 A patient with four or more mood disturbances within a single year that meet both the duration and symptom criteria for major depressive, mixed, manic, and/or hypomanic episodes, demarcated by remission or switch to opposite polarity, meets the DSM-5 criteria for which of the following disorders?

A. Bipolar disorder with rapid cycling specifier.
B. Unspecified bipolar and related disorder.
C. Cyclothymic disorder.
D. Schizoaffective disorder (bipolar type).

44 Which of the following disorders has been shown to have the greatest degree of heritability?

A. Schizophrenia.
B. Autism.
C. Bipolar disorder.
D. Alcoholism.
E. ADHD.

45 A 42-year-old man presents to a psychiatrist 6 months after a motor vehicle accident. He has difficulty sleeping because he has frequent nightmares about the accident. He has not been able to drive since the accident, and his wife usually drives for him. Even then, he finds it very difficult to be in a car, often panicking if another car is near them on the road. Which of the following medications would be the most appropriate for this man?

A. Propranolol.
B. Nortriptyline.
C. Clonazepam.
D. Olanzapine.
E. Sertraline.

46 A patient presents with involuntary frowning, blinking, grimacing, and choreoathetoid movements of the upper extremities after several years of antipsychotic medication treatment. Which one of the following is the most likely diagnosis?

A. Akinesia.
B. Akathisia.
C. Acute dystonia.
D. Parkinsonism.
E. Tardive dyskinesia.

47 Which of the following diagnoses is most common among individuals with bulimia nervosa?

A. General anxiety disorder.
B. Obsessive-compulsive disorder.
C. Alcohol use disorder.
D. Major depressive disorder.
E. Intermittent explosive disorder.

48 A 31-year-old man is admitted to an inpatient psychiatric unit after a suicide attempt. Past records show a history of dependence on multiple substances. He sleeps poorly and the next day paces around the unit, restless and grumpy. He is tachycardic at 112 beats per minutes, his palms and forehead are sweaty, and his hands are showing a coarse tremor. When asked, the patient says he feels anxious. The most likely diagnosis is:

A. Alcohol withdrawal.
B. Nicotine withdrawal.
C. Opioid withdrawal.
D. Cannabis withdrawal.
E. Methamphetamine withdrawal.

49 A 28-year-old woman with an identical twin is diagnosed with major depressive disorder. She asks you to comment on the chance her sister will develop the same illness. Which of the following is the best response regarding the genetic basis of depression?

A. "Major depression is a genetic illness. Your sister will definitely develop it as well."
B. "While schizophrenia is quite heritable, there is only a slightly increased risk that your sister will become depressed."
C. "The likelihood of identical twins sharing an affective illness is high."
D. "Although there may be some genetic basis for affective illness, it is one's childhood environment that determines whether illness will manifest."
E. "Your sister's risk of developing depression is the same as any other sibling."

50 For the detection and identification of delirium in medically ill patients, the best strategy to employ is:

A. Enhanced EEG monitoring.
B. Serum and urine lab tests.
C. Revised Mini Mental State Exam.
D. Specific neuroimaging.
E. Observation and rating scales.

51 A 58-year-old man with a history of alcohol dependence and mild dementia presents to the hospital for a liver biopsy because of suspected alcoholic hepatitis. He complains of severe anxiety about having the procedure done and requests "something for my nerves." Which of the following benzodiazepines is safest to administer?

A. Alprazolam.
B. Chlordiazepoxide.
C. Diazepam.
D. Oxazepam.
E. Clonazepam.

52 A 35-year-old patient with schizophrenia has had four serious suicide attempts over the past year despite consistent treatment with haloperidol decanoate. Given the patient's recent suicide attempts, what would be the BEST next medication trial?

A. Olanzapine.
B. Quetiapine.
C. Fluphenazine decanoate.
D. Long-acting risperidone.
E. Clozapine.

53 Cognitive-behavioral therapy (CBT) is an effective, specific treatment for generalized anxiety disorder (GAD). Emerging evidence suggests that which ONE of the following is similarly effective in treatment for GAD?

A. Dialectical behavioral therapy (DBT).
B. Interpersonal psychotherapy (IPT).
C. Psychoanalysis.
D. Short-term psychodynamic psychotherapy.
E. Supportive psychotherapy.

54 A 13-year-old boy is seen for outbursts of aggression when he is denied access to food. He is known to have an intellectual disability. His mother reports that as an infant he had poor muscle tone and a weak suck reflex. He is morbidly obese, is short for his age, and has significantly underdeveloped genitalia. His mother reports that he constantly eats to the point that they have put locks on the kitchen cabinets and refrigerator. Despite this, he will search for food in garbage cans. Lately, when he is denied food, he will have outbursts of anger in which he hits himself or others and throws objects. Which of the following BEST describes the genetic abnormality responsible for this boy's condition?

A. Williams syndrome.
B. Angelman's syndrome.
C. Prader-Willi syndrome.
D. Klinefelter's syndrome.
E. Down syndrome.

55 Which of the following statements represents the most reasonable conclusion that can be drawn from the National Institute of Mental Health's (NIMH) Clinical Antipsychotic Trials of Intervention Effectiveness (CATIE) study?

A. Second-generation antipsychotics offer no benefit in schizophrenia over first-generation antipsychotics.
B. Clinicians should consider both first- and second-generation antipsychotics when treating schizophrenia.
C. Antipsychotic medications appear to be less efficacious than previously thought.
D. Second-generation antipsychotics demonstrate little difference from one another.
E. When given in idealized settings, most antipsychotics are roughly equivalent in efficacy.

56 Poststroke depression is most commonly associated with cerebrovascular disease involving the:

A. Anterior communicating artery.
B. Anterior cerebral artery.
C. Middle cerebral artery.
D. Posterior communicating artery.
E. Basilar artery.

57 Which symptom of PTSD has shown promise of improvement by medications that suppress noradrenergic activity?

A. Hypervigilance.
B. Inability to recall an important aspect of the trauma.
C. Markedly diminished interest.
D. Feelings of detachment.
E. Avoidance of activities related to the trauma.

58 A 19-year-old college student comes to the clinic with a complaint of feeling "depressed and worried." He states that he may fail his English class because he is nervous about the public-speaking assignment. When he thinks about it, he feels nervous, his heart races, his palms become sweaty, and he becomes short of breath. He endorses a depressed mood because "I feel like I'm wasting my parents' money." He skipped his last three English classes because he knew it would be his turn to give a speech. He attends his other classes with no difficulty. The most likely diagnosis is:

A. Panic disorder.
B. Normal shyness.
C. Social anxiety disorder.
D. Agoraphobia.
E. Major depressive disorder.

59 A 47-year-old woman is brought for a psychiatric evaluation to assess recent changes in her behavior. Over the past 6 months, she has become increasingly disinhibited and impulsive in her behavior. Physical examination reveals mild dysarthria, dysphagia, and drooling. Slit lamp examination of the eyes indicates the presence of Kayser-Fleischer rings. Which of the following BEST describes the genetic basis for her illness?

A. Autosomal recessive.
B. Codominant.
C. Mitochondrial.
D. Polygenetic.
E. X-linked dominant.

60 A patient unconsciously perceives the therapist as having attributes associated with unpleasant interactions in the past. However, the therapist does not respond like the figure from the past, and over time, the old feelings become muted and the patient no longer needs to replay new relationships according to the old emotional script. Which of the following terms define this positive change in psychotherapy?

A. Exposure and response prevention.
B. Corrective emotional experience.
C. Reenactment of transference.
D. Shaping.
E. Strengthening ego defenses.

61 Which of the following is a risk factor for the development of psychosis while using cocaine?

A. Being female.
B. A greater duration of use during an episode
C. Nonintravenous use.
D. An elevated body mass index.
E. Being a first-time user of cocaine.

62 A 38-year-old man presents for treatment of PTSD after surviving a bridge collapse. He was driving on the crowded bridge when it suddenly collapsed, killing over 50 individuals and seriously injuring more. As part of the treatment, the therapist asks the patient to imagine that he is safely driving over a bridge. Which of the following best describes this therapeutic intervention?

A. Aversion therapy.
B. Dialectical behavioral therapy.
C. Exposure therapy.
D. Insight-oriented psychotherapy.
E. Interpersonal therapy.

63 Which of the following characteristics is/are present in patients with locked-in syndrome?

A. Persistent vegetative state.
B. Ability to experience a range of feelings.
C. Inability to recognize objects and people.
D. Severe depression and desire to die.

64 Which of the following interventions has been empirically validated through controlled and randomized trials as effective specifically for adolescents with conduct disorder?

A. Dialectical behavioral therapy.
B. Cognitive-behavioral therapy.
C. Interpersonal therapy.
D. Multisystemic therapy.
E. Psychoeducational therapy.

---

65 Which of the following is the mechanism of action of memantine, a medication used to slow cognitive decline in Alzheimer's dementia?

A. Cholinesterase inhibitor.
B. Dopamine receptor blocker.
C. Serotonergic reuptake inhibitor.
D. NMDA receptor antagonist.
E. GABA mimetic.

---

66 Which of the following genetic syndromes is caused by a 22q deletion and is clinically manifested by learning disabilities, palatal anomalies, cardiac defects, and often schizophrenia?

A. Fragile X syndrome.
B. Velocardiofacial (DiGeorge) syndrome.
C. Down syndrome.
D. Cri du chat syndrome.
E. Angelman syndrome.

---

67 Which of the following refers to an ethical decision-making approach that involves referring to similar, prior cases including legal precedents and applying reasoning from these cases to the case at hand?

A. Casuistry.
B. Ethical principles.
C. Expert opinion.
D. General ethical theory.
E. Tradition and current practice standards.

---

68 A 38-year-old woman with treatment-resistant schizophrenia is prescribed clozapine. Two weeks after beginning the medication, the woman begins to experience episodes of tachycardia with a heart rate over 120 beats per minute. Electrocardiogram reveals sustained sinus tachycardia with nonspecific ST-T wave changes and T wave flattening while standing and supine. Which of the following medications is most likely to alleviate her tachycardia without increasing chances of a serious adverse effect?

A. Atenolol.
B. Fludrocortisone.
C. Propranolol.
D. Verapamil.

---

69 The course of dementia in individuals with 16 or more years of education differs from those with lower educational attainment in which way?

A. Lower cognitive reserve.
B. Ability to maintain higher levels of cognitive functioning in early dementia.
C. Lower levels of cognitive function in early dementia.
D. Less disease burden when dementia is diagnosed.
E. Gentler slope of decline after dementia is diagnosed.

---

70 A 34-year-old woman with bipolar disorder has a body mass index of 31.2. To minimize the risk of aggravating this factor, which of the following medications would be most appropriate?

A. Lithium.
B. Clozapine.
C. Lamotrigine.
D. Olanzapine.
E. Divalproex.

71 According to the ethics primer of the American Psychiatric Association, which one of the following scenarios would most likely be considered a violation of the psychotherapeutic frame?

A. A patient is late to his psychotherapy session due to an upcoming deadline at work, but the therapist still charges the full amount for the session.
B. The therapist loses his office keys, but he lives across the street. Rather than cancel his appointments, he asks his wife and children to stay out for the day and sets up a temporary office in his living room.
C. A patient does not bring his check book to his final session of the month, when payment is due. The therapist interprets this act as an expression of ambivalence about the treatment and suggests this to the patient.
D. The therapist is diagnosed with end-stage cancer and informs his patient that owing to serious illness, he will be terminating his practice over the next month.
E. A grateful former patient wishes to donate money to the hospital with which his therapist is affiliated. Not wanting to handle the transaction himself, the therapist refers the patient to the hospital's development office.

72 Genetic linkage analysis studies provide information about which one of the following aspects of a gene:

A. Post-transitional processing.
B. Location.
C. Function.
D. Endophenotype.
E. Population frequency.

73 A 17-year-old man is brought to the emergency department after fighting with his girlfriend and ingesting a bottle of alprazolam. En route to the hospital, the girlfriend lost control of the car, causing the patient to hit his head against the windshield with loss of consciousness. Examination reveals the patient to be in stupor, with respiratory depression and coma. He has a 4-cm laceration over the right frontal area that is profusely bleeding. Which of the facts of the patient's presentation represents the greatest contraindication to the use of flumazenil?

A. Age of patient.
B. Central nervous system (CNS) depression.
C. Benzodiazepine use.
D. Possible traumatic brain injury.

74 A 42-year-old man is started on pharmacotherapy for treatment of major depressive disorder. Two weeks later, he presents with complaints of dry mouth, impaired ability to focus at close range, constipation, urinary hesitation, tachycardia, and sexual dysfunction. Which of the following medications is most likely to have caused this presentation?

A. Duloxetine.
B. Fluoxetine.
C. Imipramine.
D. Mirtazapine.
E. Venlafaxine.

75 Which of the following medications has been the only one to demonstrate a decrease in suicide risk?

A. Valproic acid.
B. Lithium.
C. Carbamazepine.
D. Lamotrigine.
E. Gabapentin.

76 A 34 year-old woman, who has been treated with an antidepressant for the past month, complains that she no longer gets relief from her back pain when she takes codeine, which has been prescribed by her orthopedist. Which one of the following antidepressants would be most likely to produce such an effect?

A. Escitalopram.
B. Sertraline.
C. Paroxetine.
D. Mirtazapin.
E. Buproprion.

77 Children of European descent with an early history of abuse have been found to be more likely to develop subsequent depression when they have a genetic polymorphism of which of the following neurotransmitter transporters?

A. Norepinephrine.
B. Dopamine.
C. Serotonin.
D. Glutamate.
E. GABA.

78 A 45-year-old woman was a witness to a motor vehicle accident that resulted in a number of fatalities. The images and the sounds of the accident greatly distressed her. The day after the accident she was seen by her family physician. The most appropriate next treatment step is:

A. Education and support about possible reactions that may occur.
B. Immediate referral to a mental health treatment program.
C. Treatment with an antidepressant.
D. Benzodiazepines as needed for sleep.
E. Critical incident debriefing.

79 A 48-year-old man with depression has been resistant to treatment with a variety of antidepressants. The decision is made to try him on a monoamine oxidase inhibitor (MAOI). In order to avoid serotonin syndrome, a washout period of at least 5 weeks is MOST indicated if he has been taking which antidepressant?

A. Bupropion.
B. Clomipramine.
C. Fluoxetine.
D. Paroxetine.
E. Venlafaxine.

80 Which of the following medications used to treat excessive daytime sleepiness associated with narcolepsy has also been abused as a "date rape" drug?

A. Sodium oxybate.
B. Modafinil.
C. Methylphenidate.
D. Selegiline.
E. Dextroamphetamine.

81 A patient recounts a story about getting angry with a store clerk. The therapist asks a factual question about the circumstance, inspiring rage in the patient, who finds him to be uncaring and seeking to blame her. The therapist says, "I wonder if what you're feeling right now is just like the feeling you had in the store, when you attributed the same uncaring attitude toward the clerk. These kinds of misreadings seem to make you very upset in many different settings." Which of the following most accurately describes this type of intervention?

A. Genetic interpretation.
B. Transference interpretation.
C. Clarification.
D. Observation.
E. Empathic validation.

82 Consideration of genotyping for human leukocyte antigen allele HLA-B 1502 has been recommended by the FDA prior to starting carbamazepine on patients with which of the following ancestries?

A. European.
B. African.
C. Asian.
D. Hispanic.
E. Native American.

83 An 84-year-old woman with a history of Alzheimer's disease presents to an emergency department after a fall. She had been experiencing difficulty sleeping at night for several months and was increasingly combative and suspicious of her daughter, with whom she lived. In developing a plan of treatment for this patient, which of the following principles is most appropriate to incorporate?

A. Adjust doses of medication slowly with long intervals between dose increments.
B. Prescribe small doses of several different medications rather than using one medication.
C. Use a long-acting injectable medication to aid adherence.
D. Use an initial loading dose of medication to speed response.

84 A 28-year-old woman with bipolar I disorder is pregnant for the first time. Throughout the pregnancy, she has been maintained on a mood stabilizer. At the time of birth, the baby is noted to have a cardiovascular defect consistent with Ebstein's anomaly. The mood stabilizer the woman was taking was most likely:

A. Carbamazepine.
B. Haloperidol.
C. Lithium.
D. Lorazepam.
E. Valproate.

85 According to simple Mendelian inheritance, if a disease gene is recessive, what is the likelihood of developing the disease if one parent has two dominant genes and the other two recessive genes?

A. 0%.
B. 25%.
C. 50%.
D. 75%.
E. 100%.

86 Which of the following is the medication most often associated with an increased risk of falls in persons age 80 or older?

A. Antihypertensives.
B. Benzodiazepines.
C. Antidepressants.
D. Histamine H_1 receptor antagonists.
E. Atypical antipsychotics.

87 Patients who are being treated with exposure therapy for anxiety disorders are:

A. Encouraged to think about nonthreatening situations during the treatment.
B. Encouraged to focus on their fears and allow feelings of anxiety to occur.
C. Required to conduct the therapy in real-life or fully realistic situations.
D. Required to develop a protocol and start with the most feared stimulus first.
E. Required to be on an appropriate type and dose of antianxiety medication.

88 What were the findings of the Treatment for Adolescents with Depression Study (TADS), with regard to efficacy of treatment?

A. Fluoxetine alone was most effective.
B. Cognitive-behavioral therapy (CBT) alone was most effective.
C. Fluoxetine plus cognitive-behavioral therapy was most effective.
D. Interpersonal therapy alone was most effective.
E. Fluoxetine plus interpersonal therapy was most effective.

89 A 76-year-old woman with a long history of generalized anxiety disorder presents to a psychiatrist. She is interested in the possibility of pharmacotherapy for this disorder. She has a history of hypertension, for which she takes amlodipine, but otherwise is in good health. The most accurate advice regarding the use of pharmacotherapy for this patient is that medications are:

A. Generally not effective in treating anxiety in elderly patients.
B. Contraindicated due to the increased side effects in older adults.
C. Less effective than psychotherapy for anxiety in older adults.
D. Not recommended owing to the high potential for drug-drug interactions.
E. A first-line treatment for anxiety in the elderly.

90 You are treating a 16-year-old patient for ADHD who has multiple café au lait spots visible on both arms and legs. A diagnosis of neurofibromatosis is made by a neurology consultant. Which one of the following modes of genetic transmission is seen in this illness?

A. Autosomal dominant.
B. Autosomal recessive.
C. Non-Mendelian inheritance.
D. X-linked recessive.
E. X-linked dominant.

91 Which of the following combination treatments has the best evidence for producing a short-term benefit of more rapid stabilization for the acute symptom treatment of panic disorder?

A. CBT and SSRI.
B. Benzodiazepine and SSRI.
C. CBT and benzodiazepine.
D. SSRI and buspirone.

92 A 22-year-old man presents repeatedly over a year with concerns that he is suffering from AIDS. He has never been found to be HIV positive, but he is not convinced despite having negative tests. He does not meet the criteria for major depressive disorder, generalized anxiety disorder, or obsessive-compulsive disorder. Which of the following is the most likely diagnosis?

A. Body dysmorphic disorder.
B. Illness anxiety disorder.
C. Conversion disorder.
D. Somatic symptom disorder.
E. Unspecified somatic symptom disorder.

93 Which of the following neurotransmitters has the largest body of evidence associating it with the reinforcing effects of various types of drugs of abuse?

A. Acetylcholine.
B. Dopamine.
C. GABA.
D. Glutamate.
E. Serotonin.

94 Which of the following is the preferred method to confirm a clinical diagnosis of narcolepsy?

A. Functional magnetic resonance imaging (fMRI).
B. Apnea monitoring.
C. Multiple sleep latency test (MSLT).
D. Human leukocyte antigen (HLA) testing.
E. Cerebrospinal fluid (CSF) hypocretin levels.

95 Which of the following psychotherapeutic interventions represents the best approach for a patient with germ obsessions who washes his hands every time he touches something he considers dirty?

A. Having the patient place his hands in a container of mud.
B. Having the patient snap his wrist with a rubber band when he washes his hands.
C. Pointing out to the patient that the germ phobia is an example of distorted thinking.
D. Having the patient touch a dirty object, then not allowing him to wash his hands.
E. Providing the patient with coping cards to remind him that the hand washing is unnecessary.

---

96 A military veteran is diagnosed with PTSD after his wife encourages him to seek treatment because of problems adjusting to civilian life. It is clear that survivor guilt is a major source of distress. Which of the following is the best intervention for this issue?

A. Vocational counseling.
B. Couples therapy.
C. Individual psychotherapy.
D. Fluoxetine.
E. Risperidone.

---

97 Which of the following cultural groups is most likely to want to be informed of a terminal prognosis?

A. Mexican Americans.
B. Korean Americans.
C. African Americans.
D. Japanese Americans.
E. Navajo Americans.

---

98 When diagnosing major depressive disorder in young children, which of the following signs or symptoms is MORE likely to be present than would be expected in an adolescent or adult?

A. Diurnal variation in mood.
B. Hypersomnia.
C. Melancholia.
D. Poor self-esteem.
E. Somatic complaints.

---

99 A mutation on which of the following chromosomes has been associated with early-onset Alzheimer's dementia?

A. Chromosome 2.
B. Chromosome 19.
C. Chromosome 21.
D. Y chromosome.
E. X chromosome.

---

100 A 16-year-old girl is brought by her parents for an evaluation as part of the admission process for a weight reduction program. The adolescent agrees that she is overweight and that she would like to lose weight. Which of the following would be MOST indicative that she will be successful in the program?

A. BMI <30.
B. No family history of eating disorders.
C. Mother successfully lost weight.
D. She is willing to take medication.
E. She is willing to change her eating habits.

---

101 A 25-year-old woman complains about shortness of breath, chest pain, and diaphoresis. She has had multiple attacks in the past 3 weeks. Her medical workup is negative. Which of the following medications is the best choice considering efficacy and side-effect profile?

A. Propranolol.
B. Desipramine.
C. Bupropion.
D. Sertraline.
E. Alprazolam.

102 The "parent of origin" effect is defined as transmission of a risk for disease based on whether an autosome has been transmitted by the mother or father. As one example of this phenomenon in psychiatric genetics, duplications of chromosome 15q inherited from the mother, but not the father, have been found to account for a small but significant proportion of cases of which of the following disorders?

A. Schizophrenia.
B. Bipolar disorder.
C. Obsessive-compulsive disorder.
D. Alcohol dependence.
E. Autism.

---

103 A 14-year-old girl presents with significant weight loss. She reports that about 1 year ago she became concerned that she was overweight and began self-inducing vomiting. Since then, she has continued to use purgatives in addition to misusing laxatives, diuretics, and enemas as a means of weight control after binging. She is intensely afraid of becoming fat. She is in the 65th percentile for weight based on height, appears cachetic, but insists she is obese. She has not experienced menses for 6 months. Which of the following symptoms will MOST likely be elicited from the patient?

A. A need for orderliness and control.
B. Competitiveness.
C. Obsessional thinking.
D. Perfectionism.
E. Comorbid impulsivity.

---

104 Cognitive deficits in schizophrenia have been associated with a decrease in $GABA_A$ receptors in which of the following brain areas?

A. Lateral amygdala.
B. Medial amygdala.
C. Dorsolateral prefrontal cortex.
D. Medial prefrontal cortex.
E. Nucleus accumbens.

---

105 A 19-year-old man presents for an outpatient evaluation of increasing concerns about germs and contamination that are now resulting in several hours per day of hand washing and cleaning rituals to relieve anxiety. He is started on sertraline, the dose of which is increased 50 mg every other day until reaching 200 mg daily. After 1 week of treatment at this dose, he has not experienced any relief of the symptoms. However, the medication is well tolerated without significant side effects. In developing further plan of treatment, which of the following is the appropriate total length of time to continue sertraline before changing to another pharmacologic agent?

A. 2 weeks.
B. 4 weeks.
C. 6 weeks.
D. 8 weeks.
E. 10 weeks.

---

106 A psychiatric consult is requested for a patient who has burns over 60% of his body. The patient has begun refusing dressing changes despite pretreatment with morphine. Pain control is adequate except during dressing changes. Upon examination, the patient reports that the pain is too severe to tolerate, and he does not feel that the morphine is adequately controlling his pain. The psychiatrist should recommend which of the following agents as an additional medication prior to dressing changes?

A. Long-acting morphine.
B. Methadone.
C. Meperidine.
D. Fentanyl.
E. Codeine.

107 A 36-year-old moderately obese man is seen for evaluation of depressed mood, difficulty falling asleep, poor appetite, and diminished concentration at work, all of which have been worsening over the past few weeks. When treatment options are discussed, he reports particular concerns about sexual side effects. Considering the patient's concerns, which one of the following medications would be most appropriate to suggest as an initial treatment?

A. Bupropion.
B. Fluoxetine.
C. Mirtazapine.
D. Nortriptyline.
E. Venlafaxine.

108 Which of the following disorders has the most evidence supporting familial aggregation of the disorder?

A. Posttraumatic stress disorder.
B. Adjustment disorder, mixed features.
C. Panic disorder.
D. Social phobia.
E. Specific phobia.

109 Which of the following medical complications is most likely to be seen in a patient with bulimia nervosa?

A. Decreased serum amylase.
B. Hyperchloremia.
C. Metabolic acidosis.
D. Hypokalemia.
E. Hyperthyroxinemia.

110 Evidence to date from OCD genetic studies indicates that its inheritance is best characterized by which pattern?

A. Automsomal dominant.
B. Autosomal recessive.
C. Sex-linked recessive.
D. Complex.
E. Mendelian.

111 A 72-year-old woman is referred to a psychiatrist because the family has noticed increasing apathy. In evaluating the patient, which of the following would be the most useful first step for revealing the likely underlying pathology?

A. An empirical trial of an antidepressant.
B. An MRI of the brain.
C. History and a full mental status examination.
D. Thyroid function testing.
E. Neuropsychological evaluation.

112 Which of the following is believed to be the chief factor in predicting outcome of psychodynamic psychotherapy?

A. Transference.
B. Countertransference.
C. Therapeutic alliance.
D. Resistance.
E. On-time payments.

113 An adolescent girl becomes anxious and "panicky" at the thought of spiders. She cannot join her high school classmates for lunch outside because of the fear that she "will run into a spider." The most appropriate diagnosis is:

A. Agoraphobia.
B. Acute stress disorder.
C. Generalized anxiety disorder.
D. Specific phobia.
E. Social phobia.

114 A 31-year-old female describes dramatic fluctuations in mood and self-esteem. Which one of the following features would be most helpful in distinguishing bipolar II disorder from borderline personality disorder during a period of elevated mood?

A. Suicidal ideation with depressed mood.
B. Psychosis while mood is elevated or irritable.
C. Impulsivity while mood is elevated or irritable.
D. A history of continued functioning through mood fluctuations.
E. Mood fluctuations are observed by others.

115 Which of the following psychiatric conditions is most commonly associated with self-neglect in the geriatric population?

A. Depression.
B. Generalized anxiety disorder.
C. Panic disorder.
D. Schizophrenia.
E. Personality disorder.

116 According to the AMA Code of Medical Ethics, which of the following educationally related gifts from a pharmaceutical company is ethically acceptable?

A. Money to help defray hotel costs during a CME event.
B. Scholarships awarded to individual residents to attend educational conferences.
C. Reimbursement of travel for a guest faculty speaker.
D. Money to compensate a psychiatrist for time spent at a CME event.

117 Which of the following statements best describes the association between PTSD and the subsequent emergence of drug use problems?

A. Young adults with PTSD due to earlier lifetime traumas, with no prior drug use disorders, are about five times more likely to develop drug-related problems subsequently compared with traumatized young adults without PTSD.
B. Experiencing significant trauma without the presence of PTSD is sufficient to subsequently increase the prevalence of drug use disorders substantially.
C. After controlling for factors such as sex, age, and ethnicity, PTSD confers no additional increased risk of subsequent drug use disorders.
D. After controlling for factors such as childhood conduct problems and risk taking, PTSD confers no additional increased risk of subsequent drug use disorders.
E. After controlling for factors such as family socioeconomic status (SES) and years of education, PTSD confers no additional increased risk of subsequent drug use disorders.

118 Borderline personality disorder is marked by pervasive instability of self-image, emotions, and impulsivity. Which of the following is a DSM diagnostic criteria for this diagnosis?

A. Consistent irresponsibility.
B. Lack of remorse after injuring others.
C. Requiring excessive admiration.
D. Sense of entitlement.
E. Unstable sense of self.

119 Which of the following should be the initial treatment of a patient with illness anxiety?

A. Cognitive-behavioral therapy.
B. Treatment of incidental physical exam findings.
C. Scheduling regular physical examinations.
D. Discussing the false nature of the illness pharmacotherapy with SSRIs.

120 A 33-year-old man with schizophrenia and alcohol dependence acknowledges that when he drinks beer the police tend to arrest him and bring him to the psychiatric hospital. He agrees to "take medicine to help [him] not drink so much." Owing to issues of noncompliance, his current medication is a long-acting injectable antipsychotic. He lives on his own and keeps his clinic appointments but has had difficulties adhering to oral medication regimens. The best medication to augment the treatment of his alcohol dependence would be:

A. Acamprosate.
B. Clozapine.
C. Disulfiram.
D. Naltrexone.
E. Ondansetron.

121 Avoidant personality disorder is marked by social inhibition, sense of inadequacy, and hypersensitivity. Which of the following is a DSM criterion for this disorder?

A. Requiring excessive admiration.
B. Difficulty making everyday decisions.
C. Excessive devotion to work to the exclusion of friendships.
D. Preoccupation with being socially criticized.
E. Reluctance to delegate tasks or to work with others.

122 Which of the following statements gives the most appropriate guidance for patients and their families regarding driving by patients with neurocognitive disorders?

A. Families have no responsibility for getting involved in driving decisions of patients with mild cognitive impairment.
B. All patients with mild cognitive impairment should be reported to their state motor vehicle departments for mandatory tracking.
C. Clinicians should advise all patients with mild cognitive impairment to stop driving and to turn in their driver's licenses.
D. Mildly impaired patients should be advised to stop driving at night.
E. Patients and families should be informed that even mild neurocognitive disorders increase the risk of vehicular accidents.

123 An 8-year-old boy presents with a 1-month history of stomachaches and headaches every morning just before going to school. When interviewed, he reports having persistent nightmares of being kidnapped and worries about his father having an accident. The most likely diagnosis is:

A. Normal childhood.
B. Agoraphobia.
C. Separation anxiety.
D. Generalized anxiety disorder.
E. Panic disorder.

124 A 65-year-old man has metastatic head-and-neck cancer that leaves him with a ptosis, facial nerve palsy, and an inability to eat solid foods. He complains of feeling hopeless, that life has lost all meaning, and that he wants to die immediately. He does not meet criteria for major depression. The best descriptor for this triad of symptoms is:

A. Anticipatory grief.
B. Demoralization.
C. Mourning.
D. Denial.
E. Bargaining.

125 A 73-year-old woman was prescribed 10 mg/day of paroxetine for anxiety 1 week ago. She now presents to the physician's office with confusion. Laboratory workup reveals low serum sodium and low plasma osmolarity. Her urine sodium and osmolarity are high. The physician should consider a diagnosis of:

A. Hypothyroidism.
B. Syndrome of Inappropriate Antidiuretic Hormone (SIADH).
C. Hyperparathyroidism.
D. Renal failure.
E. Dehydration.

126 A 37-year-old male software designer is brought to the psychiatrist's office by his brother, who reports that the patient has become increasingly suspicious over the last year. Last week, a shopping mall security guard observed him recording license plate numbers. The guard inquired, the patient explained that he was doing statistical research on license plates, and there was no further incident. He told his brother later that he thought he had noticed these cars parked in front of his home, and they might be part of scoping the neighborhood in advance of a crime. The brother is now concerned that it is only a matter of time for the patient to get into his first legal skirmish as a result of this kind of behavior. The patient reports that since his teens, he has needed to be very observant of others to protect himself. He says he has never been a victim of assault or theft only because of his constant vigilance. He experienced several days of auditory hallucinations when he was about 20 years old; "voices" were making deprecatory comments, but he cannot recall further details. These symptoms remitted entirely, and he reports no other psychotic symptoms.

He has worked at the same software company for 10 years, and although he has been promoted several times, most recently 3 months ago, he thinks he was slighted by his supervisor who gave a better position to a colleague. He is satisfied with his single status. Which ONE of the following disorders is the most likely diagnosis?

A. Paranoid personality disorder.
B. Delusional disorder.
C. Schizoid personality disorder.
D. Schizophrenia, paranoid type.
E. Schizotypal personality disorder.

127 A 6-year-old girl is referred by her teacher because of "acting out" behaviors at school, including inappropriate touching of peers and insistence on sitting on adults' laps. During the session, she tells the psychiatrist that her father touches her "secret place." The father explains that he bathes the girl at night and is simply making sure she is clean everywhere. Which of the following is the most appropriate action for the psychiatrist?

A. Advise the father not to give baths and see if the behavior resolves.
B. Tell the teacher to call child protective services.
C. Relay the findings to the teacher and tell her child protective services will not be necessary.
D. Try to gather more history to see if this constitutes sexual abuse.
E. Make a call to child protective services.

128 Patients with acute stress disorder have been shown in controlled trials to be least likely to subsequently develop posttraumatic stress disorder when treated with:

A. Cognitive-restructuring therapy.
B. Exposure therapy.
C. Systematic debriefing.
D. Couples therapy.
E. Internet-based CBT.

129 According to the results of the Clinical Antipsychotic Trials of Intervention Effectiveness (CATIE) study, approximately what percentage of patients had continued on their initial antipsychotic medications by 18 months?

A. 10%.
B. 25%.
C. 50%.
D. 75%.
E. 90%.

130 Temperament traits of Harm Avoidance, Novelty Seeking, Reward Dependence, and Persistence are defined as heritable differences underlying automatic responses to danger, novelty, social approval, and intermittent reward, respectively. Which of the following statements about the temperament traits in the general population is MOST accurate?

A. The phenotypic expression of these traits is primarily due to the experiences of the individual.
B. They are normally distributed quantitative traits.
C. They are modifiable based on the goodness of fit with the parent.
D. They are inconsistently manifested in different cultures.
E. They are similar to fluid intelligence in that they show demonstrable changes with aging.

131 A 37-year-old single man's sex life centers on donning women's lingerie before engaging in sexual activities with willing female partners. He considers himself heterosexual and has never had any interest in having sex with men. He is distressed about his sexual behavior and is now seeking treatment. Which of the following best describes his behavior?

A. Transvestic disorder.
B. Gender dysphoria.
C. Frotteurism.
D. Exhibitionism.

132 A 28-year-old woman presents to the clinic concerned about having ADHD. She has noticed that for the last 3 days she has been "hyper." She stays up until 4 A.M. to rehearse her presentations and awakens easily at 7 A.M. She also now works as late as 9 P.M., whereas she would usually stop at 6 P.M. She finds herself easily distracted and strays from her routine presentation. She experiences these symptoms about three times a year. Talking with her husband reveals that these periods are always followed by a deep depression during which she will rarely get out of bed, does not eat, and will not see clients for about 2 weeks. Her presentation is most consistent with:

A. Cyclothymia.
B. Bipolar I disorder.
C. Bipolar II disorder.
D. ADHD–inattentive type.
E. ADHD–hyperactive/impulsive type.

133 A 19-year-old woman with anorexia presents with shortness of breath and symptoms consistent with heart failure. She admits to using large amounts of ipecac. Which of the following test results would be most consistent with ipecac-induced toxicity?

A. Decrease in the serum CK value.
B. Decrease in lactate dehydrogenase.
C. Shortening of the QTc interval.
D. Enlarged heart.
E. Bradycardia.

134 An assessment of a 25-year-old woman as a candidate for psychotherapy reveals that she is able to delay gratification in order to attain personal goals but remains egocentric and defensive. She is noted to have frequent distress when attachments and desires are frustrated. She functions well under good conditions but frequently experiences problems under stress. On the basis of the *stages in the development of self-awareness and well-being*, this woman is MOST likely at what stage?

A. Stage 0: unaware.
B. Stage 1: average adult cognition.
C. Stage 2: metacognition.
D. Stage 3: contemplation.

135 Which of the following techniques or therapies has been shown, in a randomized controlled trial, to be most helpful in the treatment of acute stress disorder?

A. Cognitive restructuring.
B. Individual psychological debriefing.
C. Exposure-based therapy.
D. Eye movement desensitization and reprocessing (EMDR).
E. Group debriefing.

136 Which of the following medications should be the first-line treatment for generalized anxiety disorder?

A. Diazepam.
B. Lorazepam.
C. Buspirone.
D. Paroxetine.
E. Hydroxyzine.

137 After performing a thorough history and physical, a psychiatrist suspects that the patient has bipolar I disorder, rapid cycling. Which of the following tests should be ordered to rule out an underlying medical etiology?

A. CSF 5-HIAA.
B. 24-hour urine.
C. Thyroid function tests.
D. Liver function tests.
E. Dexamethasone suppression test.

138 The symptom domain most strongly correlated with functional impairment in schizophrenia is:

A. Positive symptoms.
B. Negative symptoms.
C. Cognitive impairment.
D. Mood disturbance.

139 A 37-year-old woman, in dynamic psychotherapy for borderline personality disorder, has been expressing an unrealistic overvaluation of the therapist. After many months of this expressed high regard, she suddenly becomes enraged after the therapist fails to return her call and now declares the therapist to be "the worst ever." Which of the following would be the most appropriate way to handle the patient's new reaction?

A. Avoid directly responding and instead encourage the patient to further express her emotions.
B. Apologize for the missed call and then suggest they move on with the current work.
C. Acknowledge the failing and then question how the patient's opinion could change so dramatically.
D. Propose that they clarify an appropriate call-back policy to avoid future mishaps.
E. Suggest to the patient that such inevitable mistakes are an important part of the therapy.

140 Which of the following is the most accurate information to give families regarding the risk of using antipsychotics to treat agitation in elderly patients with moderate dementia of the Alzheimer's type?

A. There is an increased risk of mortality but only for the antipsychotics risperidone and olanzapine.
B. Increased mortality in the elderly has been associated with both atypical and conventional antipsychotics.
C. Although suggested by earlier studies, subsequent studies have not found a significant risk of mortality with atypical antipsychotics.
D. The risk is unknown, as inadequate data exist to make any conclusive statements.
E. Although newer antipsychotics may have a risk, typical antipsychotics appear to be safe.

141 The use of stimulants to treat ADHD is relatively contraindicated if the child has which of the following comorbid conditions?

A. Tic disorder.
B. Preexisting cardiovascular disease.
C. Seizure disorder.
D. Anxiety disorder.
E. Bipolar disorder.

142 A patient describes a dinner party at which he felt increasing anxiety and a sense that people were avoiding him. He discussed this with his wife and she became irritated with him, noting that it would help if he could look people in the eye and not wear the same worn-out suit jacket to every party. He tried to explain that this was his lucky jacket and it protected them both from car accidents, but she just shook her head. On the basis of this, which of the following personality disorders is most likely?

A. Schizoid.
B. Schizotypal.
C. Antisocial.
D. Borderline.
E. Narcissistic.

143 What is the leading cause of disability in the world for persons 15–44 years of age?

A. Bipolar disorder.
B. Schizophrenia.
C. Self-inflicted injuries.
D. Unipolar major depression.
E. Alcohol use.

144 A busy 33-year-old female executive decides that she will end 10 years of smoking. She tried once before but was unsuccessful. She travels several times a month and agrees to use a nicotine inhaler, along with brief telephone counseling appointments. When is she most likely to relapse?

A. On the quit date.
B. During the first few days of the quit date.
C. 1 week after the quit date.
D. 2 weeks after the quit date.

145 Clinical efficacy of typical (first-generation) antipsychotic medications is highly correlated with binding to which of the following receptors?

A. Dopamine, D_1.
B. Dopamine, D_2.
C. Serotonin, 5-HT_{2a}.
D. Muscarinic, M_4.
E. Adrenoceptors, α_2.

146 Which of the following is a single-locus (monogenic) disorder?

A. Alzheimer's disease.
B. Bipolar disorder.
C. Autism.
D. Huntington's disease.
E. Obsessive-compulsive disorder.

147 The absence of which of the following features differentiates social communication disorder from autism spectrum disorder in DSM-5?

A. Deficits of nonverbal communicative behaviors.
B. Deficits in developing relationships appropriate to the developmental level.
C. Deficits in social-emotional reciprocity.
D. Symptoms present in the early developmental period.
E. Restrictive and repetitive behavior, interests, or activities.

148 Medications from which one of the following classes have the greatest potential for worsening symptoms of borderline personality disorder?

A. Selective serotonin reuptake inhibitors.
B. Monoamine oxidase inhibitors.
C. Anticonvulsants.
D. Atypical antipsychotics.
E. Benzodiazepines.

149 In order to be given the diagnosis of mild neurocognitive disorder (NCD), a patient must have:

A. A memory impairment.
B. A cognitive decline in at least one domain.
C. Cognitive complaints in multiple domains.
D. Compromised general cognitive function.
E. Cognitive and memory complaints meeting criteria for mild dementia.

150 A 42-year-old patient requests treatment for anxiety and interpersonal difficulties. The patient reports feelings of social inadequacy and sensitivity to rejection for the past 20 years. The patient does not attend social events or interact with others as a result of this anxiety, worries excessively about being criticized by others, and feels inferior to others. This has caused occupational problems since the patient is only able to function in jobs that have virtually no social interaction. The patient is unhappy that he has no friends and has never been romantically involved. Which of the following is the most likely diagnosis?

A. Schizoid personality disorder.
B. Generalized anxiety disorder.
C. Avoidant personality disorder.
D. Social anxiety disorder.
E. Obsessive-compulsive disorder.

151 The parents of a 10-year-old boy who has had both motor and vocal tics for over a year are wondering whether he will remain symptomatic as an adult. Which of the following statements MOST accurately describes the probable outcome of children with these symptoms?

A. By age 18, 50% of children are not symptomatic.
B. Symptoms continue to increase in adolescence and adulthood.
C. The motor tics resolve but the vocal tics persist.
D. The tics decrease in adolescence but then increase again in adulthood.

152 Increased risk of developing diabetes mellitus and dyslipidemia have most commonly been linked to:

A. Perphenazine.
B. Quetiapine.
C. Risperidone.
D. Ziprasidone.
E. Olanzapine.

153 Patients in a study were asked to exert behavioral inhibition when confronted with negative stimuli. fMRI investigations demonstrated decreased activation of the subgenual anterior cingulate cortex and the posterior medial orbitofrontal cortex and increased activity in the left and right extended amygdala and ventral striatum relative to controls. These fMRI findings were associated with which of the following diagnoses?

A. Narcissistic personality disorder.
B. Attention-deficit/hyperactivity disorder.
C. Paranoid personality disorder.
D. Borderline personality disorder.
E. Schizophrenia.

154 Binge-eating disorder is characterized by:

A. Feelings of being unable to control one's intake of food.
B. Consumption of a large amount of food over a 24-hour period.
C. Purging after eating a large amount of food.
D. Increasing amounts of exercise.
E. Progressive weight loss.

155 A patient who has been diagnosed with PTSD reports nightmares and sleep disruption. Which one of the following medications has been shown to be effective for the treatment of trauma-related nightmares and sleep disruption in patients with PTSD?

A. Topiramate.
B. Sertraline.
C. Prazosin.
D. Gabapentin.
E. Propranolol.

156 A 3-day-postpartum mother with no prior psychiatric diagnosis is concerned about feeling depressed. She endorses a decrease in energy, difficulty sleeping despite being tired, decreased appetite, and frequent mood swings saying, "One minute I'm fine, the next minute I'm crying." Which of the following is the most appropriate treatment?

A. Psychoeducation.
B. Cognitive-behavioral therapy.
C. Pharmacotherapy.
D. Hospitalization.
E. Psychodynamic psychotherapy.

157 A 44-year-old woman presents with a general history of alcohol abuse and significant depressive and anxiety symptoms over 20 years. It is unclear whether the substance use was in response to the affective symptoms or if the affective symptoms were substance-induced. Which of the following procedures would help make this determination?

A. Administer the MacAndrew Alcoholism Scale–Revised (MAC-R).
B. Conduct a detailed mental status exam, focusing on form of thought.
C. Draw a timeline of all substances used and all psychiatric symptoms.
D. Measure the percent carbohydrate-deficient transferrin.
E. Obtain serial urine toxicology tests.

158 A depressed 62-year-old man being treated with an SSRI is admitted to the hospital with motoric immobility, posturing, grimacing, echolalia, and echopraxia. Intravenous administration of lorazepam and amobarbital leads to no relief. Which of the following treatments should be considered?

A. Add a second antidepressant.
B. Begin a mood stabilizer.
C. Initiate electroconvulsive therapy.
D. Add dantrolene.
E. Administer intravenous haloperidol.

159 Which of the following antidepressants is the best choice for a patient who wants to avoid orgasm dysfunction as a side effect?

A. Bupropion.
B. Sertraline.
C. Venlafaxine.
D. Escitalopram.
E. Fluoxetine.

160 A 20-year-old female college student presents to the counseling center with concerns about her alcohol use. She describes two occasions in the past year when she attended parties and had "way too much to drink." Following these occasions she feels "lousy," postpones studying, and then must stay up late to study for tests. When she's gone to most other parties, she's had four or five drinks with no ill effects. There are no other substance-related symptoms. She expresses some concern about her drinking and asks for recommendations. The best intervention at this point would be to:

A. Provide a brief intervention.
B. Prescribe disulfiram.
C. Recommend attending Alcoholics Anonymous.
D. Prescribe naltrexone.
E. Prescribe acamprosate.

161 Which of the following medications has the greatest body of evidence supporting its use as a monotherapy for acute bipolar depression?

A. Bupropion.
B. Lamotrigine.
C. Valproate.
D. Olanzapine.
E. Quetiapine.

162 A patient reports feeling that he has always had to please others and that if he is not liked by everyone, he will never be successful. Which of the following statements would be characteristic of a cognitive-behavioral approach to the patient's problem?

A. "Let's draw out your circle of friends and examine which ones you feel you must please."
B. "Feeling you must please others is acting more out of an emotional mind than a rational mind."
C. "Tell me about your experience that you can only be successful by pleasing others."
D. "Is it possible that feeling you're not being liked by everyone is a way to ease the pressure of having to be successful?"

---

163 A 32-year-old woman presents with a history of frequent, unanticipated panic attacks. Which of the following medications is most likely to be of benefit for treating her disorder?

A. Bupropion.
B. Aripiprazole.
C. Gabapentin.
D. Clonazepam.
E. Buspirone.

---

164 Which of the following is the best established psychosocial intervention for the treatment of panic disorder?

A. Dialectical behavioral therapy.
B. Interpersonal psychotherapy.
C. Psychodynamic psychotherapy.
D. Marital and family therapy.
E. Cognitive-behavioral therapy.

---

165 A patient with a history of substance dependence and depression treated with tranylcypromine presents to the emergency room with hypertension, tachycardia, chest pain, and severe occipital headache. The patient says he had a relapse of his drug use. Which of the following substances is the most likely contributor to his clinical presentation at this time?

A. Vodka.
B. Methamphetamine.
C. PCP.
D. Marijuana.
E. Inhalants.

---

166 Trazodone exerts its hypnotic effects by interaction with which of the following neurotransmitter receptors?

A. Dopamine.
B. GABA.
C. Histamine.
D. α_2.
E. Acetylcholine.

---

167 Based on the results of Phase 1 of the Clinical Antipsychotic Trials of Intervention Effectiveness (CATIE) study, which of the following antipsychotic medications is most likely to be associated with the development of metabolic complications?

A. Olanzapine.
B. Quetiapine.
C. Risperidone.
D. Ziprasidone.
E. Perphenazine.

---

168 Which of the following SSRIs is designated as FDA pregnancy category D?

A. Fluoxetine.
B. Paroxetine.
C. Sertraline.
D. Citalopram.
E. Escitalopram.

169 According to the National Comorbidity Survey (NCS), which of the following experiences is most frequently associated with PTSD in women in the United States?

A. Being in a life-threatening accident.
B. Combat exposure.
C. Being involved in a natural disaster.
D. Sexual assault.
E. Witnessing someone being badly injured or killed.

170 The core techniques of open-ended questions, affirmation, reflective statements, and summary statements (OARS) are central to which one of the following therapies?

A. Cognitive-behavioral.
B. Interpersonal.
C. Motivational interviewing.
D. Twelve-step facilitation.
E. Prolonged exposure.

171 Which of the following is the most common sleep problem in persons with major depressive disorder?

A. Vivid mood congruent dreams.
B. Hypersomnia.
C. Restless leg syndrome.
D. Insomnia.
E. Sleep phase disorder.

172 Which of the following psychotherapeutic techniques has the greatest body of evidence supporting it as a first-line treatment for PTSD?

A. Hypnosis.
B. Eye movement desensitization and reprocessing (EMDR).
C. Prolonged exposure therapy.
D. Stress inoculation training.
E. Systematic desensitization.

173 Which of the following is most characteristic of symptoms of PTSD?

A. Persist long after the precipitating event is over.
B. Exist only while the trauma is present.
C. Directly proportional to the magnitude of the trauma.
D. Occur only in response to certain types of trauma.
E. Develop immediately upon experiencing the trauma.

174 A 38-year-old woman with a history of estrogen receptor-positive breast cancer is currently taking tamoxifen to reduce the risk of recurrence. However, she has become increasingly tearful, withdrawn, and anergic over the past month. She also notes difficulty with sleep and concentration as well as distressing hot flashes since initiating tamoxifen. Which one of the following medications is most appropriate to treat her symptoms?

A. Venlafaxine.
B. Paroxetine.
C. Gabapentin.
D. Fluoxetine.
E. Duloxetine.

175 Which of the following distinguishes acute stress disorder from PTSD?

A. Impairment in functioning.
B. Time course.
C. Dissociative symptoms.
D. Reexperiencing.

176 Which of the following symptoms meets DSM-5 criteria for alcohol use disorder?

A. Consuming enough alcohol to become intoxicated.
B. Daily drinking.
C. Repeatedly driving while intoxicated.
D. Recent ingestion of alcohol.
E. Slurred speech.

177 A psychiatrist is asked by the local school to consult on a 13-year-old boy who has exhibited problems with compulsive eating and failure to make academic progress. The boy's parents report that he has always eaten "everything in sight" and has been delayed in his development. Medical history is remarkable for poor muscle tone and failure to thrive as an infant. Physical examination reveals hypotonia, obesity, hypogonadism, a narrow-appearing forehead, down-slanting palpebral fissures, small-appearing hands and feet, and downturning of the corners of the mouth. Intelligence testing is consistent with mental retardation. What is the MOST LIKELY cause of the patient's signs and symptoms?

A. Childhood degenerative disorder.
B. Congenital rubella infection.
C. Homocystinuria.
D. Prader-Willi syndrome.
E. Tuberous sclerosis.

178 Which of the following psychosocial treatments for social phobia has the most evidence supporting effectiveness?

A. Cognitive-behavioral therapy (CBT).
B. Interpersonal psychotherapy (IPT).
C. Psychodynamic psychotherapy.
D. Family-focused therapy.
E. Group psychoeducation.

179 A 62-year-old woman presents for assessment and treatment of a 3-year history of mild but persistent depressive symptoms. One year ago, she was named board chairman of her association and also began a new relationship with a very wealthy individual. The relationship is going well emotionally and sexually, but she sometimes feels inadequate in her new social circles. She misses her former partner particularly when she feels socially awkward. After a discussion of treatment options for improving her overall level of functioning and self-satisfaction, she and her psychiatrist decide upon a structured, time-limited course of interpersonal psychotherapy (IPT). Which ONE of the following would be the most appropriate focus of the IPT?

A. Analysis of transference.
B. Delayed grief.
C. Interpersonal deficits.
D. Role dispute.
E. Role transition.

180 Which of the following congenital abnormalities is associated with maternal use of carbamazepine in the first trimester of pregnancy?

A. An increased risk of Ebstein's anomaly, the downward displacement of the tricuspid valve into the right ventricle and variable levels of right ventricular hyperplasia.
B. Craniofacial defects, fingernail hypoplasia, and developmental delay.
C. Fetal development of skin rash in a neonate who has antigen characteristics different from those of the mother.
D. Impaired temperature regulation and apnea.

181 When initiating treatment with long-acting injectable haloperidol every 4 weeks, what period of time is required to reach steady state?

A. 4 weeks.
B. 8 weeks.
C. 12 weeks.
D. 16 weeks.
E. 20 weeks.

182 In addition to pharmacotherapy, psychotherapy plays an important role in treating bipolar disorder. Which ONE of the following circumstances best describes when cognitive-behavioral therapy (CBT) is most effective in the adjunctive treatment of bipolar disorder?

A. Acutely ill, depressed.
B. Acutely ill, manic.
C. After four or more episodes.
D. Moderately or acutely ill states.
E. Recovered from acute episode.

183 Behavioral approaches such as the Semans pause maneuver, the start-stop method of Kaplan, and the pause-squeeze technique of Masters and Johnson have been employed to treat which of the following?

A. Male erectile disorder.
B. Female sexual arousal disorder.
C. Premature ejaculation.
D. Hypoactive sexual desire disorder.
E. Female orgasmic disorder.

184 A 25-year-old man with no past history of abnormal involuntary movements is being treated with haloperidol. He should be evaluated for abnormal involuntary movements every

A. 1 month.
B. 3 months.
C. 6 months.
D. 12 months.
E. 18 months.

185 A 19-year-old private in the U.S. Army loses his left leg after his vehicle drives over an improvised explosive device. Two months later he reports ongoing recurrent and intrusive recollections of the event, nightmares and flashbacks to the explosion, avoidance of any activities that remind him of the event, irritability, and disturbed sleep. Which of the following psychotherapeutic interventions is MOST likely to be effective in alleviating his symptoms?

A. Biofeedback.
B. Eye movement desensitization and reprocessing.
C. Exposure-based cognitive-behavior therapy.
D. Guided imagery therapy.
E. Hypnotherapy.

186 A 40-year-old patient is taking clozapine for treatment-resistant schizophrenia. Assuming no abnormal laboratory results, after what period of time could complete blood count monitoring be reduced to every 4 weeks?

A. 3 months.
B. 6 months.
C. 12 months.
D. 18 months.
E. 24 months.

187 For patients with functional gastrointestinal disorders, which of the following medications would be most likely to alleviate the visceral pain associated with irritable bowel syndrome?

A. Bupropion.
B. Clonazepam.
C. Fluoxetine.
D. Quetiapine.
E. Amitriptyline.

188 A 56-year old man with major depression is prescribed paroxetine. One month later, he complains of significant nausea. His dose is lowered from 20 to 10 mg/day; however, he continues to feel nauseated. He is motivated to remain on the medication if possible since he feels it has been enormously helpful for his depression. A genotyping of the cytochrome P450 2D6 gene reveals that he has one inactive copy and one partially inactive copy. Which of the following would be the most appropriate step to take?

A. Discontinue paroxetine immediately and wait 1 month.
B. Attempt even lower doses of paroxetine.
C. Discontinue paroxetine and begin fluoxetine.
D. Discontinue paroxetine and begin citalopram.
E. Continue paroxetine but add ondansetron.

189 Which symptom is characteristically seen in patients with factitious disorder?

A. Thoughts of death.
B. Pathological lying.
C. Fear of pain.
D. Perceptual disturbances.
E. Feelings of inadequacy.

190 A patient with bipolar disorder is receiving maintenance treatment with extended-release divalproex. How many hours should elapse between his last dose and drawing of the trough level of valproic acid?

A. 4 hours.
B. 8 hours.
C. 12 hours.
D. 18 hours.

191 A woman presents for help in coping with stress. During the assessment, it becomes clear that she is excessively preoccupied with her appearance, particularly her face. She spends hours a day examining and caring for her face. She is convinced that her cheekbones are uneven and make her look like a freak. Her appearance is unremarkable. After the assessment is complete, the psychiatrist's best initial approach is to:

A. Reassure the patient about her appearance.
B. Agree that the situation is quite distressing.
C. Point out that her thinking is quite distorted.
D. Agree that her appearance is a problem.
E. Explain the benefits of medication.

192 Which of the following is a common symptom of the depressive disorders specifier with seasonal pattern?

A. Light sensitivity.
B. Somatic complaints.
C. Insomnia.
D. Overeating.
E. Impulsiveness.

193 Which of the following techniques is commonly used in motivational interviewing?

A. Confrontation.
B. Interpretation of transference.
C. Identification of cognitive distortions.
D. Decision balance.
E. Relaxation training.

194 Which of the following factors best differentiates acute stress disorder from PTSD?

A. Chronicity.
B. Traumatic event severity.
C. Presence of nightmares.
D. Level of functional impairment.
E. Severity of subjective response to the event.

195 Which of the following best describes the mechanism of action of flumazenil in the treatment of benzodiazepine overdose?

A. Flumazenil blocks benzodiazepines from crossing the blood-brain barrier.
B. Flumazenil competes with benzodiazepines at central synaptic GABA receptor sites.
C. Flumazenil decreases the influx of chloride ions into GABAergic neurons preventing hyperpolarization.
D. Flumazenil increases the influx of sodium ions into GABAergic neurons causing depolarization.
E. Flumazenil increases the rate of oxidative metabolism of benzodiazepines.

---

196 A 22-year-old woman was involved in a severe motor vehicle accident in which several people were significantly injured. She had difficulty recalling portions of the accident, nightmares, and difficulty falling asleep. She refused to drive her car, had difficulty concentrating, and felt emotionally numb. She was unable to attend work. Her symptoms spontaneously resolved after a month, and she was able to return to work. The most likely diagnosis is:

A. Acute stress disorder.
B. Adjustment disorder.
C. Posttraumatic stress disorder.
D. Panic disorder.
E. Brief psychotic disorder.

---

197 Which of the following is the most common form of affective illness in families of patients with bipolar disorder?

A. Bipolar disorder.
B. Unipolar depression.
C. Dysthymia.
D. Premenstrual dysphoric disorder.
E. Cyclothymia.

---

198 The use of bright light treatment has been shown to be efficacious and safe for the treatment of:

A. Dysthymia.
B. Nonseasonal depression.
C. Bipolar disorder.
D. PTSD.

---

199 Stimulus control treatment for insomnia works by:

A. Reassuring patients that a quiet environment will help them fall asleep.
B. Reestablishing an automatic connection between going to bed and falling asleep.
C. Subtly punishing the patient for failure to fall asleep.
D. Making both bedtimes and rising times more regular.

---

200 Which of the following is one of the standards used to determine mental capacity in decision making?

A. Absence of psychosis.
B. Agreement with the medical recommendations.
C. Severity of psychiatric illness.
D. Rational decision making.
E. Presence of abstract thought.

---

201 Which of the following treatments has the best body of evidence in preventing poststroke depression in older populations?

A. Escitalopram.
B. Mianserin.
C. Sertraline.
D. Problem-solving therapy.
E. Cognitive-behavioral therapy.

202 A single mother reports that her 12-year-old child has become increasingly defiant with parental requests, at times becoming physically aggressive by kicking doors and hitting walls. She notes that the child does not exhibit these problems with the father. Which of the following is the most appropriate treatment?

A. Inoculation techniques, such as boot camp.
B. Contingency management.
C. Medication management.
D. Send the child to live with the father temporarily.
E. Brief hospitalization.

203 A 22-year-old man with chronic schizophrenia developed gynecomastia after being treated with risperidone for many months. His prolactin level is markedly elevated and you want to switch him to the antipsychotic drug that is less likely to cause this problem. Which one of the following would be the most appropriate choice?

A. Aripiprazole.
B. Olanzapine.
C. Perphenazine.
D. Haloperidol.
E. Paliperidone.

204 A 70-year-old man presents to a clinic with progressive memory loss. Which of the following findings is most representative of cortical dementia in this patient?

A. Apathy.
B. Aphasia.
C. Decreased attention.
D. Bradyphrenia.
E. Mood lability.

205 A psychiatrist is asked to determine if a very ill, delirious, and possibly senile patient has the capacity to make a new will. Which of the following features must be present to determine that the patient has the capacity?

A. Orientation to time and place.
B. Unimpaired attention span.
C. Awareness that she is making a will.
D. Choice of beneficiary that is not frivolous.
E. Ability to recognize family.

206 Which of the following types of therapy used to treat schizophrenia is based on the premise that attempting to suppress or control mental events is NOT helpful?

A. Traditional cognitive-behavioral therapy (CBT).
B. Compliance therapy.
C. Acceptance and commitment therapy (ACT).
D. Supportive psychotherapy.
E. Illness education.

207 A 45-year-old patient requests a medication to treat symptoms consistent with generalized anxiety disorder (GAD). The patient has a history of heavy drinking. Which of the following medications would be most appropriate to prescribe?

A. Clonazepam.
B. Bupropion.
C. Quetiapine.
D. Diazepam.
E. Venlafaxine.

208 A bus driver calls in sick whenever there is inclement weather such as rain or light snow. He has never had an accident while driving, nor does he know anyone personally who had an accident due to inclement weather. He also avoids driving his own car in poor weather and attempts to convince his family members to do the same. He admits he is very cautious about many things, which interferes with his sleep, causes fatigue, and makes him irritable. Which of the following is the most likely diagnosis?

A. Panic disorder.
B. Social phobia: situational.
C. Posttraumatic stress disorder.
D. OCD.
E. Generalized anxiety disorder.

209 A 20-year-old woman was brought to the emergency department by police after disrupting one of her university classes. She was agitated and demanded that her intellectual abilities be acknowledged. She had pressured speech and her affect alternated between periods of euphoria and irritability. Her roommate told the emergency staff that the patient had been very energetic, had been unable to sleep for a week, and had previously been admitted to hospital for a similar episode. Which of the following diagnoses is most likely?

A. Cocaine intoxication.
B. Cyclothymia.
C. Bipolar I disorder.
D. Bipolar II disorder.
E. Schizophrenia.

210 Children and adolescents are considered a vulnerable population in the conduct of research because they:

A. Cannot consent.
B. Suffer more adverse effects.
C. Are in riskier studies.
D. Cannot assent.
E. Do not benefit.

211 A 53-year-old man presents asking for help with problem drinking. He reports frequent swelling of his ankles and says that when he goes to the corner store, he has to walk slowly or he'll get too short of breath. He says he's supposed to be taking "some heart pills" but hasn't had any for a number of months and can't remember their names. He has attempted to quit drinking on two prior occasions and was treated with diazepam for "the shakes." He has been drinking 1–2 pints of rum daily for the past 10 months. His last drink was several hours ago. What would be the most appropriate initial referral?

A. Medical hospitalization.
B. Partial hospitalization program.
C. Intensive outpatient program.
D. Office-based program.
E. Therapeutic community.

212 A 46-year-old man is begun on citalopram 20 mg daily for a major depressive episode. After 4 weeks, he returns to his psychiatrist citing little if any change in his symptoms. Which of the following would be the most appropriate next step in the patient's treatment?

A. Increase the patient's dosage to 40 mg/day of citalopram.
B. Discontinue citalopram and begin venlafaxine.
C. Continue citalopram but add lithium.
D. Begin vagal nerve stimulation.
E. Continue citalopram and begin aripiprazole.

213 Which of the following features would be most predictive of a favorable response to lithium maintenance in bipolar disorder?

A. Euthymic intervals.
B. Rapid cycling.
C. Mixed episodes.
D. Substance abuse.
E. Psychosis.

214 Which of the following medications has shown the most evidence for reducing suicide risk in the long-term treatment of bipolar disorder?

A. Carbamazepine.
B. Divalproex.
C. Gabapentin.
D. Lithium.
E. Olanzapine.

215 A 56-year-old man with a history of cancer presents with confusion, pure amnestic syndrome, and affective symptoms. Diagnostic studies are consistent with paraneoplastic limbic encephalitis. Which of the following cancers is the most common cause of this paraneoplastic syndrome?

A. Pancreatic cancer.
B. Prostate cancer.
C. Renal cancer.
D. Small cell lung cancer.
E. Testicular cancer.

216 A 24-year-old man on lithium maintenance therapy develops severe, persistent polyuria and polydipsia. Which of the following medications is most likely to be effective in treating these side effects without requiring administration of supplemental electrolytes?

A. Amiloride.
B. Furosemide.
C. Hydrochlorothiazide.
D. Metolazone.
E. Torsemide.

217 A 17-year-old patient diagnosed with anorexia nervosa at age 14 is brought to a psychiatrist by her parents. They are concerned because she is 65% of her expected body weight. The most appropriate intervention is to:

A. Suggest a group therapy program.
B. Initiate treatment with an antidepressant.
C. Restore the patient's nutritional state.
D. Refer the patient and family for counseling.
E. Provide cognitive therapy.

218 According to the results of the Clinical Antipsychotic Trials of Intervention Effectiveness (CATIE) study, which antipsychotic medication had the lowest all-cause discontinuation rate?

A. Olanzapine.
B. Quetiapine.
C. Risperidone.
D. Ziprasidone.
E. Perphanazine.

219 Which of the following medication combinations for individuals with OCD comorbid with tic disorder is supported best by evidence?

A. Fluoxetine plus clonazepam.
B. Sertraline plus buspirone.
C. Mirtazapine plus naltrexone.
D. Fluvoxamine plus haloperidol.

220 Studies of the neurobiological correlates of borderline personality disorder have revealed hyperactivity in which one of the following?

A. Amygdala.
B. Prefrontal cortex.
C. Tegmental area.
D. Cingulate.
E. Accumbens.

221 A 38-year-old patient with major depressive disorder has had a partial response to 80 mg of citalopram. He states this is the best drug that he has been on, but he continues to experience symptoms despite being on the medication for 7 weeks. He continues to occasionally have suicidal thoughts, which frightens him because he made a suicide attempt 4 years ago. The best intervention at this time is to augment with:

A. Fluoxetin.
B. Lamotrigine.
C. Lithium.
D. Thyroid.
E. Buspirone.

222 Which of the following medications for bipolar disorder has been associated with polycystic ovarian syndrome (PCOS)?

A. Topiramate.
B. Divalproex.
C. Carbamazepine.
D. Lamotrigine.
E. Lithium.

223 The parents of a 4-year-old boy report that a few hours after he goes to sleep, their son will suddenly get up in the bed and look extremely frightened. His heart races; he is diaphoretic and cries out. He is difficult to awaken and has no recall of the event the next morning. Which of the following is the most appropriate next step in the management of this patient?

A. Administer a short-acting hypnotic for 2 weeks.
B. Have the child go to bed at a later time.
C. Obtain an electroencephalogram to rule out temporal lobe epilepsy.
D. Reassure the parents that their son will outgrow the disorder.
E. Suggest to the parents that they allow their son to sleep with them for a temporary period.

224 A 68-year-old woman being treated for bipolar disorder became semicomatose and incontinent of urine. Her serum sodium concentration was 110 mmol/L. Which of the following medications is the most likely cause?

A. Lithium.
B. Divalproex.
C. Oxcarbazepine.
D. Lamotrigine.
E. Olanzapine.

225 In bipolar disorder, which of the following characteristics BEST differentiates adult-onset bipolar disorder from childhood-onset?

A. Presence of psychotic features.
B. Prolonged early course.
C. Mixed episodes.
D. Recurrent depression.
E. Treatment resistance.

226 A psychiatrist's neighbor tells her that he is having trouble sleeping due to work-related stresses. He asks for recommendations and some medication until he can get an appointment with his internist. What ethical problem results if the psychiatrist gives the neighbor the medication?

A. Prescribing medication creates a doctor-patient relationship.
B. The assistance may be ineffective, straining the relationship.
C. Providing free care can foster resentment.
D. Assisting this neighbor creates an expectation that the psychiatrist will treat other neighbors.

227 A local radio talk show host comes to see you for psychotherapy because you were described as "the best doctor at the clinic" by one of his friends. He spends most of the hour talking about problems he is having with a workmate who he feels is treating him rudely. At the end of the session, he asks to be seen at a special time to accommodate his work schedule. When you tell him you will be unavailable at that time, he becomes dismissive and angry. These traits are suggestive of which ONE of the following personality disorders?

A. Schizoid.
B. Antisocial.
C. Obsessive-compulsive.
D. Narcissistic.
E. Borderline.

228 In DSM-5, in what way are the criteria for anorexia nervosa revised from DSM-IV?

A. The amenorrhea requirement is lifted.
B. A subtype related to atypical anorexia is added.
C. The "significantly low body weight" requirement is removed.
D. The diagnostic criteria for anorexia nervosa were not revised.

229 Which of the following traumatic events is MOST likely to induce PTSD in exposed individuals?

A. Unexpected death.
B. Natural disasters.
C. Motor vehicle accidents.
D. Witness to violence.
E. Sexual assault.

230 A 9-year-old boy is brought by his mother at the insistence of the school for the assessment of behavior problems. The diagnosis of attention-deficit/hyperactivity (ADHD) disorder is made, along with the recommendation to start stimulant medication. The mother is concerned that stimulant medication might put her son at risk for developing substance use problems. Regarding the risk of developing substance use problems, what is known about stimulant treatment for ADHD?

A. Increased risk of drug dependence only.
B. Increased risk of both alcohol and drug dependence.
C. Decreased risk of drug dependence only.
D. Decreased risk of both alcohol and drug dependence.
E. Unchanged risk for both alcohol and drug dependence.

231 Which of the following disorders must be considered specifically in the differential diagnosis of individuals with late-onset (after the age of 45 years) OCD?

A. Huntington's disease.
B. Autism spectrum disorder.
C. Delusional disorder.
D. Body dysmorphic disorder.
E. Schizophrenia.

232 A psychiatrist has been seeing a terminally ill woman in psychotherapy. The patient has become too ill to come to the office, so the psychiatrist elects to make a house call. In committing this boundary crossing, he should:

A. Act in a more social manner.
B. Discuss this variation from usual practice with a lawyer before going.
C. Discuss the implications of this change of venue with the patient.
D. Never go to the patient's home.

233 Which of the following is the most common psychiatric symptom found in patients with fibromyalgia?

A. Anorexia.
B. Psychosis.
C. Hypersomnia.
D. Mania.
E. Depression.

234 Which type of treatment program has the best short-term outcomes for cocaine dependence?

A. Voucher-based contingency management.
B. Psychodynamic group psychotherapy.
C. Interpersonal psychotherapy.
D. Twelve-step groups (without other counseling).
E. Cue exposure therapy.

235 A patient in therapy has recently been told that his psychiatrist may change jobs and will be transferring his care to another psychiatrist. He has always needed a great deal of reassurance but now calls almost daily asking for opinions on decisions he is trying to make in his life. He often worries his ill wife will die before he does. Each time he is advised to attend day treatment to get further support; he often agrees to do so but does not follow through. On the basis of this vignette, which of the following personality disorders is most likely?

A. Dependent.
B. Antisocial.
C. Paranoid.
D. Borderline.
E. Narcissistic.

236 During an initial evaluation, a patient complains of multiple episodes of having palpitations, sweating, and intense anxiety. Information that would be most supportive of panic disorder is that the episodes occur when the patient:

A. Is reminded of a past assault.
B. Must use a public bathroom.
C. Attends a large party.
D. Is in essentially any setting.
E. Must use an elevator.

237 Which of the following statements most accurately describes the benefits of SSRIs in the treatment of PTSD? SSRIs have been shown to

A. Ameliorate core PTSD and other associated symptoms.
B. Treat primarily the comorbid psychiatric disorders.
C. Improve primarily hyperarousal symptoms.
D. Improve the effectiveness of α_2-adrenergic agonists.
E. Act only to augment psychotherapy in PTSD.

238 Which of the following factors will increase the potential for toxicity with lithium?

A. Cigarette smoking.
B. Concomitant administration of mirtazapine (Remeron).
C. Drinking a lot of water.
D. Exercising outdoors on a hot day.

239 An individual with a history of opiate dependence admits to daily use of opiates, but a confirmatory urine toxicology screen is negative. Which of the following opiates is the patient most likely using?

A. Hydrocodone.
B. Morphine.
C. Codeine.
D. Heroin.
E. Opium.

240 A 72-year-old man with severe chronic obstructive airway disease complains of anxiety, muscle tension, and a general feeling of uneasiness. The most appropriate psychotropic medication for this patient's condition would be:

A. Clonazepam.
B. Diazepam.
C. Alprazolam.
D. Lorazepam.
E. Buspirone.

241 Which of the following statements best describes the mechanism of action of acamprosate thought to occur in the treatment of alcohol use disorder?

A. Acamprosate blocks the reuptake of chloride ions in central GABAergic neurons.
B. Acamprosate competes with alcohol for central GABAergic neurons in a dose-dependent fashion.
C. Acamprosate affects μ opiate receptors blocking the centrally mediated reinforcing effects of alcohol.
D. Acamprosate inhibits aldehyde dehydrogenase, resulting in the accumulation of toxic levels of acetaldehyde.
E. Acamposate reduces neuronal hyperactivity during early alcohol recovery.

242 Which of the following substances is associated with an increase in the long-term risk of developing psychotic disorder?

A. Alcohol.
B. Cannabis.
C. Nicotine.
D. Opiates.
E. Inhalants.

243 A psychiatrist may terminate care of a patient in which of the following circumstances?

A. Patient has not paid a bill.
B. Patient has failed to be cooperative in treatment.
C. Patient has consultation with another psychiatrist.
D. Patient misses two appointments and does not return the psychiatrist's calls.
E. Patient is hospitalized on an inpatient unit and care is permanently transferred.

244 Which of the following medications, commonly used in alcohol treatment to decrease craving, has been shown to be more effective if given after a period of sobriety?

A. Acamprosate.
B. Disulfiram.
C. Gabapentin.
D. Naltrexone.
E. Topiramate.

245 Which of the following is characteristic of social anxiety disorder (social phobia)?

A. Spontaneous uncued panic attacks.
B. Avoiding public speaking because of trembling.
C. Fear of humiliation when speaking in a group setting.
D. Fainting while having blood drawn.
E. Avoiding parties because of fear of contamination.

246 A patient with OCD and fears of contamination insists that his family remove their shoes when they enter his living space. Which of the following concepts best describes this behavior?

A. Repetition compulsion.
B. Displacement.
C. Ritual by proxy.
D. Projection.
E. Reaction formation.

247 A 48-year-old woman is brought to the emergency department after being found unconscious. Examination reveals respiratory depression, extreme miosis, stupor, coma, and pulmonary edema. The patient's presentation is MOST consistent with an overdose of:

A. Alcohol.
B. Cannabis.
C. Inhalants.
D. Opioids.
E. Sedative-hypnotics.

248 Patients with obsessive-compulsive disorder are most likely to respond to which of the following therapy modalities?

A. Psychoanalysis.
B. Dynamic psychotherapy.
C. Dialectical behavior therapy.
D. Motivational enhancement therapy.
E. Exposure and response prevention.

249 Which of following is the most common fear during the dying process?

A. Loneliness.
B. Abandonment.
C. Pain.
D. Uncertainty.

250 A 38-year-old woman is admitted to the hospital with a severe manic episode. On examination, she is noted to have motor excitement, mutism, and stereotypic movements. Which of the following medications would be the most appropriate in treating this patient?

A. Carbamazepine.
B. Haloperidol.
C. Lamotrigine.
D. Lorazepam.
E. Olanzapine.

251 A 35-year-old man with a history of opiate dependence is brought to the emergency department after being found unconscious. Examination reveals respiratory depression, extreme miosis, stupor, coma, and pulmonary edema. The emergency department physician administers naloxone 1 mg intravenously every 3 minutes until a maximum dosage of 10 mg has been given. However, the patient remains unresponsive. What would be the most appropriate next step?

A. Double the next intravenous dose of naloxone.
B. Increase the frequency with which the naloxone is administered.
C. Reconsider the diagnosis of an opioid overdose.
D. Start a continuous infusion of naloxone.
E. Switch from intravenous naloxone to nasogastric administration of naltrexone.

252 The concept that directs child psychiatrists and health care providers to involve children in decisions about their care commensurate with their developmental capacity is referred to as:

A. Cognitive incapacity.
B. Pediatric assent.
C. Pediatric consent.
D. Remaining autonomy.

253 Which of the following syndromes is the most common form of inherited intellectual disability?

A. Fragile X syndrome.
B. Williams syndrome.
C. Rett syndrome.
D. Prader-Willi syndrome.
E. Angelman syndrome.

254 Hypertensive paroxysms associated with diaphoresis, tachycardia, flushing, nausea, and significant apprehension suggests the presence of which of the following general medical conditions that mimics anxiety?

A. Mitral valve problem.
B. Cocaine withdrawal.
C. Coronary insufficiency.
D. Hyperthyroidism.
E. Pheochromocytoma.

255 Behavioral therapy for a patient with OCD is most difficult when which of the following symptoms are present?

A. Observable rituals.
B. Delusions.
C. Contamination fears.
D. Checking behaviors.

256 A psychiatrist is seeing a 35-year-old patient with schizophrenia who is accompanied by his mother. During a discussion about possible medication options, the psychiatrist turns to the patient and asks "What would you prefer to do?" This question is an example of which ethical principle?

A. Altruism.
B. Respect for autonomy.
C. Beneficence.
D. Nonmaleficence.

257 Which of the following defines the virtue "veracity"?

A. Saying only what is true, never misleading the patient, and pacing disclosure to the patient effectively.
B. Practicing medicine consistent with the highest intellectual and moral standards, both professional and individual.
C. Recognizing, preventing, and relieving pain, suffering, and distress and acting to prevent and relieve pain, suffering, and distress.
D. Not being excessively swayed by potential feared consequence.
E. Taking reasonable risks to one's self-interest (in time, convenience, health, and even life) to protect the interests of patients.

258 A 25-year-old man has a history of facial and truncal tics since childhood. He presents to an outpatient clinic for evaluation of anxiety and is diagnosed as having OCD. Which of the following patterns of OCD symptoms is he most likely to exhibit?

A. Obsessions and checking.
B. Cleanliness and washing.
C. Symmetry and ordering.
D. Hoarding.

259 The starting dose of lamotrigine should be reduced by half if a patient is taking which of the following medications?

A. Carbamazepine.
B. Oral contraceptive.
C. Phenobarbital.
D. Divalproex.
E. Phenytoin.

260 A 75-year-old man with a history of mild Alzheimer's disease becomes increasingly aggressive at home. In addition, he is noted to have worsening memory and word-finding difficulty, inadequate self-care, and less interest in activities. Which of the patient's symptoms is most likely to be helped by risperidone?

A. Memory.
B. Word finding.
C. Independent functioning.
D. Aggression.
E. Interest in activities.

261 Two teenagers randomly fire their guns at a 54-year-old man in their neighborhood. A week later, the patient complains that he can't "get it out of my mind" and is having frequent nightmares about this incident. He is always "on the watch" when he drives down the road and avoids going out alone. The most likely diagnosis for this patient is:

A. Generalized anxiety disorder.
B. Obsessive-compulsive disorder.
C. Acute stress disorder.
D. Social phobia.
E. Posttraumatic stress disorder.

262 A 42-year-old patient complains of a fear of crowded places. This fear is present in any situation in which the patient perceives that escape may be difficult, including riding alone in elevators and cars. As a result of this fear, the patient rarely leaves home. Which of the following is the most likely diagnosis?

A. Social phobia.
B. Agoraphobia.
C. Specific phobia.
D. Avoidant personality disorder.
E. Panic disorder.

263 Which of the following is an objective sleep disturbance that occurs in depression?

A. Shortened sleep latency.
B. Decreased nighttime arousal.
C. Increased total sleep time.
D. Shortened REM latency.
E. Increased slow-wave sleep.

264 The main factor of somatic symptom disorder that differentiates it from factitious disorder or malingering is that in somatic symptom disorder:

A. Patients seek to play the sick role.
B. There are external incentives for the behavior.
C. Complaint of symptoms is exaggerated.
D. Patients often have had multiple hospitalizations.
E. Symptoms are not under voluntary control.

265 A 38-year-old married woman presents to a psychiatrist complaining of difficulty in her sex life. She reports that for much of her married life, she has had little interest in sexual intercourse with her husband. She has not had any affairs, and she denies any discord in her relationship with her husband aside from the lack of a satisfactory sex life. She does not masturbate and rarely has any sexual fantasies. On the few occasions that she does have intercourse with her husband, she is able to enjoy sex and achieve an orgasm. Which of the following diagnoses is most appropriate?

A. Genito-pelvic pain/penetration disorder.
B. Sexual aversion disorder.
C. Female sexual interest/arousal disorder.
D. Sexual dysfunction due to a general medical condition.
E. Female orgasmic disorder.

266 The age at which a clinician should consider the possibility of early-onset Alzheimer's disease is

A. 35 years.
B. 45 years or below.
C. 55 years or below.
D. 65 years or below.
E. 75 years or below.

267 A 22-year-old woman is driving her boyfriend home. The car hits a tree and he is killed. Six months after the accident, she is still unable to drive, she reports disturbing dreams related to the event and avoids going out, jumps when she hears loud noises, and cannot feel any sadness or happiness. What is the most likely diagnosis for this patient?

A. Adjustment disorder.
B. Agoraphobia.
C. Major depressive disorder.
D. Posttraumatic stress disorder.
E. Acute stress disorder.

268 Which of the following actions is most likely to ease the fears of a dying patient and his family?

A. Postponing the discussion of pain and pain management.
B. Giving the family and patient information on a need to know basis.
C. Telling the patient that only the family's input regarding care will be sought.
D. Educating the patient that he may have discomfort that cannot be alleviated.
E. Obtaining the patient's wishes regarding treatment decisions.

269 A 26-year-old bystander of a horrific motor vehicle accident is taken to the emergency department after reporting that suddenly she had gone blind. She does not appear to focus on anyone who is talking. However, her eyes are noted to track her reflection when a mirror is waved in front of her. After hospital admission, a complete medical and neurological workup is found to be normal. What should be the first intervention for her condition?

A. Pointing out that she can see as a result of the mirror test.
B. Instituting a reward system for sight improvement.
C. Discussing the stress of the event under amobarbital.
D. Suggesting symptom improvement through hypnosis.
E. Reassuring her that her sight will soon return.

270 A 48-year-old obese man presents for an evaluation at the prompting of his wife. The wife, who has accompanied the patient to the appointment, complains that the patient snores loudly and keeps her awake at night. She states he sometimes seems to be gasping for air. On questioning, the patient admits to falling asleep easily during the day and even falling asleep while driving on occasion. He also complains of morning headaches and was recently diagnosed with hypertension. Which of the following is the best initial treatment for this patient's condition?

A. Uvulopalatopharyngoplasty.
B. Temazepam.
C. Biofeedback.
D. Modafinil.
E. Nasal continuous positive airway pressure (CPAP).

271 A 55-year-old patient with alcohol dependence treated with naltrexone 50 mg daily has been abstinent from alcohol for the past 2 months. The patient has been advised to undergo surgical knee replacement. What is the minimum duration of time prior to the surgery for which naltrexone must be discontinued in order for opiate analgesia to be effective?

A. 24 hours.
B. 72 hours.
C. 5 days.
D. 1 week.
E. 2 weeks.

272 A 35-year-old patient worries obsessively that he will kill his mother. To alleviate the anxiety, he calls her repeatedly throughout the day to hear her voice and reassure himself that he has not harmed her. He has tried adequate trials of high doses of fluoxetine, paroxetine, lorazepam, and clonazepam without improvement. Which of the following medications would be most appropriate to prescribe next?

A. Citalopram.
B. Alprazolam.
C. Bupropion.
D. Lithium.
E. Clomipramine.

273 A 60-year-old man with early Parkinson's disease presents to your office at the urging of his wife. She reports that the patient has begun "acting out" his dreams while asleep, and on at least one occasion this "acting out" led to his assaulting her. Polysomnogram is likely to demonstrate motor artifact and/or lack of complete hypotonia during which phase of sleep?

A. Stage I.
B. Stage II.
C. Stage III.
D. Stage IV.
E. REM sleep.

274 Adding which one of the following medicines can increase the risk of toxicity in a patient stabilized on lamotrigine for bipolar maintenance therapy?

A. Lithium.
B. Valproate.
C. Quetiapine.
D. Topiramate.
E. Olanzapine.

275 A 52-year-old man presents with a rapidly progressive dementia, visual symptoms, and cerebellar signs. Within a few weeks, he is mute and has myoclonus. He dies 4 months later. Light microscopy of the brain reveals spongiform changes. This presentation is most consistent with which of the following diagnoses?

A. Creutzfeldt-Jakob disease.
B. HIV infection.
C. Huntington's disease.
D. Progressive supranuclear palsy.
E. Wilson's disease.

276 A family is seen in family therapy. During the process, the therapist attempts to increase differentiation, decrease triangulations, resolve cutoffs, and improve the ability of the family to manage anxiety. This process is MOST consistent with which family therapeutic approach?

A. Behavioral/cognitive-behavioral therapy.
B. Systemic family therapy.
C. Psychodynamic-psychoanalytic psychotherapy.
D. Strategic family therapy.
E. Transgenerational family therapy.

277 Which of the following diagnoses has been eliminated in DSM-5?

A. Gender identity disorder.
B. Borderline personality disorder.
C. Gender dysphoria.
D. Pedophilic disorder.
E. Transvestic disorder.

278 A 72-year-old patient is admitted to the hospital with a fever of 101.8° F and a urinary tract infection. The patient believes that it is 1974 and that the hospital room is a kitchen. The nursing staff is concerned because the patient is agitated, trying to get out of bed, and trying to pull out the IV. Which of the following medications is the best choice for the patient's agitation?

A. Lorazepam.
B. Haloperidol.
C. Diazepam.
D. Thioridazine.
E. Valproate.

279 Which of the following stages has been identified by Kübler-Ross as a part of the process for dying patients?

A. Anger.
B. Suicidal ideation.
C. Intellectualization.
D. Visual hallucinations.
E. Disorientation.

280 In individuals who partially respond to an SSRI, which of the following is an effective adjunct to SSRIs for the core symptoms of PTSD?

A. Tricyclic antidepressants (TCAs).
B. Atypical antipsychotics.
C. Anticonvulsants.
D. Benzodiazepines.
E. Prolonged exposure therapy.

281 The treatment for body dysmorphic disorder that has been shown to be most effective includes which of the following psychotherapeutic techniques?

A. Mindfulness training.
B. Exposure and response prevention.
C. Group psychotherapy.
D. Social skills training.
E. Biofeedback.

282 A 69-year-old woman is hospitalized for pyelonephritis, which is successfully treated with antibiotics. Discharge to her home, where she lives alone, is planned. However, her daughter calls and informs the treatment team that she found several bottles of recently prescribed unused medications in the patient's home. The team wonders whether the patient can safely manage her medications at home and asks psychiatry to evaluate her capacity. Which of the following potential reasons for medication noncompliance implies that the patient lacks capacity?

A. The patient was too delirious from her infection to remember to take her medications.
B. The patient's eyesight is too impaired to read the instructions on her pill bottles.
C. The patient is unable to understand the reasons the medications were prescribed.
D. The patient has a long history of noncompliance owing to a general mistrust of doctors.
E. The patient felt too hopeless and depressed to comply with her medication regimen.

283 A 35-year-old man presents with memory deficits and emotional lability. Head computed tomography reveals atrophy of the caudate. His father died from the same disorder when he was 38 years old. This presentation is most consistent with which of the following disorders?

A. Alzheimer's disease.
B. Huntington's disease.
C. Progressive multifocal leukodystrophy.
D. Subacute sclerosing panencephalitis.
E. Whipple's disease.

284 A 21-year-old patient has been diagnosed as having panic disorder. She reports that she frequently had difficulties with side effects in starting medications in the past. For this patient, which of the following would be the best beginning daily dose of sertraline?

A. 25 mg.
B. 50 mg.
C. 75 mg.
D. 100 mg.

285 Paranoid personality disorder is marked by pervasive distrust and suspiciousness of others. For this diagnosis, distrust and suspiciousness can be manifested by which ONE of the following?

A. Choosing solitary activities most of the time.
B. Experiencing social anxiety that persists even with familiarity.
C. Experiencing unusual perceptions such as bodily illusions.
D. Reading hidden, threatening meaning into benign events.
E. Showing emotional detachment.

286 A 50-year-old man with a 20-year history of smoking 1–2 packs per day attempts to quit by using the nicotine patch. He relapses to smoking after 4 days of cessation. He comes for an appointment, saying he knew it was going to be harder than he thought and he's not sure he can go through the process again. The best response would be:

A. "Most people need more than two tries before they successfully quit."
B. "You will need to try harder next time."
C. "With persistence, about 75% of smokers successfully quit."
D. "Let's try the same thing again."
E. "Most smokers require more intensive treatment to quit."

287 In elderly patients, which of the following conditions is most important to address to prevent depressive symptoms after hip fracture surgery?

A. Postoperative pain.
B. Requiring assistance with mobility.
C. Using benzodiazepines daily.
D. Using >4 medications.

288 A 36-year-old woman with breast cancer completed radiotherapy. However, 3 months later she continues to complain of disabling fatigue. In evaluating this patient, which of the following symptoms would suggest that the fatigue was directly due to her medical condition rather than depression?

A. Late insomnia.
B. Impaired concentration.
C. Feelings of limb heaviness.
D. Decreased interest in activities.
E. Weight loss.

289 A 24-year-old woman is comatose with generalized myoclonic twitching and is found to have a serum lithium concentration of 4.2 mEq/L. The treatment of choice is:

A. Saline diuresis.
B. Hemodialysis.
C. Exchange transfusion.
D. Plasmapheresis.

290 A 72-year-old man is referred by his primary care doctor to a geriatric psychiatrist for treatment of depression. Two weeks earlier, the man had seen his primary care doctor, who started citalopram 20 mg daily. The patient continues to report severe depressive symptoms. On interview, it becomes apparent that this is the man's first episode of depression, and he has no history of any prior psychiatric disorder. The psychiatrist should advise that the patient:

A. Discontinue citalopram and begin nortriptyline.
B. Discontinue citalopram and begin venlafaxine.
C. Continue citalopram but add lithium.
D. Continue the current treatment as prescribed.
E. Increase the citalopram to 40 mg daily.

291 In addition to being effective in treating major depression, interpersonal psychotherapy (IPT) has been shown to be highly effective in the treatment of which of the following disorders?

A. Substance use disorder.
B. Bulimia nervosa.
C. Obsessive-compulsive disorder.
D. Schizophrenia.
E. Persistent depressive disorder.

292 A decrease of which neuropeptide has been linked most closely to narcolepsy?

A. Neurotensin.
B. Oxytocin.
C. Somatostatin.
D. Hypocretin.
E. Melanocyte-stimulating hormone.

293 Which of the following antidepressants could be prescribed for a depressed patient who has major concerns about the possible effects of medication on sexual functioning?

A. Sertraline.
B. Venlafaxine.
C. Paroxetine.
D. Bupropion.
E. Trazodone.

294 Which of the following disorders was previously included in DSM-IV as an anxiety disorder and is included in DSM-5 in its own chapter/category with specific criteria for children?

A. Selective mutism.
B. Separation anxiety.
C. PTSD.
D. Agoraphobia.

295 When compared with individuals with Parkinson's disease dementia (PD-D), individuals with Alzheimer's disease dementia (AD-D) typically show more severe impairment in:

A. Apraxia.
B. Visual hallucinosis.
C. Depressive symptoms.
D. Visuospatial dysfunction.

296 Generally, restraint and seclusion are considered appropriate treatment interventions when the patient is at imminent risk to harm himself or others AND:

A. The patient is refusing medication.
B. No less restrictive alternative is available.
C. The hospital prefers physical to chemical restraint.
D. The time period is expected to be brief.
E. A physician is present to write the order.

297 A bus carrying students from a local high school is swept down the side of the mountain following a mudslide. Despite rescue attempts, all the youth on the bus either die or are seriously injured. On the basis of prevalence data, which of the following groups of individuals is most likely to develop PTSD symptoms after the disaster?

A. Family members.
B. First responders.
C. Guidance counselors.
D. Classmates.
E. Teachers.

298 In association with research leading up to DSM-5, the core features of personality disorders were reexamined. Investigators assessed which characteristics were stable, trait-like, and "attitudinal" and which tend to vary with life stresses over time. For which one of the following personality disorder diagnoses were rigidity and problems delegating found to be the least changeable criteria?

A. Schizotypal personality disorder.
B. Narcissistic personality disorder.
C. Borderline personality disorder (BPD).
D. Avoidant personality disorder.
E. Obsessive-compulsive personality disorder (OCPD).

299 Which of the following antiepileptic drugs has been shown to be effective in treating binge-eating disorder associated with obesity in short-term, placebo-controlled studies?

A. Topiramate.
B. Lamotrigine.
C. Oxcarbazepine.
D. Valproate.
E. Tiagabine.

300 A 32-year-old man is admitted to the hospital with a severe episode of bipolar disorder, mixed. Which of the following would be the best first-line pharmacologic treatment for him?

A. Lithium alone.
B. Lithium plus a benzodiazepine.
C. Lithium plus an antidepressant.
D. Lithium plus an antipsychotic.
E. Lithium plus valproate.

301 Which of the following medications has the strongest body of evidence for the treatment of bulimia nervosa?

A. Bupropion.
B. Fluoxetine.
C. Duloxetine.
D. Paroxetine.
E. Venlafaxine.

302 Which of the following patterns is most likely to be seen on an EEG of a delirious patient?

A. Generalized slowing.
B. Increased alpha.
C. Decreased theta.
D. Triphasic sharp waves.
E. Focal high-frequency spikes.

303 Which of the following types of psychotherapy focuses on a patient's current social functioning within one of four problem areas (reaction, interpersonal disputes, role transition, or interpersonal deficits)?

A. Supportive psychotherapy.
B. Interpersonal psychotherapy.
C. Cognitive therapy.
D. Psychodynamic psychotherapy.
E. Psychoanalytic psychotherapy.

304 A patient with a long history of successful treatment with 20 mg of fluoxetine has been found to be HIV+ and has begun antiretroviral therapy. The patient sees you because of a return of symptoms of depression. Which of the following is the most likely pharmacologic cause?

A. As the patient gained weight from an increased appetite, more of the fluoxetine became bound to fat cells.
B. The protease inhibitor caused lipodystrophy, which decreased fluoxetine levels.
C. The protease inhibitor began to compete with fluoxetine for protein-binding sites.
D. The protease inhibitor induced the activity of an enzyme that enhanced the metabolism of fluoxetine and norfluoxetine.
E. The protease inhibitor has a direct interaction on the fluoxetine, causing it to lose efficacy.

305 A 24-year-old man is arrested after repeated episodes of rubbing his genitals against women's buttocks while riding on the subway. The most likely paraphilic diagnosis is which of the following?

A. Fetishistic disorder.
B. Frotteuristic disorder.
C. Exhibitionism.
D. Voyeurism.
E. Sexual masochism.

306 Which ONE of the following is the most consistently agreed upon characteristic of supportive psychotherapy?

A. It is a form of psychodynamic psychotherapy.
B. It is based on the use of transference or other interpretation.
C. It is best for patients with Axis II disorders.
D. Its practice requires only common sense, interpersonal skills, and a capacity for empathy.
E. It serves primarily to strengthen the patient's self-esteem.

307 Which of the following treatments has the greatest body of evidence demonstrating efficacy for treatment of specific phobia?

A. Eye movement desensitization and reprocessing (EMDR).
B. In vivo exposure therapy.
C. Hypnotherapy.
D. Pharmacotherapy.
E. Imaginal exposure therapy.

308 A 23-year-old man is the sole survivor of a fire aboard a crowded plane. In the immediate aftermath of exposure to the trauma, which of the following interventions is most likely to be successful in preventing psychological sequelae?

A. Encourage him to imagine positive emotions.
B. Have the man ventilate about how he is feeling.
C. Normalize the stress reaction.
D. Prescribe a short-acting benzodiazepine.
E. Use critical incident debriefing.

309 Following survival of a tornado that killed 38 people in a local community, a woman is provided with education and training in coping skills that includes deep-muscle relaxation, breathing control, assertiveness, role-playing, covert modeling, thought stopping, positive thinking, and self-talks. The intervention described is:

A. Aversion therapy.
B. Insight-oriented psychotherapy.
C. Interpersonal therapy.
D. Stress inoculation training (SIT).

310 Which of the following symptoms is most consistent with a medication side effect of an antipsychotic medication rather than progression of Huntington's disease?

A. Flowing movements.
B. Postural instability.
C. Effects on swallowing.
D. Akathisia.
E. Facial apraxia.

311 The hormone that masculinizes the human brain during uterine life is:

A. Testosterone.
B. Dihydrotestosterone.
C. Estrone.
D. Estradiol.
E. Progesterone.

312 Which of the following cognitive abilities is preserved in normal aging?

A. Working memory.
B. Perceptual-motor skills.
C. Vocabulary.
D. Fluency.
E. Logical problem solving.

313 Explicit feelings of shame, shame proneness, and self-stigma associated with higher ratings of anger and hostility have been empirically demonstrated to be increased in patients with which of the following disorders?

A. Social phobia.
B. Borderline personality disorder.
C. Histrionic personality disorder.
D. Persistent depressive disorder.
E. Paranoid personality disorder.

314 Following a massive hurricane, the occupants of a city are placed in a temporary refugee camp until other housing can be obtained. Which of the following ways of organizing the refugee camp is likely to be most successful in preventing PTSD?

A. Bring in citizen leaders from nearby cities to run the camp.
B. Develop the camp into a village with a village council.
C. Have the military oversee operation of the camp.
D. Organize the camp along racial, religious, and ethnic divisions.
E. Provide individuals with their own tents.

315 Which of the following signs and symptoms is most reliable in distinguishing between delirium and dementia?

A. Orientation.
B. Short-term memory.
C. Long-term memory.
D. Sleep pattern.
E. Level of consciousness.

316 A 64-year-old patient is hospitalized for an injury that occurred while he was inebriated. Three days after admission, the patient is disoriented, hallucinating, and has a grand mal seizure. His blood pressure is 160/100, with a pulse of 105. Which of the following medications is most appropriate for managing this patient's condition?

A. Haloperidol.
B. Sertraline.
C. Quetiapine.
D. Lorazepam.
E. Propranolol.

317 Which of the following chromosomal abnormalities is associated with an increased risk of early-onset Alzheimer's dementia?

A. Angelman syndrome (deletion of the 15q11-q13 region of chromosome 15).
B. Down syndrome (trisomy 21).
C. Turner syndrome (monosomy X).
D. Klinefelter syndrome (46, xy/47, xxy mosaicism).

318 Which of the following is the most common psychiatric diagnosis among patients with cancer who have no prior psychiatric history?

A. Posttraumatic stress disorder.
B. Major depressive disorder.
C. Acute stress disorder.
D. Adjustment disorder.
E. Generalized anxiety disorder.

319 A 40-year-old woman with bipolar I disorder complains of a lengthy, paralyzing period of depression following an episode of mania that led to hospitalization. Her symptoms have not responded to treatment with lamotrigine alone. Which of the following medications has the best evidence for efficacy as monotherapy to treat this patient's depression?

A. Aripiprazole.
B. Haloperidol.
C. Quetiapine.
D. Valproic acid.

320 A 28-year-old man presents with the chief complaint of excessive daytime sleepiness. He reports the sudden onset of brief periods of daytime sleep that are very restful. On a few occasions, he has experienced brief muscle paralysis after laughter. Recently, he has had two episodes of temporary paralysis when he awakens during the morning accompanied by vivid visual hallucinations. A polysomnogram is most likely to show which of the following?

A. Episodes of decreased blood oxygen saturation in spite of ventilatory effort.
B. Sleep-onset REM periods (SOREMPS) within 15 minutes of falling asleep.
C. Increased sleep spindles and K-complexes in stage 2 non-REM sleep.
D. Multiple awakenings during stage 3 and 4 of non-REM sleep.
E. Prolonged episodes of REM sleep in the first half of the night.

321 Which of the following is most likely to be predictive of a good prognosis in schizophrenia?

A. Early age at onset of symptoms.
B. Presence of predominantly negative symptoms.
C. Acute onset with underlying precipitating factors.
D. Presence of neurological signs and symptoms.
E. Low IQ.

322 Which of the following medications is considered to be a first-line pharmacological treatment for delirium?

A. Lorazepam.
B. Haloperidol.
C. Quetiapine.
D. Trazodone.
E. Hydroxyzine.

323 A 67-year-old woman presents with visual hallucinations, memory loss, apathy, and extrapyramidal symptoms. The patient's extrapyramidal symptoms increase markedly when given olanzapine 2.5 mg. This presentation is most consistent with:

A. Vascular dementia.
B. Dementia of the Alzheimer's type.
C. Lewy body dementia.
D. Dementia due to HIV.
E. Dementia due to Huntington's disease.

324 A 70-year-old woman presents with a history of a fixed belief that her arms and legs are infested with bugs that are crawling and biting her. She has no known associated medical condition and is physically healthy. Which of the following is best supported as a treatment of her condition?

A. Methylphenidate.
B. Imipramine.
C. Pimozide.
D. Selegiline.
E. Fluoxetine.

325 For the treatment of genito-pelvic pain/penetration disorder (vaginismus), which of the following interventions in combination with education and counseling would be most effective?

A. A short-acting benzodiazepine prior to intercourse.
B. Guided imagery during intercourse.
C. Limiting intercourse to the female superior position.
D. Use of a vibrator applied to the clitoris to induce orgasm.
E. Vaginal dilation exercises using plastic dilators.

326 Which antidepressant group is most likely to induce significant anticholinergic side effects that should be considered when treating late-life depression?

A. Serotonin norepinephrine reuptake inhibitors.
B. Monoamine oxidase inhibitors.
C. Selective serotonin reuptake inhibitors.
D. Reversible monoamine oxidase inhibitors.
E. Tricyclic antidepressants.

327 A 69-year-old man with chronic obstructive pulmonary disease, cirrhosis of the liver, benign prostatic hypertrophy, and alcohol dependence is prescribed acamprosate as part of his comprehensive treatment plan for his alcoholism. Which of the following laboratory tests would be most appropriate to obtain in order to determine the best starting dose of acamprosate?

A. Alanine aminotransferase.
B. Electrolytes.
C. Creatinine clearance.
D. Serum osmolality.
E. Serum total protein.

328 Social rhythm therapy for bipolar disorder is based on which of the following types of psychotherapy?

A. Cognitive-behavioral therapy.
B. Family therapy.
C. Group therapy.
D. Interpersonal therapy.
E. Psychodynamic psychotherapy.

329 A 15-year-old girl is diagnosed with anorexia nervosa. She has had symptoms for 18 months. Her medical status is stable, and she maintains an acceptable weight. The treatment that would be most beneficial for ongoing care is:

A. Behavioral management.
B. Psychodynamic psychotherapy.
C. Cognitive-behavioral therapy.
D. Family therapy.
E. Dialectical behavior therapy.

330 Which one of the following medications is associated with causing Ebstein's anomaly in the newborn if taken regularly by pregnant women?

A. Lithium.
B. Valproic acid.
C. Carbamazepine.
D. Lamotrigine.
E. Aripiprazole.

331 A 42-year-old woman receiving chemotherapy for non-Hodgkin's lymphoma develops anorexia-cachexia syndrome. She is started on a medication to address her symptoms. A few weeks later she returns with reports of an increase in her sense of well-being and decreased pain and nausea. However, she has gained no weight and has new-onset muscle weakness. Which of the following agents is most likely responsible?

A. Corticosteroids.
B. Cyproheptadine.
C. Medroxyprogesterone acetate.
D. Metoclopramide.
E. Ondansetron.

332 A 42-year man is being treated with cognitive-behavior therapy (CBT) for depression. He describes several mistakes he made at work and voices the belief that "No matter what I try, I always fail." This is an example of:

A. Automatic thought.
B. Maladaptive schema.
C. Full consciousness.
D. Modified cognition.
E. Unconscious conflict.

333 Which of the following mood stabilizers is FDA-approved for acute mania in children older than 12 years?

A. Lithium.
B. Sodium valproate.
C. Carbamazepine.
D. Lamotrigine.
E. Topiramate.

334 A 66-year-old man being treated for bipolar disorder is noted to have asymptomatic hypercalcemia and elevated levels of parathyroid hormone. Which of the following medications is the most likely cause?

A. Divalproex.
B. Lamotrigine.
C. Lithium.
D. Topiramate.
E. Olanzapine.

335 A 28-year-old hospitalized patient is started on an antipsychotic medication for schizophrenia. Within 3 weeks, the patient complains of chest pain, shortness of breath, and swelling of the lower extremities. Which medication is the patient most likely taking?

A. Fluphenazine.
B. Quetiapine.
C. Risperidone.
D. Aripiprazole.
E. Clozapine.

336 A requirement in the United States for initiating hospice care is that the patient must have:

A. A cognitive-impairing terminal illness.
B. A health care power of attorney.
C. A prognosis ≤6 months to live.
D. No family members able to provide care.
E. Medicare and/or Medicaid benefits.

337 A 38-year-old patient with schizophrenia is observed holding her arms in bizarre positions for hours at a time. On interview, the patient does not answer any questions but rather repeats everything the psychiatrist says. Which of the following is the most appropriate initial treatment?

A. Lorazepam.
B. Propranolol.
C. Diphenhydramine.
D. Phenobarbital.
E. Botulinum toxin.

338 Procedural justice in the process of civil commitment refers to:

A. Physician decision making that supports a beneficial outcome for patients.
B. A style of communication that alleviates patients' experience of coercion.
C. The inclusion of a patient's family in commitment decisions.
D. Judicial decision making that takes into account patients' therapeutic options.
E. Choosing the least restrictive alternative for patients.

339 A review of the current evidence suggests that the BEST explanation for an increase in the rate of autism spectrum disorders is:

A. Exposure to childhood vaccines.
B. Rates of genetic mutations.
C. Exposure to environmental toxins.
D. Screening and diagnosis.
E. Survival of premature infants.

340 A 22-year-old male college student has a positive HIV test. History reveals he had unprotected sex with multiple partners. His complete blood count is consistent with anemia. Which of the following factors places him at highest risk for eventually developing an HIV dementia?

A. Age.
B. Anemia.
C. Educational level.
D. Gender.
E. Multiple sexual partners.

341 The symptom that is most suggestive that an individual has generalized anxiety disorder (GAD) is worrying about:

A. Specific behaviors.
B. Physical symptoms.
C. Embarrassment.
D. All experiences.
E. Past events.

342 A 7-year-old boy with an anxiety disorder is in cognitive-behavior therapy. The parents ask how they should approach getting the child to do activities that he is fearful about, such as socializing with peers and participating in competitive situations. Which of the following is the MOST appropriate response?

A. Wait until the anxiety and fearfulness have been resolved.
B. Start when the child understands his anxieties.
C. Gradually approach with reinforcement for trying.
D. Find appropriate non-anxiety-producing substitutes.
E. Make fun activities contingent on doing anxiety-provoking things.

343 A patient presents with a well-defined history of recurrent hypomanic episodes but denies ever having had depressive symptoms or full manic episodes. According to DSM-5 criteria, the most appropriate diagnosis would be:

A. Cyclothymic disorder.
B. Schizoaffective disorder.
C. Bipolar I disorder.
D. Bipolar II disorder.
E. Other specified bipolar and related disorder.

344 Which of the following is a required criterion for the diagnosis of depression with melancholic features?

A. Mood worse in the late afternoon.
B. Middle or late insomnia.
C. Significant hyperphagia or weight gain.
D. Mood changes similar to those found in bereavement.
E. Loss of pleasure in all, or almost all, activities.

345 A 10-year-old boy is referred for psychiatric assessment after setting his family's home on fire. His mother smoked cigarettes during the pregnancy. The patient grew up in an extremely impoverished neighborhood with his mother as his sole caregiver. His mother describes the boy as being extremely oppositional and defiant as a preschooler. She has primarily used corporal punishment including beating him with a belt and electric cords. Since starting school, he has had multiple suspensions for fighting with peers and teachers. Intelligence testing is consistent with borderline intellectual functioning. Which of these factors from the patient's history is MOST predictive of a poor outcome in this patient's conduct disorder?

A. Early age at onset of symptoms.
B. Exposure to toxins in utero.
C. Lack of a father figure in his life.
D. Impaired intellectual functioning.

346 During the assessment of a 3½-year-old boy who has been referred for biting other children at preschool, the mother discloses that the boy's stepfather has been physically abusive toward her. The child may have witnessed some of the abusive episodes. Which of the following MUST be done prior to the end of the session?

A. Explain that the child is at risk for PTSD.
B. Refer the mother for her own treatment.
C. Find contact information for shelters.
D. Explore whether the child has been abused.
E. Explore mother's reasons for staying with the stepfather.

347 Which of the following signs differentiates patients with cognitive symptoms of depression from patients who are severely demented?

A. Less attention to self-care.
B. Cognitive impairment.
C. Complaints of memory loss.
D. Less attention to environment.
E. Memory storage and retrieval.

348 A 32-year-old woman who does not want to take medication complains about shortness of breath, chest pain, and diaphoresis. She has had multiple attacks in the past 3 weeks. Her medical workup is negative. Which of the following treatments has the strongest evidence supporting it as first choice for this patient?

A. Dialectical behavioral therapy.
B. Family therapy.
C. Group therapy.
D. Patient support groups.
E. Cognitive-behavioral therapy.

349 A 74-year-old man with known dementia is admitted to the hospital for workup and treatment of a presumed delirium. He scores a 21 on the Mini-Mental State Examination (MMSE) on admission and a 15 two days later. Nursing notes from his hospitalization indicate that there are times when he is completely alert and other times when he is nearly stuporous. Without appearing bothered, he has occasionally described seeing brightly colored birds perching on the windowsill of his room. A thorough delirium workup reveals no cause for his waxing and waning mental status findings. This description is most consistent with which dementing process?

A. Vascular dementia.
B. Alzheimer's dementia.
C. Frontotemporal dementia.
D. Lewy body dementia.
E. Korsakoff dementia.

350 In DSM-5, which of the following disorder(s) of children and adolescents is NOT classified among the neurodevelopmental disorders?

A. Tic disorders.
B. Attention-deficit/hyperactivity disorder.
C. Disruptive mood dysregulation disorder.
D. Learning disorders.
E. Social (pragmatic) communication disorder.

351 Which of the following psychosocial treatments for depression has the most robust data supporting its use?

A. Cognitive-behavioral therapy.
B. Dialectical behavioral therapy.
C. Group therapy.
D. Psychodynamic psychotherapy.
E. Supportive therapy.

352 A 25-year-old patient with schizophrenia is admitted to the hospital with auditory hallucinations and persecutory delusions. The psychiatrist initiates haloperidol 5 mg orally twice per day. After 48 hours of receiving medication, the patient becomes increasingly irritable and agitated and is noted to be restless and pacing. The patient's blood pressure is 130/85 with a pulse of 88. The next step in management of this patient's symptoms should be to:

A. Increase the haloperidol to 10 mg orally twice per day.
B. Administer benztropine 1 mg orally twice per day.
C. Administer a one-time dose of haloperidol 5 mg intramuscularly.
D. Administer a one-time dose of diphenhydramine 25 mg intramuscularly.
E. Initiate propranolol 20 mg orally three times per day.

353 Which of the following doses of haloperidol decanoate has been shown to have the lowest rate of symptomatic exacerbation yet minimal increased risk of adverse effect or subjective discomfort?

A. 25 mg/month.
B. 50 mg/month.
C. 100 mg/month.
D. 200 mg/month.

354 Which of the following medications has the potential for a significantly increased risk of hemorrhagic pancreatitis?

A. Clozapine.
B. Divalproex.
C. Nefazodone.
D. Pemoline.
E. Thioridazine.

355 Which of the following situations is the individual with social phobia likely to avoid?

A. Crossing bridges.
B. Eating in public.
C. Being in closed spaces.
D. Proximity to spiders.
E. Sitting in movie theaters.

356 A 32-year-old woman with a history of early-childhood abuse and abandonment begins dynamic psychotherapy. Although the initial stages of treatment proceed well, after 3 months her psychiatrist notices that she is becoming more critical of the therapy and frequently questions the value of it. In addition, she is dismissive of the psychiatrist and begins to question whether the psychiatrist is adequately trained. As a result, the psychiatrist begins to dread the sessions and occasionally begins the sessions late. This mode of interaction is best described as a type of:

A. Projective identification.
B. Displacement.
C. Sublimation.
D. Paranoid-schizoid position.
E. Ambivalent/resistant pattern.

357 The parents of a 16-year-old-year boy ask if he can be treated to prevent the development of schizophrenia. For the last year, the boy has been more irritable, staying in his room most of the time playing music. His grades have declined. His uncle was diagnosed with schizophrenia at the age of 17. Which of the following statements BEST describes the current knowledge about the early identification and treatment of individuals who will become schizophrenic?

A. Many adolescents with these symptoms will not become schizophrenic.
B. Treatment with low-dose atypical antipsychotics will prevent schizophrenia.
C. Long-term use of atypical antipsychotics does not have major adverse effects.
D. Psychosocial interventions are more effective than medication treatment.

358 Which of the following is a common adverse effect of monoamine oxidase inhibitors therapy?

A. Serotonin syndrome.
B. Hypertensive crisis.
C. Priapism.
D. Orthostatic hypotension.
E. Weight loss.

359 A patient who was recently diagnosed with panic disorder complains 2 days after starting citalopram that she continues to be very anxious about having another panic attack. Even her sleep has been disrupted. Which of the following would treat her anxiety best?

A. Increase the citalopram.
B. Add lithium.
C. Lower citalopram.
D. Add clonazepam.
E. Add trazodone.

360 A 32-year-old woman presents to the emergency department after being raped. She appears confused and extremely frightened. She mentions a history of prior rapes. Which of the following psychotherapies, if administered soon after the event, has the best body of evidence in preventing the patient from progressing to PTSD?

A. Supportive psychotherapy.
B. Psychological debriefing.
C. Hypnosis.
D. Cognitive-behavioral therapy.
E. Single-session exposure therapy.

361 A 28-year-old patient with schizophrenia is prescribed an atypical antipsychotic medication. A baseline fasting plasma glucose level is obtained and is within normal limits. After what period of time should this test be repeated?

A. 2 weeks, and then quarterly.
B. 3 months, and then annually.
C. 6 months, and then annually.
D. Every 6 months.
E. Annually.

362 Which of the following reflects the APA's position on psychiatrists' participation in legally authorized executions?

A. Sanctioning of participation is determined by state associations.
B. Psychiatrists should not participate in executions.
C. Participation is left up to the discretion of the psychiatrist.
D. Psychiatrists may only perform a mental status exam prior to execution.
E. Psychiatrists may participate if they are only in a supervisory role.

363 A 20-year-old college student presents to the mental health clinic because for the past 6 months he worries constantly about things going on at his part-time job and about exams that he must take in his classes. He has chronic problems with concentration and sleep and complains that he is easily fatigued. He states that he is tired of the pressure he always feels. He adds that he has also been to the medical clinic because he feared that his frequent muscle tension meant he had a neurological disease. Which of the following is the most likely diagnosis?

A. Major depression.
B. Illness anxiety disorder.
C. Generalized anxiety disorder (GAD).
D. Adjustment disorder.
E. Somatic symptom disorder.

364 Which medication has the most evidence supporting its use as an augmenting agent for treatment-resistant major depression?

A. Divalproex sodium.
B. Lamotrigine.
C. Lithium.
D. Lorazepam.
E. Phenelzine.

365 Eye movement desensitization and reprocessing (EMDR) has several features that distinguish it from the other cognitive-behavioral treatments for PTSD. In addition to the directed eye movements, which of the following also distinguishes EMDR?

A. Having patients think about the trauma rather than verbalize it.
B. Encouraging patients to learn to identify cognitive distortions.
C. Utilizing and emphasizing exposures to the traumatic material.
D. Teaching relaxation and imaging techniques to manage anxiety.
E. Employing homework assignments to reinforce session work.

366 A 28-year-old woman with bipolar II disorder has been using an oral contraceptive for birth control. She currently presents with a hypomanic episode. Which of the following medications would be best to treat her hypomania without impairing the efficacy of the oral contraceptive?

A. Carbamazepine.
B. Lithium.
C. Oxcarbamazepine.
D. Topirimate.

---

367 Which psychotherapeutic modality involves teaching patients to tolerate distress, regulate their emotions, reduce vulnerability to cues, and avoid or distract without problem behavior, while concomitantly reducing reinforcement of maladaptive behavior?

A. Psychoanalytic psychotherapy.
B. Cognitive-behavioral therapy.
C. Interpersonal psychotherapy.
D. Dialectical behavior therapy.
E. Supportive therapy.

---

368 Which of the following drug classes is the preferred initial pharmacotherapy for social anxiety disorder?

A. Tricyclic antidepressant (TCA).
B. Monoamine oxidase inhibitor (MAOI).
C. Benzodiazepine (BDZ).
D. Selective serotonin reuptake inhibitor (SSRI).
E. Beta-blockers.

---

369 Which of the following factors is most likely to be associated with bacterial soft-tissue infections in drug users?

A. Cleaning the skin before injection.
B. Being HIV negative.
C. Being an experienced injector.
D. Intravenous injection.
E. Subcutaneous injection.

---

370 A 40-year-old patient complains of episodes of intense fear with associated somatic symptoms that have a sudden onset and peak within minutes. Which of the following is the essential feature required for a diagnosis of panic disorder?

A. Anticipatory anxiety and avoidance of public speaking.
B. Unexpected, "out-of-the-blue" nature of the episodes.
C. Presence of four or more characteristic symptoms during episodes.
D. Episodes precipitated by memories of a past trauma.
E. Episodes triggered by contact with "contaminated" objects.

---

371 A 53-year-old man with a history of alcohol dependence has been abstinent from alcohol for 3 months. Although he continues to attend peer support groups, he reports that he has recently begun drinking one to two drinks approximately every other day and is fearful that his relapse will worsen. Which of the following medications would be the most appropriate first-line pharmacological intervention for this patient?

A. Naltrexone.
B. Acamprosate.
C. Bupropion.
D. Fluoxetine.
E. Disulfiram.

---

372 A 20-year-old patient with schizophrenia receiving antipsychotic treatment complains of breast tenderness, galactorrhea, and amenorrhea. Which of the following medications is the patient most likely taking?

A. Aripiprazole.
B. Risperidone.
C. Quetiapine.
D. Clozapine.
E. Ziprasidone.

373 Which of the following statements most accurately reflects the position of the *APA's Principles of Medical Ethics* on faculty psychiatrists having sex with trainees?

A. There is no established APA position on sexual relationships with trainees.
B. Sexual relationships with trainees are absolutely unethical.
C. Sexual relationships are permissible when both parties are consenting adults.
D. Sexual behavior in faculty-trainee relationships may negatively impact patient care.

374 In which of the following situations would a high-potency benzodiazepine be the preferred initial pharmacotherapy for panic disorder?

A. Comorbid major depression.
B. Need for rapid onset of action.
C. Anticipation of long-term treatment.
D. Associated agoraphobia.
E. Comorbid cardiovascular disease.

375 Which of the following substance abuse therapist attributes has the greatest and most consistent impact on patient retention and reduced substance use?

A. Therapists skilled at limit setting.
B. Therapists who were successfully treated for substance dependence.
C. Therapists who have a first-degree relative who was substance dependent.
D. Therapists with strong interpersonal skills.
E. Therapists who are knowledgeable about both biological and psychosocial interventions.

376 The daughter of an 89-year-old man with severe dementia requests that her father be deemed incompetent. The ultimate decision to determine competence is made by the:

A. Daughter.
B. Court
C. Psychiatrist.
D. Treating physician.
E. Health care power of attorney.

377 Anger is most closely associated with which of the following temperament traits?

A. Harm avoidance.
B. Novelty seeking.
C. Reward dependence.
D. Persistence.

378 An 80-year-old man is brought to the emergency room after suffering a grand mal seizure. His serum sodium concentration is 107 mmol/L. Which of the following medications is most likely to have caused the hyponatremia?

A. Topiramate.
B. Lamotrigine.
C. Gabapentin.
D. Oxcarbazepine.
E. Valproate.

379 In children with major depressive disorder, which of the following is MORE likely to occur in boys than girls?

A. Feelings of anxiety.
B. Acting-out behaviors.
C. Poorer self-esteem.
D. Severe symptoms of depression.
E. Shorter period of recovery.

380 A 21-year-old patient dropped out of college and has been unable to attend social gatherings as a result of extreme fear of embarrassing herself. She has failed to respond to therapeutic trials of paroxetine, fluvoxamine, sertraline, clonazepam, and buspirone. Which of the following medications would be most appropriate to prescribe next?

A. Fluoxetine.
B. Propranolol.
C. Phenelzine.
D. Lithium.
E. Risperidone.

381 Which of the following psychotropic medications has been associated with polycystic ovarian syndrome?

A. Lithium.
B. Divalproex.
C. Methylphenidate.
D. Citalopram.
E. Aripiprazole.

382 A 58-year-old patient with diabetic peripheral neuropathic pain presents with major depressive disorder. Which of the following antidepressants is most likely to have beneficial effects on both conditions?

A. Bupropion.
B. Duloxetine.
C. Escitalopram.
D. Nefazodone.
E. Mirtazapine.

383 When initiating treatment with risperidone long-acting injection, oral risperidone should be concomitantly prescribed for what length of time?

A. 1 week.
B. 3 weeks.
C. 6 weeks.
D. 8 weeks.
E. 12 weeks.

384 Which of the following personality disorders most closely resembles social anxiety disorder?

A. Schizoid.
B. Borderline.
C. Avoidant.
D. Dependent.
E. Histrionic.

385 Which antidepressant has been shown to be most efficacious in the treatment of depression in patients with HIV/AIDS with chronic diarrhea?

A. Fluoxetine.
B. Mirtazapine.
C. Paroxetine.
D. Sertraline.
E. Venlafaxine.

386 Which of the following is the best predictor of a recurrence of depression in someone with major depressive disorder?

A. Family history of depression.
B. Prior episodes of depression.
C. Prior suicidal attempt.
D. Comorbid psychiatric disorder.
E. Comorbid medical condition.

387 A patient has been successfully treated with an SSRI for acute panic episodes. What is the minimum length of time recommended for maintenance pharmacotherapy for this patient?

A. 2–4 months.
B. 6–12 months.
C. 18 months.
D. Over 24 months.

388 Which of the following is a required gateway symptom for major depressive disorder?

A. Insomnia or hypersomnia.
B. Recurrent thoughts of death.
C. Feelings of worthlessness.
D. Psychomotor agitation or retardation.
E. Loss of interest or pleasure.

389 In contrast to delusional disorder, schizophrenia is characterized by which of the following?

A. Disorganized speech.
B. Grandiosity.
C. Mood episodes.
D. Paranoid beliefs.
E. Physiological effects of a general medical condition.

390 In DSM-5, which of the following symptoms of PTSD is classified as a criterion D symptom of negative alteration in cognition or mood?

A. Difficulty falling asleep.
B. Recurrent nightmares.
C. Exaggerated startle response.
D. Inability to recall important aspects of the trauma.
E. Difficulty concentrating.

391 The personality disorder most closely associated with social anxiety disorder is which of the following?

A. Schizoid.
B. Obsessive-compulsive.
C. Histrionic.
D. Avoidant.
E. Borderline.

392 In order to make a diagnosis of bulimia nervosa, the symptoms must have duration of at least:

A. 1 month.
B. 3 months.
C. 6 months.
D. 9 months.
E. 12 months.

393 A 65-year-old man whose wife died 3 months ago presents to the clinic, accompanied by his daughter. The daughter states that the couple were married for 40 years and that he now feels utterly worthless without his wife. Since her death, he has stayed in the house, letting the newspapers pile up, and he doesn't answer the phone. He stopped his weekly fishing trips with his neighbor, a pastime of his for 20 years. He denies suicidal ideation but states that he wishes to join his wife. He has lost 30 pounds over the past 3 months and has stopped taking his hypertension medications. What is the most likely diagnosis?

A. Bereavement.
B. Adjustment disorder with depressed mood.
C. Major depressive disorder.
D. Depressive disorder, not otherwise specified.
E. Persistent depressive disorder (dysthymic disorder).

394 In dialectical behavior therapy (DBT), the term *dialectical* refers to which of the following therapeutic principles?

A. Psychic integration of good and bad objects.
B. A simultaneous emphasis on validation and change.
C. Efforts to treat both the manic and depressed phases of bipolar disorder.
D. A simultaneous focus on both thoughts and behaviors.
E. A dual focus on one's feelings and their impact on others.

395 Which of the following approaches to neurotransmitter modulation would be most appropriate in treating a patient with Tourette's disorder?

A. Dopaminergic modulation at the striatum and serotonergic modulation at the orbitofrontal cortex.
B. Dopaminergic modulation at the striatum.
C. Serotonergic modulation at the orbitofrontal cortex.
D. Noradrenergic modulation.

396 Features that support the diagnosis of somatic symptom disorder include distressing somatic symptoms plus abnormal thoughts, persistently high level of anxiety, and

A. State of being symptomatic that is persistent.
B. Distinct, clearly delineated symptoms of limited duration.
C. Symptoms that are different from those of organic disorders.
D. Symptoms that do not cause functional impairment.
E. Signs that are not acknowledged or recognized by the patient.

397 Demographic and clinical factors associated with suicide in patients with schizophrenia include:

A. Older age.
B. Female gender.
C. Higher cognitive function.
D. Lower socioeconomic status.
E. Good social support.

398 Which of the following therapeutic strategies for OCD maintains treatment success for the longest period of time after active therapy is discontinued?

A. Psychoeducation.
B. Record keeping.
C. A selective serotonin reuptake inhibitor.
D. Exposure and response prevention.
E. Supportive psychotherapy.

399 The highest level of decision-making capacity is required for which of the following actions?

A. Making a will.
B. Appointing a substitute decision maker.
C. Agreeing to participate in a research study.
D. Making a decision about treatment.
E. Consenting to phlebotomy.

400 Which of the following agents has been shown to be effective in the treatment of trauma-related nightmares and sleep disruption?

A. Phenelzine.
B. Prazosin.
C. Bupropion.
D. Cyproheptadine.
E. Diphenhydramine.

SECTION 2
Answers and Explanations

1 An 18-year-old woman is brought to the emergency department after collapsing at a party. She appears delirious and confused, with a temperature of 104°F. The friends who brought her to the emergency room say that she might have taken some pills. She was talking about feeling blissful and dancing a lot until she collapsed. Which of the following is the most likely drug ingested?

A. Methylenedioxymethamphetamine (MDMA).
B. Ketamine.
C. Flunitrazepam.
D. Gamma-hydroxybutyrate (GHB).

The correct response is option A: Methylenedioxymethamphetamine (MDMA).

MDMA, ketamine, and GHB, commonly known as "club drugs," are frequently used at rave parties. They are also known as Ecstasy, Special K, and liquid Ecstasy, respectively. MDMA intoxication can produce severe adverse effects, including altered mental status, convulsions, hypotherma or hyperthermia, cardiovascular instability, hepatotoxicity, and even death. This severity of intoxication is uncommon, however, in community settings.

Ketamine has a high therapeutic index and typically produces distorted perceptions of time, surroundings, and one's body. GHB can produce a sense of disinhibition, somewhat like alcohol. While overdose can produce an altered mental status, hyperthermia is rare. Flunitrazepam, a short-acting benzodiazepine, can induce amnesia and has been called a "date rape drug."

McDowell DM: MDMA, Ketamine, GHB and the "Club Drug" Scene, in The American Psychiatric Publishing Textbook of Substance Abuse Treatment. Edited by Galanter M, Kleber HD. Washington, DC, American Psychiatric Press, 2004, pp 321–333

Weaver MF, Schnoll SH: Hallucinogens and Club Drugs, in The American Psychiatric Publishing Textbook of Substance Abuse Treatment. Edited by Galanter M, Kleber HD. Arlington, VA, American Psychiatric Publishing, 2008, pp 191–200

2 Which one of these terms defines the most common form of genetic variation observed in the genome?

A. Short tandem repeat.
B. Single nucleotide polymorphism (SNP).
C. Haplotype.
D. Allele.
E. Variable number of tandem repeat.

The correct response is option B: Single nucleotide polymorphism (SNP).

SNPs are DNA sequence variations occurring when a single nucleotide (A, T, C, or G) in the genome (or other shared sequence) differs between members of a species or between paired chromosomes in an individual. An SNP, therefore, involves a single base difference at a particular site in the genome. In two-thirds of the cases, a cytosine (C)-to-thymidine (T) exchange occurs. Although many SNPs do not produce physical changes in people, scientists believe that other SNPs may predispose people to disease and even influence their response to drug regimens. A haplotype is the sequence of alleles along an adjacent series of polymorphic sites on a single chromosome. An allele is one member of a pair of genes located at a specific position on a specific chromosome.

SNPs: Variations on a theme. http://www.ncbi.nlm.nih.gov/About/primer/snps.html
Burmeister M: Genetics of Psychiatric Disorders: A Primer. Focus 2006 4:324–325

3 In adults, which of the following disorders is diagnosed in nearly equal numbers in men and women?

A. Generalized anxiety disorder.
B. Panic disorder.
C. Specific phobia.
D. Obsessive-compulsive disorder (OCD).
E. Agoraphobia.

The correct response is option D: Obsessive-compulsive disorder (OCD).

OCD is diagnosed in nearly equal numbers in adult men and women. Although it is slightly higher in adult women than men, males are more commonly affected in childhood. Females are twice as likely as males to be diagnosed with generalized anxiety disorder. Panic disorder has a 2:1 female:male ratio. Twice as many women are diagnosed with specific phobia and twice as many with agoraphobia as men.

American Psychiatric Association: Diagnostic and Statistical Manual of Mental Disorders, 5th Edition. Arlington, VA, American Psychiatric Association, 2013. pp 239, 681

4 Which of the following selective serotonin reuptake inhibitors (SSRIs) is most likely to be "self-tapering," thereby decreasing the chances of withdrawal effects?

A. Citalopram.
B. Escitalopram.
C. Fluoxetine.
D. Paroxetine.
E. Sertraline.

The correct response is option C: Fluoxetine.

Fluoxetine has a half-life of 4–6 days, citalopram 35 hours, escitalopram 27–32 hours, and sertraline 26 hours. Paroxetine has the shortest half-life of 21 hours and is most the common SSRI associated with a discontinuation syndrome. The withdrawal symptoms resemble "flu-like" syndrome. The elimination half-life of norfluoxetine, the main metabolite of fluoxetine, is even longer (4–16 days).

Sadock BJ, Sadock VA, Ruiz P (eds): Kaplan & Sadock's Comprehensive Textbook of Psychiatry, 9th ed. Philadelphia, Lippincott Williams & Wilkins, 2009, p 3199
Sadock BJ and Sadock VA (eds): Kaplan & Sadock's Synopsis of Psychiatry, 10th ed. Philadelphia, Lippincott Williams & Wilkins, 2007, 1090–1091
Rosenbaum JF & Tollefson GD. In Schatzberg AF Nemeroff CB (eds). Essentials of Clinical Psychopharmacology. 2nd ed. Washington, DC: American Psychiatric Publishing, 2006. p 33

5 Dialectical behavior therapy (DBT) was developed specifically for the treatment symptoms associated with which one of the following personality disorders?

A. Antisocial.
B. Borderline.
C. Avoidant.
D. Obsessive-compulsive.
E. Histrionic.

The correct response is option B: Borderline.

DBT was developed initially by Marsha M. Linehan, Ph.D., as a treatment for parasuicidal behaviors associated with borderline personality disorder. Subsequently, it has been used to treat a variety of conditions including emotional disregulation associated with eating disorders, adult attention-deficit/hyperactivity disorder, and major depressive disorder. DBT involves skills training, individual therapy, telephone consultation, and use of a consultation team.

Sadock BJ, Sadock VA (eds): Kaplan & Sadock's Comprehensive Textbook of Psychiatry, 9th ed. Philadelphia, Lippincott Williams & Wilkins, 2009, pp 2884–2893

Robins CJ, Chapman AL: Dialectical behavior therapy: current status, recent developments, and future directions. J Pers Disord. 2004; 18:73–89

Linehan MM: Dialectical behavior therapy for borderline personality disorder. Theory and method. Bull Menninger Clin. 1987; 51: 261–76

6 The most common cause of treatment failure in HIV/AIDS patients on antiretroviral medications is that most patients:

A. Have infections that are resistant to most available medications.
B. Fail to maintain the required adherence to the medication regime.
C. Do not start treatment until the infection is in the terminal stages.
D. Refuse to participate in medical treatment and take medications.
E. Have such severe side effects that medications cannot be used.

The correct response is option B: Fail to maintain the required adherence to the medication regime.

A major approach to the prevention of HIV disease progression is the optimization of adherence to antiretroviral regimens. Despite the considerable advances in the treatment of HIV/AIDS, treatment regimes remain complicated and difficult to maintain with many patients having inadequate responses because of a lack of adherence to the medications.

Forstein M, Cournos F, Douaihy A, Goodkin K, et al: Guideline Watch: Practice Guideline for the Treatment of Patients with HIV/AIDS. American Psychiatric Association; 2006. p 3 http://www.psychiatryonline.com/content.aspx?aid=147976

Goodkin K. Psychiatric aspects of HIV spectrum disease. FOCUS. 2009; 3:303–310

7 Advanced paternal age is a well-established risk factor for which of the following psychiatric illnesses?

A. Schizophrenia.
B. Substance dependence.
C. Major depressive disorder.
D. Generalized anxiety disorder.

The correct response is option A: Schizophrenia.

Studies have linked schizophrenia, as well as autism and bipolar disorder, to advanced paternal age, defined differently in different studies but generally between ages 40 and 50.

Brown AS et al: Paternal age and risk of schizophrenia in adult offspring, Am J Psychiatry 2002; 159:1528–1533

Dalman C: Advanced paternal age increases risk of bipolar disorder in offspring, Evid. Based Ment. Health 2009; 12;59 doi:10.1136/ ebmh.12.2.59

Reichenberg A et al: Advancing paternal age and autism, Arch Gen Psychiatry. 2006; 63:1026–1032

Sipos A et al: Paternal age and schizophrenia: a population based cohort study, BMJ, doi:10.1136/ bmj.38243.672396.55 (published 22 October 2004)

8 A 21-year-old woman presents with questions about her risk of developing schizophrenia. She is worried because her 18-year-old brother has recently been diagnosed with schizophrenia and required hospitalization for psychosis. There are no other family members who have a history of schizophrenia. Having a sibling with schizophrenia increases a person's risk of developing schizophrenia by approximately what amount?

A. The sibling is no more likely to develop schizophrenia.
B. The risk of developing schizophrenia for a sibling is 50%.
C. The risk of developing schizophrenia for a sibling is 10-fold.
D. The risk of developing schizophrenia is 30-fold.
E. It is almost certain the sibling will develop schizophrenia.

The correct response is option C: The risk of developing schizophrenia is 10-fold.

The risk of developing schizophrenia for a sibling of a patient with schizophrenia is estimated at 10%. More than 25 studies have consistently reported elevated risk for schizophrenia in first-degree relatives of individuals with schizophrenia (parents, mean=5.6%; sibs, 10.1%; children, 12.8%). This is a 10-fold increase above the general population lifetime risk of 1%.

Hales RE, Yudofsky SC (eds): The American Psychiatric Publishing Textbook of Psychiatry, 5th ed. Washington, DC, American Psychiatric Publishing, 2008, p 208

Shih RA, Belmonte PL, Zandi PP. A review of the evidence from family, twin and adoption studies for a genetic contribution to adult psychiatric disorders. International Review of Psychiatry 2004.16:4,260–283 open access http://dx.doi.org/10.1080/09540260400014401

NIMH Genetics Workgroup. Report of the NIMH Genetic's Workgroup: Summary of Research. Biological Psychiatry. 1999; 45:573–602

9 An 18-year-old female has high scores on scales of the personality traits of Harm Avoidance and Reward Dependence. On the basis of these personality traits, she is at HIGHEST risk for developing which one of the following disorders?

A. Anorexia nervosa.
B. Major depressive disorder.
C. Obsessive-compulsive disorder.
D. Schizophrenia.
E. Social anxiety disorder.

The correct response is option E: Social anxiety disorder.

Personality traits are consistently associated with different clinical disorders that a clinician may use the information in the differential diagnostic process. Anorexia nervosa is associated with high Harm Avoidance and Persistence; major depressive disorder with high Harm Avoidance and low Self-Directedness; obsessive-compulsive disorder with high Harm Avoidance and low Novelty Seeking; and social anxiety disorder with high Harm Avoidance and Reward Dependence.

Sadock BJ, Sadock VA (eds): Kaplan and Sadock's Comprehensive Textbook of Psychiatry, 9th ed. Philadelphia, Lippinicott Williams & Wilkins, 2009, pp 2211–2212

Faytout M, Tignol J, Swendsen J, Grabot D, et al: Social phobia, fear of negative evaluation and harm avoidance. Eur Psychiatry. 2007 Mar;22(2):75–9. Epub 2006 Nov 13

Mörtberg E, Bejerot S, Aberg Wistedt A. Temperament and character dimensions in patients with social phobia: patterns of change following treatments? Psychiatry Res. 2007 Jul 30;152(1):81–90. Epub 2007 Feb 27

10 A 40-year-old man with a 20-year history of heroin dependence and high tolerance is admitted to the hospital for IV antibiotic treatment of bacterial endocarditis. To prevent opioid withdrawal, considering his opioid tolerance, he is prescribed a moderately high dose of buprenorphine. He is just beginning to experience withdrawal symptoms before the first buprenorphine dose, but shortly thereafter, his anxiety, muscle aches, and rhinorrhea worsen. At this point, the best option would be to:

A. Increase the dose of buprenorphine.
B. Decrease the dose of buprenorphine.
C. Change to methadone.
D. Add a benzodiazepine.
E. Add naltrexone.

The correct response is option C: Change to methadone.

B-cause buprenorphine is only a partial agonist at the μ opioid receptor, when given in high doses to someone with high tolerance in early withdrawal, it can induce withdrawal. Increasing the dose may worsen withdrawal, whereas decreasing the dose may not provide adequate μ coverage. The best option is to change to the full agonist methadone, which has a linear dose-response curve, allowing for easier dose titration and alleviation of withdrawal symptoms. Naltrexone, a full μ antagonist, will worsen the withdrawal symptoms. The benzodiazepine is likely to have minimal effect, having no activity at the μ receptor.

Center for Substance Abuse Treatment: Clinical Guidelines for the Use of Buprenorphine in the Treatment of Opioid Addiction. Treatment Improvement Protocol (TIP) Series 40. DHHS Publication No. (SMA) 04-3939. Rockville, MD: Substance Abuse and Mental Health Services Administration, 2004. http://www.buprenorphine.samhsa.gov/publications.html
Pechnick RN, Glasner-Edwards S, Hrymoc M, Wilkins, JN. Preclinical development and clinical implementation of treatments for substance abuse disorders. FOCUS: Substance Abuse: Spring 2007; 2:151–162

11 A 35-year-old man with obsessive-compulsive disorder presents for treatment. He would prefer not using medication because of possible side effects. Which of the following psychotherapies would be the treatment of choice for his disorder?

A. Supportive psychotherapy.
B. Exposure with response prevention.
C. Hypnotherapy.
D. Interpersonal therapy.
E. Psychodynamic psychotherapy.

The correct response is option B: Exposure with response prevention.

Exposure with response prevention (ERP) is the psychotherapeutic treatment of choice for obsessive-compulsive disorder. In ERP, patients are exposed to the feared stimuli and obsessions while rituals that typically serve to reduce anxiety are prevented.

Sadock BJ, Sadock VA, Ruiz P (eds): Kaplan and Sadock's Comprehensive Textbook of Psychiatry, 9th ed. Philadelphia, Lippincott Williams & Wilkins, 2009, p 2790
Koran LM: Obsessive-compulsive disorder: An update for the clinician. Focus 2007; 5(3):299–313
American Psychiatric Association Practice Guideline for the Treatment of Patients with Obsessive-Compulsive Disorder. 2007. http://psychiatryonline.org/guidelines.aspx

12 An adolescent with mild intellectual disability continues to be significantly depressed despite actively participating in psychotherapy for several months. Which of the following is the best clinical option?

A. Start treatment with an atypical antipsychotic.
B. Start treatment with an SSRI.
C. Change psychotherapeutic approaches.
D. Implement intense behavioral management.

The correct response is option B: Start treatment with an SSRI.

Generally, symptoms in individuals with intellectual disability are treated with the same medications that are used in individuals who have no intellectual disability. Children and adolescents with intellectual disability may have less of a response or have more side effects. For depression, an SSRI would be the first choice with ongoing monitoring for adverse effects. Starting an antidepressant as an adjunct to psychotherapy after the adolescent has failed to respond to psychotherapy alone is a standard approach to the treatment of adolescent depression.

AACAP practice parameter for the assessment and treatment of children and adolescents with depressive disorders. J Am Acad Child Adolesc Psychiatry. 2007. Reprinted in FOCUS: Child and Adolescent Psychiatry. Summer 2008; 6(3):387

AACAP practice parameter for the assessment and treatment of children, adolescents, and adults with mental retardation and comorbid mental disorders. J Am Acad Child Adolesc Psychiatry. 1999; 38:1609

Handen B, Gilchrist R. Practitioner review: psychopharmacology in children and adolescents with mental retardation. Journal of Child Psychology & Psychiatry and Allied Disciplines. 2006; 47:871–82

13 Personalities characterized by the traits of persistence, perfectionism, and decreased flexibility in "set shifting" (i.e., the ability to move back and forth between tasks, operations, or mental sets) are associated with which of the following disorders?

A. Alcohol dependence in full-sustained remission.
B. Delusional disorder.
C. Anorexia nervosa.
D. Early Alzheimer's disease.
E. Traumatic brain injury.

The correct response is option C: Anorexia nervosa.

Persistence and perfectionism are associated with obsessive-compulsive personality traits and disorders, occurring in many patients with anorexia nervosa. When patients with anorexia nervosa were compared with control subjects without anorexia nervosa on neuropsychological tests of "set shifting," functions primarily linked to the prefrontal cortex, patients with anorexia nervosa and their healthy sisters both took significantly longer on set-shifting tasks than the control subjects without anorexia nervosa and did not differ from each other. Recovered women did not differ from unrecovered women on these tasks. Specifically in reaction to tasks requiring behavioral response shifts, these patients showed brain patterns that differed significantly from the comparison. These findings are consistent with other features of obsessive-compulsive personalities found in these populations. Such features have been linked to abnormalities in the serotonergic system, implicated in the regulation of impulsivity and cognitive inflexibility, reported in anorexia nervosa.

Zastrow A, Kaiser S, Stippich C, Walther S, et al: Neural correlates of impaired cognitive-behavioral flexibility in anorexia nervosa. Am J Psychiatry. 2009 May; 166(5):608–16

Holliday J, Tchanturia K, Landau S, Collier D, Treasure J.: Is impaired set-shifting an endophenotype of anorexia nervosa? Am J Psychiatry, December 2005; 162:2269–2275

14 Which of the following treatments is considered the best approach to managing a patient with panic disorder, unresponsive to initial treatments with an SSRI and a benzodiazepine?

A. Serotonin-norepinephrine reuptake inhibitor (SNRI).
B. Buspirone.
C. Atypical antipsychotic.
D. Another SSRI.
E. Cognitive-behavioral therapy (CBT).

The correct response is option E: Cognitive-behavioral therapy (CBT).

On the basis of the current evidence, CBT is the psychosocial treatment that would be indicated most often. According to The American Psychiatric Association Practice Guideline for the Treatment of Patients with Panic Disorder, the effects of CBT have been shown to be at least as efficacious as those of first-line pharmacotherapies. CBT for panic disorder has continued to demonstrate short- and long-term efficacy in clinical trials and may present less risk of relapse than pharmacological treatment.

Bystritsky A. Diagnosis and treatment of anxiety. FOCUS Summer 2004; 3:333–342

American Psychiatric Association Practice Guideline for the Treatment of Patients with Panic Disorder (2009). http://psychiatryonline.org/guidelines.aspx

15 A 27-year-old man has borderline personality disorder, primarily manifested by an inability to control his urges to hurt himself. As a result, when frustrated, he will frequently superficially cut his wrists. Which of the following medications has been found to be most helpful in curbing this behavior?

A. Olanzapine.
B. Fluoxetine.
C. Clonazepam.
D. Divalproex.
E. Naloxone.

The correct response is option B: Fluoxetine.

Although psychotherapy remains the primary treatment for borderline personality disorder, an increasing body of literature suggests that pharmacotherapy may have a role. Pharmacotherary should be symptom-focused; the symptomatic targets of therapy are grouped into three clusters: cognitive-perceptual symptoms, affective dysregulation, and impulsive behavioral dyscontrol. For impulsive behavioral dyscontrol such as that exhibited by the patient in this question, SSRIs have the strongest data for efficacy; among the SSRIs, fluoxetine has been most often studied. Low-dose neuroloeptics have some efficacy as well and are considered second-line treatment, often in conjunction with an SSRI. Although atypical neuroleptics are becoming more commonly used in clinical practice, they have rarely been studied, and the bulk of data are for typical neuroleptics. Among the anticonvulsants, divalproex has been most often studied—it has shown some efficacy for affective instability, but the results for impulsivity have been equivocal. Benzodiazepines, although widely employed, have little evidence to support their use, and although some preliminary case studies have reported good results with opiate antagonists, the only controlled trial so far showed no difference from placebo.

Oldham JM, Bender DS, Skodol AE, Dyck IR, et al: Testing an APA practice guideline: Symptom-targeted medication utilization for patients with borderline personality disorder. J Psychiatr Pract 2004 May;10(3):156–61. Reprinted in FOCUS 2005;3:484–488

American Psychiatric Association. Practice guideline for the treatment of patients with borderline personality disorder. 2001. http://psychiatryonline.org/guidelines.aspx

16 A visibly pregnant 29-year-old woman presents seeking treatment for oxycodone dependence. Because of her pregnancy, she wants to stop using all drugs and does not want to take any medications. She went through untreated opiate withdrawal in the past when she couldn't get any pills, and although it was very uncomfortable, she thinks she could do it again with intensive social support and counseling. At this point, the best treatment recommendation would be to initiate:

A. Methadone maintenance.
B. Methadone-assisted withdrawal.
C. Clonidine-naltrexone-assisted withdrawal.
D. Buprenorphine maintenance.
E. Daily clinic visits to provide support.

The correct response is option A: Methadone maintenance.

Notwithstanding the patient's initial thoughts of avoiding medications, opioid withdrawal should be avoided in pregnancy because of the greater risk of adverse fetal outcomes compared with methadone maintenance. Withdrawing the mother completely from opioids raises the risk of relapse and that the fetus will be harmed. Nonpharmacological treatment alone will likely expose the fetus to continued illicit drug use and multiple withdrawals. Naltrexone should never be given to a pregnant woman because of the risk of spontaneous abortion, stillbirth, and other adverse events. There is a long history of the safety of methadone maintenance for both mother and fetus/neonate. Early clinical experience suggests that buprenorphine may have similar safety, but there is insufficient evidence to recommend its initiation in known pregnancy.

American Psychiatric Association Practice Guideline for the Treatment of Patients with Substance Use Disorders, 2nd ed (2006), http://psychiatryonline.org/guidelines.aspx

Galanter M, Kleber HD (eds): Textbook of Substance Abuse Treatment, 4th ed. Arlington, VA, American Psychiatric Publishing, 2008, pp 281–82

17 A 38-year-old female patient with schizophrenia has been treated with haloperidol and risperidone at different times in the past. Currently, she exhibits a nonrhythmical hyperkinetic movement disorder of the lips and jaw. The movement disorder most likely consistent with this finding is:

A. Akathisia (motor restlessness).
B. Parkinsonian's tremor.
C. Tardive dyskinesia.
D. Tardive dystonia.

The correct response is option C: Tardive dyskinesia.

Tardive dyskinesia is a nonrhythmical movement disorder first presenting in the mouth area. Parkinson's tremor is a perioral tremor (and therefore is rhythmical). Akathisia usually manifests in the lower limbs, leg shifting from one foot to the other or pacing. Tardive dystonia usually presents in the head and neck (e.g., sideways movement of the head associated with hypertonicity of muscles).

Kay J, Tasman A. Essentials of Psychiatry. John Wiley and Sons, Hoboken, NJ, 2006, pp 952–954

18 Which one of the following dimensions assessed on the Temperament and Character Inventory (TCI) is MOST likely to increase with age?

A. Cooperativeness.
B. Harm avoidance.
C. Persistence.
D. Reward dependence.
E. Self-transcendence.

The correct response is option A: Cooperativeness.

Personality disorder is associated with younger age. This indicates maturation with increasing age. In general, three dimensions of personality change substantially with age. Novelty Seeking decreases; Cooperativeness increases; and Self-Directedness increases.

Sadock BJ, Sadock VA (eds): Kaplan and Sadock's Comprehensive Textbook of Psychiatry, 9th ed. Philadelphia, Lippincott Williams & Wilkins, 2009, p 2233

19 A 74-year-old man presents with a history of rapidly progressive cognitive decline with ataxia, multifocal myoclonic jerks, and visual field cut. MRI reveals increased T2 and FLAIR signal intensity in the basal ganglia. Which of the following is the most likely diagnosis?

A. Alzheimer's dementia.
B. Huntington's chorea.
C. Creutzfeldt-Jakob disease.
D. Vascular dementia.
E. Lewy body disease.

The correct response is option C: Creutzfeldt-Jakob disease.

Creutzfeldt-Jakob disease is the most common among the prion-related neurodegenerative disorders and is characterized by rapid cognitive decline with ataxia, multifocal myoclonic jerks, and startle myoclonus. Other clinical features include weakness, neuropathy, chorea, hallucinations, visual field cuts, language disturbances, and seizures. MRI of the head can show very specific abnormalities and can aid in the diagnosis. Increased T2 and FLAIR signal intensity in the basal ganglia is reported. Alzheimer's disease is characterized by a gradual onset of cognitive decline along with impairment of executive function or ataxia, apraxia, or agnosia. Vascular dementia is often associated with a stepwise deterioration and presence of strokes. Lewy body dementia is often characterized by progressive cognitive decline, extrapyramidal symptoms, and visual hallucinations. Huntington's chorea is characterized by choreiform, dyskinetic movements, and may be associated with cognitive decline.

Yudofsky SC, Hales RE (eds): The American Psychiatric Publishing Textbook of Neuropsychiatry and Behavioral Sciences, 5th ed. Washington DC: American Psychiatric Publishing, 2008. pp 955–957

20 Genome-wide association studies (GWAS) have implicated regions of which chromosome in autism spectrum disorders (ASD)?

A. Chromosome 1.
B. Chromosome 5.
C. Chromosome 8.
D. Chromosome 22.

The correct response is option B: Chromosome 5.

The first published GWAS of ASD found evidence of a genome-wide significant association signal on chromosome 5p14. This original genome-wide association signal was replicated in a large case-control sample. The second association data identified genome-wide significant association on chromosome 5p15.

Collectively, the two reported ASD GWAS studies point to regions of chromosome 5p that may include common genetic variants that contribute to ASD risk. Additional studies will be required.

Campbell DB: Advances and challenges in the genetics of autism. FOCUS Summer 2010 8(3):339–349

21 A 16-year-old woman presents with fatigue and dehydration. On physical examination, she is noted to have swollen salivary glands and calluses on her knuckles. She is also hypokalemic. These findings are most consistent with which of the following diagnoses?

A. Chronic fatigue syndrome.
B. Bulimia nervosa.
C. Obsessive-compulsive disorder.
D. Anorexia nervosa.
E. Rumination disorder.

The correct response is option B: Bulimia nervosa.

No specific diagnostic test for bulimia nervosa currently exists. Bulimia nervosa, purging type, is characterized by frequent episodes of binge eating and "self-induced vomiting or the misuse of laxatives, diuretics, or other medications." Swollen salivary glands, calluses on knuckles, and hypokalemia are complications of excessive self-induced vomiting.

American Psychiatric Association: Diagnostic and Statistical Manual of Mental Disorders, 5th Edition. Arlington, VA, American Psychiatric Association, 2013, pp 345–348
Mehler PS. Bulimia nervosa. N Engl J Med. 2003; 349:875–881
Hales RE, Yudofsky SC, Gabbard GO (eds): The American Psychiatric Publishing Textbook of Psychiatry, 5th ed. Washington, DC, American Psychiatric Publishing, 2008. pp 983–984

22 A 21-year-old college student is seen in the university counseling center because of relationship problems. He has had one serious relationship with a woman that lasted about 6 months. He terminated the relationship because he discovered that the woman was seeing someone else. Although he wants to engage in a new relationship, he is extremely reluctant, stating: "Women just can't be trusted." Which of the following BEST describes this thinking error?

A. Arbitrary inference.
B. Dichotomous thinking.
C. Magnification.
D. Overgeneralization.
E. Selective abstraction.

The correct response is option D: Overgeneralization.

Overgeneralization is the process that occurs when someone believes in and follows a general rule on the basis of limited examples. *Arbitrary inference* is reaching a conclusion in the absence of any evidence that would support the idea (e.g., assuming you will lose your job because your boss sends you an e-mail asking to meet). *Dichotomous thinking* is "all or nothing" thinking in which a person reduces situations to "black versus white." *Magnification* is when an individual assigns subjective "weights" to his or her interpretation of situations, resulting, for example, in giving negative events greater weight than positive occurrences. Last, *selective abstraction* is focusing on a detail taken out of context.

Sadock BJ, Sadock VA, Ruiz P (eds): Kaplan and Sadock's Comprehensive Textbook of Psychiatry, 9th ed. Philadelphia, Lippinicott Williams & Wilkins, 2009, pp 2858–2859

Textbook of Psychotherapeutic Treatments.Gabbard GO (ed). Arlington, VA, American Psychiatric Publishing, 2009, p 173

23 A 40-year-old patient is diagnosed with Alzheimer's disease (AD). Which of the following genes is associated with this very early form of Alzheimer's disease?

A. Presenilin 1.
B. Presenilin 2.
C. Apo E2.
D. Apo 3.
E. Apo 4.

The correct response is option A: Presenilin 1.

Only 10% of Alzheimer's cases are considered to be hereditary. Of these, 70%–80% are attributable to mutations in the presenilin 1 gene, found on chromosome 14, which causes onset of symptoms at 40–50 years of age. Mutations in presenilin 2 are rare causes of early-onset familial AD. A mutation in presenilin 2 is associated with onset at approximately age 50. Apolipoprotein E2 (Apo E2) protects Tau protein from phosphorylation and thus from the neurofibrillary tangles associated with the disease, whereas Apo E3 and Apo E4 are not associated as strongly with this protection. The E3 and E4 alleles account for 10%–50% of the risk of sporadic AD with onset of symptoms at 60 years of age.

Sadock BJ, Sadock VA (eds): Kaplan & Sadock's Synopsis of Psychiatry: Behavioral Sciences/Clinical Psychiatry, 10th ed. Philadelphia, Lippincott Williams & Wilkins, 2007, p 129

Alzheimer's Disease Genetics Fact Sheet, NIH Publication No. 08-6424, November 2008, http://www.nia.nih.gov/alzheimers/publications/geneticsfs.htm

Bettens K, Sleegers K, Van Broeckhoven C: Current status on Alzheimer disease molecular genetics: from past, to present, to future. Hum Mol Genet. 2010 Apr 15;19(R1):R4–R11. Epub 2010 Apr 13

Jayadev S, Leverenz JB, Steinbart E, Stahl J, et al: Alzheimer's disease phenotypes and genotypes associated with mutations in presenilin 2. Brain. 2010 Apr;133(Pt 4):1143–54

24 During an interview of a patient with a substance use disorder, the therapist asks the patient about the pros and cons of specific behaviors, explores the patient's goals and associated ambivalence about reaching those goals, and listens reflectively to the patient's response. This treatment approach is most consistent with:

A. Cognitive-behavioral therapy.
B. Contingency management.
C. Interpersonal therapy.
D. Motivational enhancement therapy.
E. Psychodynamic psychotherapy.

The correct response is option D: Motivational enhancement therapy.

Motivational enhancement therapy (MET) combines techniques from cognitive, client-centered, systems, and social-psychological persuasion approaches. MET is characterized by an empathic approach in which the therapist helps to motivate the patient by exploring readiness for change. This treatment modality is effective even for patients who are not highly motivated to change.

American Psychiatric Association Practice Guideline for the Treatment of Patients with Substance Use Disorders, 2nd Edition (2006), http://psychiatryonline.org/guidelines.aspx

25 Which of the following antidepressants has the greatest body of evidence for efficacy in treating major depressive disorder in children and adolescents?

A. Citalopram.
B. Fluoxetine.
C. Fluvoxamine.
D. Sertraline.
E. Paroxetine.

The correct response is option B: Fluoxetine.

Fluoxetine has the greatest body of evidence for treating child and adolescent depression (ages 8 to ≤18). Studies have shown mixed results for other SSRIs. Studies have also shown some evidence of efficacy in other SSRIs, but the strongest evidence of efficacy in RTC exists for fluoxetine.

Cheung AH, Emslie GJ, Mayes TL. The use of antidepressants to treat depression in children and adolescents. Can Med Assoc J 2006; 174:193–200

Boylan K, Romero S, Birmaher B. Psychopharmacologic treatment of pediatric major depressive disorder. Psychopharmacol 2007; 191:27–38

Vasa RA, Carlino AR, Pine DS. Pharmacotherapy of depressed children and adolescents: current issues and potential directions. Biol Psychiatry 2006; 59:1021–1028

AACAP practice parameter for the assessment and treatment of children and adolescents with depressive disorders. J Am Acad Child Adolesc Psychiatry. 2007. Reprinted in FOCUS. 2008; 6(3):389

26 A city is attacked by terrorists intermittently over a 3-week period. There is no indication that the attacks will stop. Which of the following interventions is most likely to be effective in lowering the risk of developing posttraumatic stress disorder (PTSD) in the months following exposure?

A. Educating the public about symptoms of PTSD.
B. Evacuating the most vulnerable population.
C. Limiting exposure to media coverage of the attacks.
D. Providing psychological debriefing to survivors.
E. Reestablishing a relative sense of safety.

The correct response is option E: Reestablishing a relative sense of safety.

Negative posttrauma reactions tend to persist under conditions of ongoing threat or danger, as studies in a variety of cultures have shown. To the extent that safety is introduced, these reactions show a gradual reduction over time. Moreover, even where threat continues, those who can maintain or reestablish a relative sense of safety have considerably lower risk of developing PTSD in the months following exposure than those who do not.

Hobfoll SE, Watson P, Bell CC, Bryant RA, et al: Five essential elements of immediate and mid-term mass trauma intervention: empirical evidence. Psychiatry. 2007; 70(4):283–315. Reprinted in FOCUS. 2009; 2:221–242

27 Defining high-risk situations, covert antecedents, and stimulus control techniques are a focus of which of the following therapeutic modalities?

A. Brief psychodynamic psychotherapy.
B. Cognitive-behavioral therapy.
C. Supportive therapy.
D. Interpersonal therapy.
E. Relapse prevention therapy.

The correct response is option E: Relapse prevention therapy.

Relapse prevention therapy focuses on factors or situations that can precipitate or contribute to relapse to substance use. These factors include immediate determinants, such as high-risk situations, and covert antecedents, such as seemingly irrelevant decisions. Stimulus control techniques are employed to help with management of cravings and/or urges. Brief psychodynamic psychotherapy focuses on the role unconscious processes play in the patient's present behavior. Cognitive-behavioral therapy focuses on patterns of thinking and underlying beliefs that are maladaptive. Supportive therapy encompasses a variety of techniques but tends to focus on maximizing a patient's adaptive coping mechanisms. Interpersonal psychotherapy focuses on the connections between a person's symptoms and their interactions with others.

Larimer ME, Palmer RS, Marlatt GA: Relapse prevention: an overview of Marlatt's cognitive-behavioral model. Alcohol Research and Health 1999; 23:151–60

28 A 42-year-old patient with schizophrenia presents to the emergency department with confusion and agitation following an overdose of antipsychotic medication. The patient has a temperature of 101.7 degrees Fahrenheit, blood pressure of 140/80 mm Hg, and pulse of 112. Physical examination reveals hot, dry skin, dilated pupils, and decreased bowel sounds. This patient's symptoms are most likely caused by medication effects at which of the following receptors?

A. Muscarinic cholinergic.
B. Nicotinic cholinergic.
C. α_1-adrenergic.
D. Histaminergic.
E. Dopaminergic.

The correct response is option A: Muscarinic cholinergic.

Antipsychotic medications have effects at muscarinic cholinergic, α_1-adrenergic, histaminergic, and dopaminergic receptors. This patient's symptoms are most consistent with anticholinergic toxicity and therefore are most likely to be caused by blockade at the muscarinic cholinergic receptors.

Schatzberg AF, Nemeroff CB (eds): Essentials of Clinical Psychopharmacology, 2nd ed. Arlington, VA, American Psychiatric Publishing, 2006. p 218

29 Which of the following therapies for borderline personality disorder incorporates psychoeducation about the illness, emotional management skills training, and behavior skills training?

A. Mentalization-based therapy.
B. Schema-focused therapy.
C. Trauma-focused cognitive-behavior therapy.
D. Eye movement desensitization and reprocessing.
E. Systems Training for Emotional Predictability and Problem Solving (STEPPS).

The correct response is option E: Systems Training for Emotional Predictability and Problem Solving (STEPPS).

The STEPPS program combines cognitive-behavioral elements with skills training. It is done only in groups and is meant to complement ongoing therapy. Mentalization-based therapy, although useful in borderline personality disorder, is a psychoanalytic treatment. Schema-focused therapy is a cognitive therapy for borderline personality disorder. Trauma-focused cognitive-behavior therapy and eye movement desensitization and reprocessing are treatments for PTSD.

Blum N et al: Systems Training for Emotional Predictability and Problem Solving (STEPPS) for outpatients with borderline personality disorder: A randomized controlled trial and 1-year follow-up. Am J Psychiatry 2008; 165:469
Hales RE, Yudofsky SC, Gabbard GO: The American Psychiatric Publishing Textbook of Psychiatry, 5th ed, Arlington, VA: American Psychiatric Publishing, 2008, pp 580, 842

30 When managing a chronically suicidal patient, respecting the patient's preference to remain at home and not be admitted to the psychiatric unit for additional care reflects which of the following ethical principles?

A. Autonomy.
B. Beneficience.
C. Nonmaleficence.
D. Egalitarianism.

The correct response is option A: Autonomy.

A decision to respect a patient's preference reflects a decision to respect a patient's decision making or *autonomous* judgment of the possible benefits and adverse consequences for the decisions made. Beneficence-based obligations seek to provide beneficial outcomes to patients and to avoid possible adverse consequences of patients' decision making. Physicians have obligations of beneficence and obligations to respect patients' autonomy or preferences. Many chronically suicidal patients are safely managed at home. Nonmaleficence refers to not causing harm by a decision made. Justice-based considerations are less relevant here. Egalitarian justice is an obligation to provide benefits in equal proportion to individual's needs.

Roberts LW. Ethical principles and skills in the care of mental illness. FOCUS: Forensic and Ethical Issues Fall 2003; 4:340.
Sadock BJ, Sadock VA, Ruiz P (eds): Kaplan & Sadock's Comprehensive Textbook of Psychiatry, 9th ed. Philadelphia, Lippincott Williams & Wilkins, 2009, p 4441

31 A 12-year-old boy is hospitalized after a serious suicide attempt. His parents report that they noticed a difference in his behavior about a year ago. He became increasingly withdrawn; he was preoccupied with mythical creatures; his academic performance declined significantly; and he had difficulty sleeping and a decreased appetite. Over the past 2 months, he has seemed progressively worse. He has demonstrated both persecutory and somatic delusions and has reported he hears voices telling him to "beware—they are watching you—you're a naughty little boy." Today he heard a voice telling him that he was "rotting inside," and in response, he attempted to hang himself. On examination, he denies a mood disturbance. His thinking is illogical and nonlinear. What is the most likely diagnosis?

A. Bipolar disorder.
B. Attention-deficit/hyperactivity disorder.
C. Schizophrenia.
D. Major depressive disorder.
E. Autism spectrum disorder.

The correct response is option C: Schizophrenia.

Auditory hallucinations are the most frequently reported positive symptom of childhood-onset schizophrenia. It is estimated that 80%–100% of children with schizophrenia age 13 years or younger report hallucinations. The other symptoms in the vignette occur less frequently. The lack of mood disturbance eliminates the possibility of bipolar disorder or major depressive disorder. This patient's symptoms (e.g., delusions, auditory hallucinations) and presentation (onset of symptoms at 11 years old) are inconsistent with attention-deficit/hyperactivity disorder (ADHD) and autism spectrum disorder.

Dulcan MK, Weiner JM. Essentials of Child and Adolescent Psychiatry. Arlington (VA): American Psychiatric Publishing, 2006. pp 238–240, 238–240

Hales RE, Yudofsky SC, and Gabbard GO (eds). The American Psychiatric Publishing Textbook of Psychiatry. 5th ed. Arlington (VA), American Psychiatric Publishing, 2008. pp 836, 882–892

---

32 Individuals with two copies of which one of the following genes develop Alzheimer's disease (AD) eight times more frequently than those without it?

A. APOE E1.
B. APOE E2.
C. APOE E3.
D. APOE E4.
E. APOE E5.

The correct response is option D: APOE E4.

Of the three allelic varieties of the APOE gene, APOE E2 may provide some protection against developing AD. The most common allele, APOE E3, may be risk neutral, while APOE E4 is associated with increased susceptibility to the disease. Individuals with a single copy of the E4 gene may have AD three times more frequently compared to individuals with no E4 gene. Furthermore, individuals with two E4 genes have the disease eight times more frequently than do those with no E4 gene. According to NIH, "APOE E4 occurs in about 40% of all people who develop late-onset AD and is present in about 25% to 30% of the population. People with AD are more likely to have an APOE E4 allele than people who do not develop AD. However, many people with AD do not have an APOE E4 allele." Diagnostic testing for this gene is not currently recommended because it is found in persons without dementia.

Alzheimer's Disease Genetics Fact Sheet, NIH Publication No. 08-6424, November 2008, http://www.nia.nih.gov/alzheimers/publications/geneticsfs.htm

Sadock BJ, Sadock VA (eds): Kaplan & Sadock's Comprehensive Textbook of Psychiatry, 9th ed. Philadelphia, Lippincott Williams & Wilkins, 2009, pp 4059–4060

33 In the Alternative DSM-5 Model for Personality Disorders (DSM-5 Section III), personality disorder trait domains of psychopathology and their polar opposites are described with a listing of personality facets under each domain. In addition to negative affectivity (vs. emotional stability), detachment (vs. extraversion), disinhibition (vs. conscientiousness), and psychoticism (vs. lucidity), which of the following is included as the trait domain polar opposite of antagonism?

A. Agreeableness.
B. Brightness.
C. Happiness.
D. Humor.
E. Optimism.

The correct response is option A: Agreeableness.

In DSM-5 in the Alternative DSM-5 Model for Personality Disorders, the clinical utility of the personality trait model lies in its ability to focus attention on multiple relevant areas of personality variation in the individual patient. These five broad domains are maladaptive variants of the five domains of the validated and replicated model known as the five-factor model of personality. The DSM-5 trait model focuses on personality traits associated with psychopathology; there are healthy adaptive and resilient personality traits identified as the polar opposites of these traits. Their presence can greatly mitigate the effects of mental disorders and facilitate coping and recovery. *Antagonism* is defined as behaviors that put the individual at odds with other people, including an exaggerated sense of self-importance.

Rottman BM, Ahn W, Sanislow CA, Kim NS: Can clinicians recognize DSM-IV personality disorders from five-factor model descriptions of patient cases? Am J Psychiatry 2009; 166:427–433

Clark LA: Assessment and diagnosis of personality disorder: perennial issues and emerging reconceptualization. Annu Rev Psychol 2007; 58:227–257

American Psychiatric Association: Diagnostic and Statistical Manual of Mental Disorders, 5th Edition. Arlington, VA, American Psychiatric Association, 2013, Alternative DSM-5 Model for Personality Disorders, pp 770–781

34 A 32-year-old man with a history of bipolar I disorder has been off all medication for more than 6 months. He currently presents with symptoms consistent with a moderately severe major depressive episode. Which of the following has the best evidence as a pharmacologic treatment for him?

A. Clonazepam and lithium.
B. Olanzapine and fluoxetine.
C. Lithium and paroxetine.
D. Valproate and fluoxetine.
E. Bupropion alone.

The correct response is option B: Olanzapine and fluoxetine.

Of the pharmacological options given, only the olanzapine and fluoxetine combination has substantial evidence for efficacy in randomized placebo-controlled, double-blind trials. In general, antidepressant monotherapy is not recommended because of a potential increase in the likelihood of hypomanic, manic, or mixed episodes occurring. However, some studies have supported the use of paroxetine, venlafaxine, or quetiapine alone. Although some clinicians will initiate simultaneous treatment with lithium and an antidepressant, this is generally reserved for more severely ill patients or when other approaches, such as initiation and optimization of lithium, have not produced a clinical response.

American Psychiatric Association Practice Guideline for the Treatment of Patients with Bipolar Disorder, 2nd ed (2002). http://psychiatryonline.org/guidelines.aspx.

Hirschfeld RMA: "Guideline Watch: Practice Guideline for the Treatment of Patients with Bipolar Disorder, 2nd Edition" APA Practice Guidelines November 2005. http://psychiatryonline.org/guidelines.aspx.

Selle V, Schalkwijk S, Vázquez GH, Baldessarini RJ: Treatments for acute bipolar depression: meta-analyses of placebo-controlled, monotherapy trials of anticonvulsants, lithium and antipsychotics. Pharmacopsychiatry 2014; 47(2):43–52

35 Which of the following psychiatric disorders confers the highest genetic relative risk for first-degree relatives?

A. Panic disorder.
B. Alcoholism.
C. Major depression.
D. Bipolar disorder.
E. Schizophrenia.

The correct response is option D: Bipolar disorder.

All of the above disorders have a significant relative risk (the risk to a relative of an affected individual compared to the overall incidence of the disorder). However, bipolar disorder has the highest at 24.5, followed by schizophrenia at 18.5, panic at 9.6, alcoholism at 7.4, and major depression at 3.0.

Hales RE, Yudofsky SC, Gabbard GO (eds): The American Psychiatric Publishing Textbook of Psychiatry, 5th ed, 2008 pp 196–197

36 A 35-year-old woman began taking citalopram, 20 mg, daily about 3 months ago when she presented with symptoms consistent with panic disorder. On the current regimen, her symptoms are under control. Until her recent episode of illness, she has had no other history of psychiatric symptoms, and there is no family history of psychiatric illness. How long should she continue this medication?

A. 4 weeks.
B. 3 months.
C. 1 year.
D. 3 years.
E. Indefinitely.

The correct response is option C: 1 year.

Pharmacotherapy should generally be continued for 1 year or more after acute response to promote further symptom reduction and decrease risk of recurrence. Incorporating maintenance treatment (e.g., monthly "booster" sessions focused on relapse prevention) into psychosocial treatments for panic disorder also may help maintain positive response, although more systematic investigation of this issue is needed.

American Psychiatric Association Practice Guideline for the Treatment of Patients with Panic Disorder (2009). http://psychiatryonline.org/guidelines.aspx

37 On the basis of the results of the National Institute of Mental Health funded multisite Multimodal Treatment Study of Children with Attention Deficit-Hyperactivity Disorder (MTA), which of the following interventions was proven to be the MOST effective in treating the majority of children with ADHD?

A. Medication alone.
B. Medication with an intensive summer treatment program.
C. Medication with community referral.
D. Medication with parent training.
E. Medication with school consultation.

The correct response is option A: Medication alone.

Although it would seem logical that combined treatments would improve outcomes for the child with ADHD, this was not supported by the MTA study. The MTA study randomly assigned children ages 7–9 years with ADHD (combined type) to either 1) medication treatment (primarily psychostimulants), 2) a comprehensive psychosocial treatment package including parent training, intensive summer treatment program, and school consultation, 3) the combined psychosocial package and medication, or 4) community referral as a control group. Children randomly assigned to the medication treatment arm overall had significantly improved outcomes compared with children receiving psychosocial treatment alone or those referred out for community care. Subjects receiving the combined medication and psychosocial treatment fared little better in general than subjects receiving medication treatment alone. The advantage of combination therapy over medication treatment alone was small.

AACAP practice parameter for the assessment and treatment of children and adolescents with attention-deficit/hyperactivity disorder. J Am Child Adolesc Psychiatry. 2007. Reprinted in FOCUS. 2008; 6(3):409

Dulcan MK, Weiner JM. Essentials of Child and Adolescent Psychiatry. Arlington, VA, American Psychiatric Publishing, 2006. pp 341–342

The MTA Cooperative Goup. A 14-month randomized clinical trial of treatment strategies for attention-deficit/hyperactivity disorder. Arch Gen Psychiatry 1999; 56(12):1073–86

---

38 Which of the following personality disorders (PDs) is most common in the biological relatives of patients with schizophrenia?

A. Schizoid.
B. Paranoid.
C. Schizotypal.
D. Histrionic.
E. Antisocial.

The correct response is option C: Schizotypal.

There is a greater presence of schizotypal patients in families with a history of schizophrenia than in control groups. There is less correlation between paranoid or schizoid PD in families with schizophrenia. Cluster B disorders, including histrionic and antisocial PD, have different genetic associations. Specifically, antisocial PD is associated with alcohol use disorders, and histrionic is associated with somatization disorder (Briquet's syndrome).

Sadock BJ, Sadock VA (eds): Kaplan & Sadock's Synopsis of Psychiatry: Behavioral Sciences/Clinical Psychiatry, 10th ed. Philadelphia, Lippincott Williams & Wilkins, 2007, p 791

---

39 Which of the following symptoms is a diagnostic feature of atypical depression?

A. Insomnia.
B. Weight loss.
C. Suicidal ideation.
D. Mood reactivity.
E. Inappropriate guilt.

The correct response is option D: Mood reactivity.

The atypical features specifier in DSM-5 can be applied to major depressive episodes in depression or bipolar disorder or to persistent depressive disorder. But the criteria that differentiate atypical depression from those disorders require mood reactivity as well as two or more of the following: weight gain or appetite increase, hypersomnia, leaden paralysis, and rejection sensitivity (a long-standing pattern).

American Psychiatric Association: Diagnostic and Statistical Manual of Mental Disorders, 5th Edition. Arlington, VA, American Psychiatric Association, 2013, pp 185–186

40 A 33-year-old man whose bipolar I disorder has been well controlled on medication presents to the emergency department with severe left upper quadrant pain radiating to his back, nausea, and vomiting. Which medication is most likely contributing to these symptoms?

A. Lamotrigine.
B. Lithium.
C. Olanzapine.
D. Valproate.
E. Ziprasidone.

The correct response is option D: Valproate.

Rare, idiosyncratic, but potentially fatal, adverse events with valproate include irreversible hepatic failure, hemorrhagic pancreatitis, and agranulocytosis. Thus, patients taking valproate should be instructed to contact their psychiatrist or primary care physician immediately if they develop symptoms of these conditions. The symptoms and laboratory findings are consistent with a diagnosis of acute pancreatitis. On the basis of reports of pancreatitis associated with valproate use, a black box warning was added to its package insert in 2000. Although routine monitoring of pancreatic function is not necessary, clinical manifestations suggestive of acute pancreatitis should be evaluated promptly and fully.

American Psychiatric Association Practice Guideline for the Treatment of Patients with Bipolar Disorder, 2nd Edition (2002). Reprinted in FOCUS: Bipolar Disorder, 2003; 1:84–85. http://psychiatryonline.org/guidelines.aspx
Pellock JM, Wilder BJ, Deaton R, Sommerville KW: Acute pancreatitis coincident with valproate use: a critical review. Epilepsia 2002; 43:1421–1424
Yazdani K, Lippmann M, Gala I: Fatal pancreatitis associated with valproic acid. Medicine 2002; 81:305–310

41 A sniper attacks a city hall building, killing 13 individuals and significantly injuring another 12 before he takes his own life. Therapists from the local mental health clinic are dispatched to the scene to provide psychological debriefing to prevent PTSD symptoms. Using an evidence-based framework, what is the most likely impact of this intervention on direct survivors?

A. It will be ineffective or harmful to the direct survivors.
B. It will decrease the probability of developing PTSD symptoms.
C. It will decrease the severity of PTSD symptoms.
D. It will decrease the time period for recovery from PTSD symptoms.
E. It will delay the onset of PTSD symptoms.

The correct response is option A: It will be ineffective or harmful to the direct survivors.

Restoring social and behavioral functioning after disasters and situations of mass casualty has been extensively explored over the last few decades. No evidence-based consensus has been reached to date with regard to effective interventions. Recent findings indicate that commonly utilized interventions, such as psychological debriefing, do not prevent PTSD, may not be effective in preventing long-term distress and dysfunction, and may even be harmful to direct survivors of disasters.

Hobfoll SE, Watson P, Bell CC, Bryant RA, et al: Five essential elements of immediate and mid-term mass trauma intervention: empirical evidence. Psychiatry. 2007; 70(4):284. Reprinted in FOCUS. 2009; 2:221–242

42 You are asked to write 22 questions for a board-type examination in less than 4 weeks. Your first thought is, "I will never be able to get all those questions written in such a short time!" You ignore the fact that you seem to have been able to be successful at this several times before. From a cognitive therapy perspective, what is the best description of this type of thinking?

A. Magnification.
B. Minimization.
C. Personalization.
D. Selective abstraction.
E. Catastrophic thinking.

The correct response is option E: Catastrophic thinking.

Catastrophic thinking involves predicting the worst possible outcome while ignoring more likely eventualities. *Magnification* is overvaluing and *minimization* is undervaluing the significance of a personal attribute, a life event, or a future possibility. *Personalization* is linking external occurrences to oneself when there is little reason to do so. *Selective abstraction* is drawing a conclusion based only on a small portion of available data.

Hales RE, Yudofsky SC, Gabbard GO (eds): The American Psychiatric Publishing Textbook of Psychiatry, 5th ed. Arlington, VA, American Psychiatric Publishing, 2008, p 1214

43 A patient with four or more mood disturbances within a single year that meet both the duration and symptom criteria for major depressive, mixed, manic, and/or hypomanic episodes, demarcated by remission or switch to opposite polarity, meets the DSM-5 criteria for which of the following disorders?

A. Bipolar disorder with rapid cycling specifier.
B. Unspecified bipolar and related disorder.
C. Cyclothymic disorder.
D. Schizoaffective disorder (bipolar type).

The correct response is option A: Bipolar disorder with rapid cycling specifier.

The rapid cycling specifier, the presence of four or more distinct mood episodes per year, can be applied to both bipolar I and bipolar II disorder. *Cyclothymic disorder* is characterized by numerous periods of hypomanic symptoms that do not meet criteria for manic episode and numerous periods of depressive symptoms that do not meet criteria for major depressive episode. *Unspecified bipolar and related disorder* refers to patients that do not meet criteria for any specific mood disorder. *Schizoaffective disorder (bipolar type)* meets the full criteria for schizoaffective disorder, and a manic episode is part of the presentation. Major depressive episodes may also occur.

American Psychiatric Association: Diagnostic and Statistical Manual of Mental Disorders, 5th Edition. Arlington, VA, American Psychiatric Association, 2013, pp 106, 139, 149–150

Schneck CD, Miklowitz DJ, Calabrese JR, Allen MH, et al: Phenomenology of rapid-cycling bipolar disorder: data from the first 500 participants in the Systematic Treatment Enhancement Program Am J Psychiatry 2004; 161:1902–1908

44 Which of the following disorders has been shown to have the greatest degree of heritability?

A. Schizophrenia.
B. Autism.
C. Bipolar disorder.
D. Alcoholism.
E. ADHD.

The correct response is option B: Autism.

Heritability is the proportion of variance in familial risk attributed to genes. It is 90% for autism compared to at least 75% for bipolar disorder and schizophrenia, 60% for ADHD, and 40% for alcoholism.

Sadock BJ, Sadock VA (eds): Kaplan & Sadock's Comprehensive Textbook of Psychiatry, 9th ed. Philadelphia, Lippincott Williams & Wilkins, 2009, pp 304

45 A 42-year-old man presents to a psychiatrist 6 months after a motor vehicle accident. He has difficulty sleeping because he has frequent nightmares about the accident. He has not been able to drive since the accident, and his wife usually drives for him. Even then, he finds it very difficult to be in a car, often panicking if another car is near them on the road. Which of the following medications would be the most appropriate for this man?

A. Propranolol.
B. Nortriptyline.
C. Clonazepam.
D. Olanzapine.
E. Sertraline.

The correct response is option E: Sertraline.

Although a number of medications have shown some efficacy for posttraumatic stress disorder, the American Psychiatric Association's Practice Guideline for the Treatment of Patients with Acute Stress Disorder and Posttraumatic Stress Disorder and the 2009 Guideline Watch recommend selective serotonin reuptake inhibitors as the first-line medication treatment for patients with PTSD. The other medications listed are generally not considered first-line medications as they have fewer data to support their use.

American Psychiatric Association Practice Guideline for the Treatment of Patients With Acute Stress Disorder and Posttraumatic Stress Disorder. Am J Psychiatry. 2004; 161(11 Suppl):3–31. http://psychiatryonline.org/guidelines.aspx

Benedek DM, Friedman MJ, Zatzick D, Ursano RJ. Guideline Watch (March 2009): Practice Guideline for the Treatment of Patients with Acute Stress Disorder and Posttraumatic Stress Disorder. FOCUS. 2009; 2:204–213. http://psychiatryonline.org/guidelines.aspx

46 A patient presents with involuntary frowning, blinking, grimacing, and choreoathetoid movements of the upper extremities after several years of antipsychotic medication treatment. Which one of the following is the most likely diagnosis?

A. Akinesia.
B. Akathisia.
C. Acute dystonia.
D. Parkinsonism.
E. Tardive dyskinesia.

The correct response is option E: Tardive dyskinesia.

Tardive dyskinesia is characterized by involuntary movements of the face, trunk, or extremities and usually occurs after prolonged exposure to dopamine-blocking agents. Symptoms include facial and oral movements, extremity movements, and trunk movements. The Abnormal Involuntary Movement Scale is used to examine for these side effects.

Hales RE, Yudofsky SC, Gabbard GO (eds.): The American Psychiatric Publishing Textbook of Psychiatry, 5th ed. Arlington, VA, American Psychiatric Publishing, 2008, pp 1090–91

47 Which of the following diagnoses is most common among individuals with bulimia nervosa?

A. General anxiety disorder.
B. Obsessive-compulsive disorder.
C. Alcohol use disorder.
D. Major depressive disorder.
E. Intermittent explosive disorder.

The correct response is option D: Major depressive disorder.

High rates of co-occurring psychiatric illness are found in patients seeking treatment for anorexia and bulimia. Lifetime co-occurring major depression or dysthymia has been reported in 50%–75% of patients with anorexia and bulimia. Although the other disorders may co-occur with bulimia nervosa, the prevalence rates are much lower.

Sadock BJ, Sadock VA, Ruiz P (eds): Kaplan & Sadock's Comprehensive Textbook of Psychiatry, 9th ed. Philadelphia, Lippincott Williams & Wilkins, 2009, pp 2140–41

American Psychiatric Association Practice Guideline for the Treatment of Patients with Eating Disorders, 3rd ed. (2005), http://psychiatryonline.org/guidelines.aspx

---

48 A 31-year-old man is admitted to an inpatient psychiatric unit after a suicide attempt. Past records show a history of dependence on multiple substances. He sleeps poorly and the next day paces around the unit, restless and grumpy. He is tachycardic at 112 beats per minutes, his palms and forehead are sweaty, and his hands are showing a coarse tremor. When asked, the patient says he feels anxious. The most likely diagnosis is:

A. Alcohol withdrawal.
B. Nicotine withdrawal.
C. Opioid withdrawal.
D. Cannabis withdrawal.
E. Methamphetamine withdrawal.

The correct response is option A: Alcohol withdrawal.

The symptoms described are characteristic of alcohol withdrawal. Whereas anxiety, insomnia, and diaphoresis are nonspecific symptoms common with several withdrawal syndromes, a coarse tremor observable in the hands would make this patient's presentation most likely alcohol withdrawal. Opioid withdrawal resembles a severe flu-like illness characterized by rhinorrhea, sneezing, yawning, lacrimation, abdominal cramping, leg cramping, piloerection (gooseflesh), nausea, vomiting, diarrhea, and dilated pupils. Tachycardia can be a symptom of opioid withdrawal, whereas mild bradycardia would be more characteristic of nicotine withdrawal. Methamphetamine withdrawal more typically presents with hypersomnia, whereas the symptoms of cannabis withdrawal are somewhat less specific.

American Psychiatric Association: Diagnostic and Statistical Manual of Mental Disorders, 5th Edition. Arlington, VA, American Psychiatric Association, 2013, pp 499–500, 517–518

---

49 A 28-year-old woman with an identical twin is diagnosed with major depressive disorder. She asks you to comment on the chance her sister will develop the same illness. Which of the following is the best response regarding the genetic basis of depression?

A. "Major depression is a genetic illness. Your sister will definitely develop it as well."
B. "While schizophrenia is quite heritable, there is only a slightly increased risk that your sister will become depressed."
C. "The likelihood of identical twins sharing an affective illness is high."
D. "Although there may be some genetic basis for affective illness, it is one's childhood environment that determines whether illness will manifest."
E. "Your sister's risk of developing depression is the same as any other sibling."

The correct response is option C: "The likelihood of identical twins sharing an affective illness is high."

Both genetic and environmental factors likely contribute to the emergence of affective illness. Twin studies compare resemblance for a condition within types of twin pairs: monozygotic twins (MZ), who share close to 100% of their DNA, and dizygotic twins (DZ), who share DNA like other sibling pairs. Meta-analysis of data reports a summary heritability of 37%. For published studies since 1985, MZ concordance ranged from 30% to 50% and DZ concordance from 12% to 40%.

Hettema JM: Genetics of depression, FOCUS Summer 2010; 8:316–322

Smoller JW, Sheidley BR, Tsuang MT. Psychiatric Genetics: Applications in Clinical Practice. American Psychiatric Publishing, 1st edition, 2008, p 145

---

50 For the detection and identification of delirium in medically ill patients, the best strategy to employ is:

A. Enhanced EEG monitoring.
B. Serum and urine lab tests.
C. Revised Mini Mental State Exam.
D. Specific neuroimaging.
E. Observation and rating scales.

The correct response is option E: Observation and rating scales.

Delirium remains a condition that is often not detected or diagnosed. There have been improvements in screening due to the development of sensitive observation and rating scales such as Delirium Rating Scale–Revised-98, including a version for use with children; the Delirium Observation Screening Scale; and the Confusion Assessment Method for the Intensive Care Unit.

Cook IA. Guideline Watch: Practice Guideline for the Treatment of Patients with Delirium. Washington, DC: American Psychiatric Association; 2004. http://psychiatryonline.org/guidelines.aspx

Fearing MA, Inouye SK: Delirium, in The American Psychiatric Publishing Textbook of Geriatric Psychiatry. Edited by Blazer DG, Steffens DC. Washington, DC, American Psychiatric Publishing, 2009, pp 229–241. Reprinted in FOCUS 2009; 7:53–63

---

51 A 58-year-old man with a history of alcohol dependence and mild dementia presents to the hospital for a liver biopsy because of suspected alcoholic hepatitis. He complains of severe anxiety about having the procedure done and requests "something for my nerves." Which of the following benzodiazepines is safest to administer?

A. Alprazolam.
B. Chlordiazepoxide.
C. Diazepam.
D. Oxazepam.
E. Clonazepam.

The correct response is option D: Oxazepam.

For patients who have severe hepatic disease, who are elderly, or have delirium, dementia, or another cognitive disorder, short-acting benzodiazepines such as oxazepam or lorazepam are preferred. Oxazepam, temazepam, and lorazepam do not require multistep biotransformation; they are metabolized by phase II enzymes (glucuronidation) that are not affected by alcohol-related hepatitis.

American Psychiatric Association Practice Guideline for the Treatment of Patients with Substance Use Disorders, 2nd Edition, (2006). p 380–381. http://psychiatryonline.org/guidelines.aspx

---

52 A 35-year-old patient with schizophrenia has had four serious suicide attempts over the past year despite consistent treatment with haloperidol decanoate. Given the patient's recent suicide attempts, what would be the BEST next medication trial?

A. Olanzapine.
B. Quetiapine.
C. Fluphenazine decanoate.
D. Long-acting risperidone.
E. Clozapine.

The correct response is option E: Clozapine.

Clozapine has been shown to have the greatest therapeutic effect on suicidal behavior associated with schizophrenia, possibly reducing the suicide rate by as much as 75%–85%. For these reasons, clozapine should be preferentially considered for patients with schizophrenia who have a history of chronic and persistent suicidal ideation or behaviors.

Clozaril® package insert, Novartis Pharmaceuticals Corporation, East Hanover, NJ, 2005. http://www.pharma.us.novartis.com/product/pi/pdf/Clozaril.pdf.

American Psychiatric Association Practice Guideline for the Treatment of Patients with Schizophrenia, 2nd ed (2004). pp 576. http://psychiatryonline.org/guidelines.aspx

---

53 Cognitive-behavioral therapy (CBT) is an effective, specific treatment for generalized anxiety disorder (GAD). Emerging evidence suggests that which ONE of the following is similarly effective in treatment for GAD?

A. Dialectical behavioral therapy (DBT).
B. Interpersonal psychotherapy (IPT).
C. Psychoanalysis.
D. Short-term psychodynamic psychotherapy.
E. Supportive psychotherapy.

The correct response is option D: Short-term psychodynamic psychotherapy.

As Leichsenring et al. (2009) report in their prospective, randomized study of 57 patients with generalized anxiety disorder (GAD), subjects were treated with cognitive-behavioral therapy (CBT) or short-term psychodynamic psychotherapy. Both groups improved significantly in measures of anxiety and depression. However, CBT was more effective in reducing the level of worrying. CBT often targets worrying as a symptom.

Leichsenring F, Salzer S, Jaeger U, Kächele H, et al: Short-term psychodynamic psychotherapy and cognitive-behavioral therapy in generalized anxiety disorder: a randomized, controlled trial. Am J Psychiatry 2009; 166:875–881

---

54 A 13-year-old boy is seen for outbursts of aggression when he is denied access to food. He is known to have an intellectual disability. His mother reports that as an infant he had poor muscle tone and a weak suck reflex. He is morbidly obese, is short for his age, and has significantly underdeveloped genitalia. His mother reports that he constantly eats to the point that they have put locks on the kitchen cabinets and refrigerator. Despite this, he will search for food in garbage cans. Lately, when he is denied food, he will have outbursts of anger in which he hits himself or others and throws objects. Which of the following BEST describes the genetic abnormality responsible for this boy's condition?

A. Williams syndrome.
B. Angelman's syndrome.
C. Prader-Willi syndrome.
D. Klinefelter's syndrome.
E. Down syndrome.

The correct response is option C: Prader-Willi syndrome.

The patient's presentation is consistent with Prader-Willi syndrome. Prader-Willi syndrome represents an important genetic principle known as genomic imprinting. The majority of individuals have deletions of a segment of chromosome 15. Prader-Willi syndrome emerges most frequently from deletions or absence of 15q12 from paternal origin.

Sadock BJ, Sadock VA (eds): Kaplan and Sadock's Comprehensive Textbook of Psychiatry, 9th ed. Philadelphia, Lippinicott Williams & Wilkins, 2009, p 583

55 Which of the following statements represents the most reasonable conclusion that can be drawn from the National Institute of Mental Health's (NIMH) Clinical Antipsychotic Trials of Intervention Effectiveness (CATIE) study?

A. Second-generation antipsychotics offer no benefit in schizophrenia over first-generation antipsychotics.
B. Clinicians should consider both first- and second-generation antipsychotics when treating schizophrenia.
C. Antipsychotic medications appear to be less efficacious than previously thought.
D. Second-generation antipsychotics demonstrate little difference from one another.
E. When given in idealized settings, most antipsychotics are roughly equivalent in efficacy.

The correct response is option B: Clinicians should consider both first- and second-generation antipsychotics when treating schizophrenia.

The CATIE study was designed to compare various antipsychotic medications in real-world treatment settings. The primary outcome concerned time until a switch in medication, thus it is not a study of efficacy. The finding that outcomes were similar for the first-generation antipsychotic perphenazine and the second-generation antipsychotics was unexpected; however, this does not imply that second-generation antipsychotic medication may not have unique benefits. In some patients, individual differences were found in outcome and side effects between the different medications. The best conclusion that can be drawn from these data is that there are significant differences between the medications and that patients may benefit from either first- or second-generation medications.

Lieberman JA, Hsiao JK: Interpreting the results of the CATIE study. Psychiatr Serv 2006 Jan;57(1):139
Ragins M: Should the CATIE study be a wake-up call? Psychiatric Services 56: 1489, 2005
Lieberman JA, Stroup TS, McEvoy JP, et al: Effectiveness of antipsychotic drugs in patients with chronic schizophrenia. New England Journal of Medicine 353:1209–1223, 2005

56 Poststroke depression is most commonly associated with cerebrovascular disease involving the:

A. Anterior communicating artery.
B. Anterior cerebral artery.
C. Middle cerebral artery.
D. Posterior communicating artery.
E. Basilar artery.

The correct response is option C: Middle cerebral artery.

Poststroke depression is highly prevalent among elderly patients with hypertension and coronary artery disease. It often involves the vascular territory of the middle cerebral artery and is seen most commonly after left hemispheric stroke. The larger the size of the ischemic area, the more depression is refractory to standard treatment approaches.

Yudofsky SC, Hales RE (eds): The American Psychiatric Publishing Textbook of Neuropsychiatry and Behavioral Sciences, 5th ed. Washington DC: American Psychiatric Publishing, 2008, pp 708–722

57 Which symptom of PTSD has shown promise of improvement by medications that suppress noradrenergic activity?

A. Hypervigilance.
B. Inability to recall an important aspect of the trauma.
C. Markedly diminished interest.
D. Feelings of detachment.
E. Avoidance of activities related to the trauma.

The correct response is option A: Hypervigilance.

Treatment with adrenergic-blocking agents, such as propranolol, has been studied to decrease symptoms of hyperarousal and intrusive recollections. The findings with propranolol enhancement are promising, but placebo-controlled randomized clinical trials on propranolol enhancement in PTSD patients are needed.

Hales RE, Yudofsky SC, Gabbard GO (eds). The American Psychiatric Publishing Textbook of Psychiatry, 5th ed. Arlington, VA, American Psychiatric Publishing, 2008, p 577

Stein DJ, Hollander E. Textbook of Anxiety Disorders. Washington, DC. American Psychiatric Publishing, 2002. pp 396–397

Raskind MA, Peskind ER, Kanter ED, Petrie EC, et al: Reduction of nightmares and other PTSD symptoms in combat veterans by prazosin: a placebo-controlled study. Am J Psychiatry. 2003 Feb;160(2):371–3

de Kleine RA, Rothbaum BO, van Minnen A. Pharmacological enhancement of exposure-based treatment in PTSD: a qualitative review. Eur J Psychotraumatol. 2013 Oct 17; 4

---

58 A 19-year-old college student comes to the clinic with a complaint of feeling "depressed and worried." He states that he may fail his English class because he is nervous about the public-speaking assignment. When he thinks about it, he feels nervous, his heart races, his palms become sweaty, and he becomes short of breath. He endorses a depressed mood because "I feel like I'm wasting my parents' money." He skipped his last three English classes because he knew it would be his turn to give a speech. He attends his other classes with no difficulty. The most likely diagnosis is:

A. Panic disorder.
B. Normal shyness.
C. Social anxiety disorder.
D. Agoraphobia.
E. Major depressive disorder.

The correct response is option C: Social anxiety disorder.

Panic disorder is unlikely, as the symptoms are limited to the specific situation of the speech. This is more than normal shyness as it is significantly interfering with occupational functioning. It is not agoraphobia because he has no difficulty going to his other classes. His depressive mood is limited to thinking about the current situation, and he shows no other symptoms of depression.

Sadock BJ, Sadock VA, eds: Kaplan & Sadock's Synopsis of Psychiatry, 9th ed. Philadelphia, Lippincott Williams & Wilkins, 2003, p 614

American Psychiatric Association: Diagnostic and Statistical Manual of Mental Disorders, 5th Edition. Arlington, VA, American Psychiatric Association, 2013, pp 202, 206

---

59 A 47-year-old woman is brought for a psychiatric evaluation to assess recent changes in her behavior. Over the past 6 months, she has become increasingly disinhibited and impulsive in her behavior. Physical examination reveals mild dysarthria, dysphagia, and drooling. Slit lamp examination of the eyes indicates the presence of Kayser-Fleischer rings. Which of the following BEST describes the genetic basis for her illness?

A. Autosomal recessive.
B. Codominant.
C. Mitochondrial.
D. Polygenetic.
E. X-linked dominant.

The correct response is option A: Autosomal recessive.

The patient's presentation is consistent with Wilson's disease. Wilson's disease is an autosomal recessive disorder caused by mutations in a copper transporting ATPase encoded by the *ATP7B* gene on chromosome 13. A characteristic feature is Kayser-Fleischer rings due to copper deposition in the outer ring of the cornea. The most common reasons for psychiatric referral are behavioral and personality changes, with disinhibition, bizarre, or impulsive behavior being present in about a quarter of patients.

Sadock BJ, Sadock VA (eds): Kaplan and Sadock's Comprehensive Textbook of Psychiatry, 9th ed. Philadelphia, Lippincott Williams & Wilkins, 2009, p 605

Smoller JW, Sheidley BR, Tsuang MT. Psychiatric Genetics: Applications in Clinical Practice. American Psychiatric Publishing, 1st edition, 2008, p 212

60 A patient unconsciously perceives the therapist as having attributes associated with unpleasant interactions in the past. However, the therapist does not respond like the figure from the past, and over time, the old feelings become muted and the patient no longer needs to replay new relationships according to the old emotional script. Which of the following terms define this positive change in psychotherapy?

A. Exposure and response prevention.
B. Corrective emotional experience.
C. Reenactment of transference.
D. Shaping.
E. Strengthening ego defenses.

The correct response is option B: Corrective emotional experience.

The term *corrective emotional experience* was introduced by Alexander and French as the fundamental therapeutic principle of all psychotherapy. In their definition, the term implies "to re-expose the patient, under more favorable circumstances, to emotional situations which he could not handle in the past. The patient, in order to be helped, must undergo a corrective emotional experience suitable to repair the traumatic influence of previous experiences." Such experiences may occur at any point of the continuum of psychotherapy.

Winston A, Rosenthal RN, Pinsker H: Introduction to Supportive Psychotherapy (Core Competencies in Psychotherapy), 1st ed.. Washington DC, American Psychiatric Publishing, 2004, p 19
Textbook of Psychotherapeutic Treatments. Gabbard GO (ed). Arlington VA, American Psychiatric Publishing, 2009, p 401

61 Which of the following is a risk factor for the development of psychosis while using cocaine?

A. Being female.
B. A greater duration of use during an episode
C. Nonintravenous use.
D. An elevated body mass index.
E. Being a first-time user of cocaine.

The correct response is option B: A greater duration of use during an episode.

Those who develop psychosis with cocaine are likely to be men, have a greater duration and amount of use, and have a lower body mass index. Intravenous abusers have more paranoia and hallucinations than nonintravenous abusers, and users are sensitized so that psychosis becomes more severe and occurs more rapidly with repeated cocaine use.

Thirthalli J, Benegal V. Psychosis among substance users. Curr Opin Psychiatry. 2006 May;19(3):239–45

62 A 38-year-old man presents for treatment of PTSD after surviving a bridge collapse. He was driving on the crowded bridge when it suddenly collapsed, killing over 50 individuals and seriously injuring more. As part of the treatment, the therapist asks the patient to imagine that he is safely driving over a bridge. Which of the following best describes this therapeutic intervention?

A. Aversion therapy.
B. Dialectical behavioral therapy.
C. Exposure therapy.
D. Insight-oriented psychotherapy.
E. Interpersonal therapy.

The correct response is option C: Exposure therapy.

Studies of exposure therapy have found that a key to therapeutic success is to interrupt the posttraumatic stimulus generalization that links harmless images, people, and things to dangerous stimuli associated with the original traumatic threat. This is done through both imagined exposure and real-world, in vivo exposures in ways that re-link those images, people, and events with safety. Dialectical behavior therapy is used to treat borderline personality disorder and has not been studied in the area of traumatic stress.

Hobfoll SE, Watson P, Bell CC, Bryant RA, et al: Five essential elements of immediate and mid-term mass trauma intervention: empirical evidence. Psychiatry. 2007; 70(4):283–315. Reprinted in FOCUS. 2009; 2:221–242

63 Which of the following characteristics is/are present in patients with locked-in syndrome?

A. Persistent vegetative state.
B. Ability to experience a range of feelings.
C. Inability to recognize objects and people.
D. Severe depression and desire to die.

The correct response is option B: Ability to experience a range of feelings.

It is important to appreciate that locked-in syndrome has very different clinical and ethical implications than a persistent vegetative state. Locked-in syndrome is typically caused by an injury to the brain stem (e.g., infarct, trauma, hemorrhage). Patients retain full consciousness and can recognize objects and people. The fact that the patient is conscious, however, is unrecognizable to everybody except the person concerned and except perhaps to those particularly attuned to the patient. A patient in locked-in syndrome cannot interact with others because he or she has lost control of the body except perhaps the ability to move the eyes up or down. Patients experience a range of feelings, especially tremendous frustration at being unable to convey feelings, and loneliness. In a persistent vegetative state, however, patients do not retain consciousness. It is important to realize that despite profound disabilities, a patient in a locked-in state does not necessarily want to die. Early goals of management include establishing effective lines of communications.

Smith E, Delargy M. Locked-in syndrome. BMJ 2005; 331:406–409

Chisholm N, Gillett G. The patient's journey: living with locked-in syndrome. BMJ 2005; 331:94–97

64 Which of the following interventions has been empirically validated through controlled and randomized trials as effective specifically for adolescents with conduct disorder?

A. Dialectical behavioral therapy.
B. Cognitive-behavioral therapy.
C. Interpersonal therapy.
D. Multisystemic therapy.
E. Psychoeducational therapy.

The correct response is option D: Multisystemic therapy.

The goal of multisystemic therapy is to empower parents with skills and resources and to empower their teenage children with conduct disorder to cope with a variety of problems. Dialectical behavioral therapy is useful for borderline personality disorder. Interpersonal therapy is often used for depression. Cognitive-behavioral and psychoeducational therapy are used for a wide range of diagnoses.

Martin A, Volkmar FR (eds): Lewis's Child and Adolescent Psychiatry, 4th ed. Philadelphia, Lippincott Williams & Wilkins, pp 859–860, 2007

65 Which of the following is the mechanism of action of memantine, a medication used to slow cognitive decline in Alzheimer's dementia?

A. Cholinesterase inhibitor.
B. Dopamine receptor blocker.
C. Serotonergic reuptake inhibitor.
D. NMDA receptor antagonist.
E. GABA mimetic.

The correct response is option D: NMDA receptor antagonist.

Memantine is an NMDA antagonist that blocks glutamate-medicated excitotoxicity. It is used in moderate to severe Alzheimer's dementia. The initial dose is 5 mg/day, which is increased in 5-mg/day increments over 4 weeks to the final dose of 10 mg twice per day. Side effects include dizziness, headache, constipation, falls, and confusion. It may be effective in reducing caregiver distress, and it may help delay institutionalization.

Spar JE, La Rue A (eds): Clinical Manual of Geriatric Psychiatry, 1st ed. Washington, DC: American Psychiatric Publishing, 2006. pp 213–214

Meeks TW, Lanouette N, Vahia I, Dawes S, Jeste DV, Lebowitz B. Psychiatric assessment and diagnosis in older adults. FOCUS. 2009 winter; 7(1):3–13

66 Which of the following genetic syndromes is caused by a 22q deletion and is clinically manifested by learning disabilities, palatal anomalies, cardiac defects, and often schizophrenia?

A. Fragile X syndrome.
B. Velocardiofacial (DiGeorge) syndrome.
C. Down syndrome.
D. Cri du chat syndrome.
E. Angelman syndrome.

The correct response is option B: Velocardiofacial (DiGeorge) syndrome.

Velocardiofacial syndrome, also known as 2q11.2 deletion syndrome and DiGeorge syndrome, is caused by a large deletion from chromosome 22, produced by an error in recombination at meiosis. It is clinically manifested by learning disabilities, palatal anomalies, cardiac defects, and often schizophrenia.

Jolin EM, Weller RA, Weller EB. Psychosis in children with velocardiofacial syndrome (22q11.2 deletion syndrome). Curr Psychiatry Rep. 2009 Apr;11(2):99–105
DiGeorge Syndrome. http://ghr.nlm.nih.gov/condition=22q112deletionsyndrome
Smoller JW, Sheidley BR, Tsuang MT. Psychiatric Genetics: Applications in Clinical Practice. American Psychiatric Publishing, 1st edition, 2008, pp 200–212

67 Which of the following refers to an ethical decision-making approach that involves referring to similar, prior cases including legal precedents and applying reasoning from these cases to the case at hand?

A. Casuistry.
B. Ethical principles.
C. Expert opinion.
D. General ethical theory.
E. Tradition and current practice standards.

The correct response is option A: Casuistry.

Casuistry refers to an appeal to relevantly similar cases including legal precedents and the application of the reasoning about these cases to the case at hand. *Ethical principles* include respect for autonomy and beneficence. *General ethical theory* refers to consequentialism (the justification of a course of action is grounded on whether consequences of the right sort result from it) and deontological approaches (the justification of a course of action is grounded in considerations other than consequences). The quality of current practice standards in ethics is judged by the ethical analysis and argument that support them.

DeGrazia D, Beauchamp TL. Philosophy, in Methods in Medical Ethics. Edited by Sugarmen J, Sulmasy DP. Washington D.C., Georgetown University Press; 2001, pp 31–46
Roberts LW, Dyer AR. Concise Guide to Ethics in Mental Health Care. American Psychiatric Publishing, Washington D.C., 2004 p 11

68 A 38-year-old woman with treatment-resistant schizophrenia is prescribed clozapine. Two weeks after beginning the medication, the woman begins to experience episodes of tachycardia with a heart rate over 120 beats per minute. Electrocardiogram reveals sustained sinus tachycardia with nonspecific ST-T wave changes and T wave flattening while standing and supine. Which of the following medications is most likely to alleviate her tachycardia without increasing chances of a serious adverse effect?

A. Atenolol.
B. Fludrocortisone.
C. Propranolol.
D. Verapamil.

The correct response is option A: Atenolol.

The cardiovascular side effects most frequently observed with clozapine are tachycardia and postural hypotension. The tachycardia is probably a direct effect of the vagolytic properties of the drug. It can present in the supine position and is thus not the result of orthostatic changes. Therefore, administration of fludrocortisone would not be beneficial. The patient would best benefit from a beta-blocker. Propranolol should not be prescribed because it may increase the risk of agranulocytosis. Verapamil would be indicated for supraventricular tachycardia.

Sadock BJ, Sadock VA (eds): Kaplan and Sadock's Comprehensive Textbook of Psychiatry, 9th ed. Philadelphia, Lippincott Williams & Wilkins, 2009, pp 3071, 3211

---

69 The course of dementia in individuals with 16 or more years of education differs from those with lower educational attainment in which way?

A. Lower cognitive reserve.
B. Ability to maintain higher levels of cognitive functioning in early dementia.
C. Lower levels of cognitive function in early dementia.
D. Less disease burden when dementia is diagnosed.
E. Gentler slope of decline after dementia is diagnosed.

The correct response is option B: Ability to maintain higher levels of cognitive functioning in early dementia.

The most commonly used screening tool for measuring cognitive function is the Mini-Mental State Examination (MMSE). A score of < 24 out of 30 is the usual cut point for detecting dementia. For highly educated individuals, defined as having 16 or more years of education, a score of < 27 has been shown to have optimal sensitivity and specificity for pursuing a more extensive dementia workup. More highly educated individuals have a higher cognitive reserve and a greater ability to maintain cognitive function in the face of neurological insults. They function at a higher cognitive level early in dementia, show a greater disease burden before dementia is diagnosed, and show a steeper slope of cognitive decline and swifter mortality once dementia is finally diagnosed.

O'Bryant SE, Humphreys JD, Smith GE, Ivnik RJ, et al: Detecting dementia with the Mini-Mental State Examination in highly educated individuals. Arch Neurol. 2008; 65:963–967

---

70 A 34-year-old woman with bipolar disorder has a body mass index of 31.2. To minimize the risk of aggravating this factor, which of the following medications would be most appropriate?

A. Lithium.
B. Clozapine.
C. Lamotrigine.
D. Olanzapine.
E. Divalproex.

The correct response is option C: Lamotrigine.

Lamotrigine is a weight-neutral medication, while all of the others are associated with weight gain as a side effect. Weight neutrality does not exclude the possibility of weight gain in individual patients, but it reduces the likelihood considerably.

Bowden CL, Calabrese JR, Ketter TA, Sachs GS, et al: Impact of lamotrigine and lithium on weight in obese and nonobese patients with bipolar I disorder. Am J Psychiatry 2006; 163:1199–1201

Merideth CH: A single-center, double-blind, placebo-controlled evaluation of lamotrigine in the treatment of obesity in adults. J Clin Psychiatry 2006; 258–262

Taylor V, MacQueen G: Associations between bipolar disorder and metabolic syndrome: a review. J Clin Psychiatry 2006;67:1034–1041

---

71 According to the ethics primer of the American Psychiatric Association, which one of the following scenarios would most likely be considered a violation of the psychotherapeutic frame?

A. A patient is late to his psychotherapy session due to an upcoming deadline at work, but the therapist still charges the full amount for the session.

B. The therapist loses his office keys, but he lives across the street. Rather than cancel his appointments, he asks his wife and children to stay out for the day and sets up a temporary office in his living room.

C. A patient does not bring his check book to his final session of the month, when payment is due. The therapist interprets this act as an expression of ambivalence about the treatment and suggests this to the patient.

D. The therapist is diagnosed with end-stage cancer and informs his patient that owing to serious illness, he will be terminating his practice over the next month.

E. A grateful former patient wishes to donate money to the hospital with which his therapist is affiliated. Not wanting to handle the transaction himself, the therapist refers the patient to the hospital's development office.

The correct response is option B: The therapist loses his office keys, but he lives across the street. Rather than cancel his appointments, he asks his wife and children to stay out for the day and sets up a temporary office in his living room.

The Ethics Primer of the American Psychiatric Association states that psychotherapy necessarily takes place within a frame, which consists of mutually agreed upon constants of the relationship, as well as human elements of the therapeutic situation. Standard fees and billing practices are one of the mutually agreed upon constants, as is the location of the sessions. Changing the location from the office to the home would be a clear violation of this aspect of the frame, as well as many others including the therapist's relative anonymity. Efforts to understand all aspects of the therapist-patient relationship are included among the human elements that compose the therapeutic situation. Finally, while accepting large gifts is typically viewed as exploiting of patients, the Ethics Primer specifically states that unsolicited institutional donations from former patients should be directed toward third parties uninvolved in the psychotherapy.

Gruenberg P: Boundary Violations, in Ethics Primer of the American Psychiatric Association. Washington DC, American Psychiatric Association, 2001

---

72 Genetic linkage analysis studies provide information about which one of the following aspects of a gene:

A. Post-transitional processing.
B. Location.
C. Function.
D. Endophenotype.
E. Population frequency.

The correct response is option B: Location.

Linkage analysis is a method of positional cloning and relies on the fact that when DNA segments or loci are near each other on a chromosome, they tend to be inherited together. Thus, it is an indirect method of tracking an unknown gene. It can be done without any knowledge of the nature of the gene itself or of the mechanism by which the gene might influence a particular disorder.

Burmeister M. Genetics of psychiatric disorders: a primer. FOCUS 2006;4:317–326

---

73 A 17-year-old man is brought to the emergency department after fighting with his girlfriend and ingesting a bottle of alprazolam. En route to the hospital, the girlfriend lost control of the car, causing the patient to hit his head against the windshield with loss of consciousness. Examination reveals the patient to be in stupor, with respiratory depression and coma. He has a 4-cm laceration over the right frontal area that is profusely bleeding. Which of the facts of the patient's presentation represents the greatest contraindication to the use of flumazenil?

A. Age of patient.
B. Central nervous system (CNS) depression.
C. Benzodiazepine use.
D. Possible traumatic brain injury.

The correct response is option D: Possible traumatic brain injury.

The characteristic of the patient that represents the greatest contraindication to the use of flumazenil is the possible traumatic brain injury. Flumazenil can affect cerebral hemodynamics and is not recommended for situations in which intracranial pressure may already be increased, such as in head injury. Flumazenil should be administered carefully to benzodiazepine-dependent patients and patients who have ingested mixed substances to avoid the production of withdrawal seizures. None of the other characteristics of the patient represent contraindications.

Hales RE, Yudofsky SC: Substance use disorders in, The American Psychiatric Publishing Textbook of clinical psychiatry. Washington DC, American Psychiatric Publishing, 2003, pp 343–4

---

74 A 42-year-old man is started on pharmacotherapy for treatment of major depressive disorder. Two weeks later, he presents with complaints of dry mouth, impaired ability to focus at close range, constipation, urinary hesitation, tachycardia, and sexual dysfunction. Which of the following medications is most likely to have caused this presentation?

A. Duloxetine.
B. Fluoxetine.
C. Imipramine.
D. Mirtazapine.
E. Venlafaxine.

The correct response is option C: Imipramine.

Imipramine is a tertiary amine tricyclic antidepressant. These medications block muscarinic receptors, producing anticholinergic effects such as the symptoms that the patient is describing. All tricyclic antidepressants have some degree of anticholinergic action. The other medications listed have much less anticholinergic activity and therefore are more widely used now. This difference in side effects improves patient compliance with taking the medicine.

Schatzberg AF, Nemeroff CB (eds). Essentials of Clinical Psychopharmacology, 2nd ed. Arlington, VA, American Psychiatric Publishing, 2006. p 19

---

75 Which of the following medications has been the only one to demonstrate a decrease in suicide risk?

A. Valproic acid.
B. Lithium.
C. Carbamazepine.
D. Lamotrigine.
E. Gabapentin.

The correct response is option B: Lithium.

Initial studies as well as a meta-analysis have demonstrated that lithium decreases suicide and that abrupt discontinuation increases suicide. A meta-analysis of 31 studies of major affective disorders found a fivefold reduction in suicides and attempted suicides during lithium treatment compared to those not taking the drug. Other studies suggest that the antisuicidal effect of lithium extends beyond its mood stabilizing property.

Kessing LV et al: Suicide risk in patients treated with lithium. Arch Gen Psychiatry 2005; 62:860–866

Sadock BJ, Sadock VA: Kaplan & Sadock's Comprehensive Textbook of Psychiatry, 9th ed. Philadelphia, Lippincott Williams & Wilkins, 2009, p 3135

American Psychiatric Association: Practice Guideline for the Assessment and Treatment of Patients with Suicidal Behaviors. 2003. http://psychiatryonline.org/guidelines.aspx

---

76 A 34 year-old woman, who has been treated with an antidepressant for the past month, complains that she no longer gets relief from her back pain when she takes codeine, which has been prescribed by her orthopedist. Which one of the following antidepressants would be most likely to produce such an effect?

A. Escitalopram.
B. Sertraline.
C. Paroxetine.
D. Mirtazapin.
E. Buproprion.

The correct response is option C: Paroxetine.

Paroxetine is a potent inhibitor of cytochrome P450 2D6 (CYP2D6). The analgesic effect of codeine depends on it being metabolized by CYP2D6 to its active metabolite morphine. The other antidepressant medications in this example are not potent inhibitors of the CYP2D6 system.

Sindrup SH, Brosen K: The pharmacogenetics of codeine hypoalgesia. Pharmacogenetics 1995; 5:335–346

Mannheimer B, Wettermark B, Lundberg M, Pettersson H, et al: Nationwide drug-dispensing data reveal important differences in adherence to drug label recommendations on CYP2D6-dependent drug interactions. Br J Clin Pharmacol 2010 Apr; 69(4):411–7

---

77 Children of European descent with an early history of abuse have been found to be more likely to develop subsequent depression when they have a genetic polymorphism of which of the following neurotransmitter transporters?

A. Norepinephrine.
B. Dopamine.
C. Serotonin.
D. Glutamate.
E. GABA.

The correct response is option C: Serotonin.

In studies replicated in children, adolescents, and young adults with a history of abuse, those with a short allele of 5-HTTLPR, the serotonin transporter, exhibited more depression than those with a long allele.

Kendler KS, Kuhn JW, Vittum J, Prescott CA, Riley B. The interaction of stressful life events and a serotonin transporter polymorphism in the prediction of episodes of major depression: a replication. Arch Gen Psychiatry 2005; 62:529–35

Uher R, Caspi A, Houts R, et al: Serotonin transporter gene moderates childhood maltreatment's effects on persistent but not single-episode depression: replications and implications for resolving inconsistent results. J Affect Disord. 2011 December; 135(0):56–65

---

78 A 45-year-old woman was a witness to a motor vehicle accident that resulted in a number of fatalities. The images and the sounds of the accident greatly distressed her. The day after the accident she was seen by her family physician. The most appropriate next treatment step is:

A. Education and support about possible reactions that may occur.
B. Immediate referral to a mental health treatment program.
C. Treatment with an antidepressant.
D. Benzodiazepines as needed for sleep.
E. Critical incident debriefing.

The correct response is option A: Education and support about possible reactions that may occur.

It is important not to pathologize all emotional responses to disaster. The initial response may represent what has been called "a normal response to an abnormal situation." Education about the normal course following a traumatic event and support are the most useful first step in addressing a patient's concerns after a trauma.

Disaster Psychiatry Handbook, American Psychiatric Association Committee on Psychiatric Dimensions of Disaster, 2004, pp 21–22. http://www.psychiatry.org/practice/professional-interests/disaster-psychiatry

American Psychiatric Association Practice Guideline for the Treatment of Patients with Acute Stress Disorder and PosttraumaticStress Disorder. Am J Psychiatry. 2004. p 11. http://psychiatryonline.org/guidelines.aspx

---

79 A 48-year-old man with depression has been resistant to treatment with a variety of antidepressants. The decision is made to try him on a monoamine oxidase inhibitor (MAOI). In order to avoid serotonin syndrome, a washout period of at least 5 weeks is MOST indicated if he has been taking which antidepressant?

A. Bupropion.
B. Clomipramine.
C. Fluoxetine.
D. Paroxetine.
E. Venlafaxine.

The correct response is option C: Fluoxetine.

MAOIs must not be prescribed with serotoninergic medications to avoid serotonin syndrome. Because of the shorter half-life of clomipramine, paroxetine, and venlafaxine, an MAOI may be started 2 weeks after washout. The same applies to bupropion as it does not have serotonergic properties. However, because of the longer half-life of fluoxetine, MAOIs must not be administered for 5 weeks after discontinuation.

Pocket Handbook of Clinical Psychiatry, 4th ed, Sadock BA and Sadock VA, Lippinicott, Williams and Wilkins, 2005. p 161

---

80 Which of the following medications used to treat excessive daytime sleepiness associated with narcolepsy has also been abused as a "date rape" drug?

A. Sodium oxybate.
B. Modafinil.
C. Methylphenidate.
D. Selegiline.
E. Dextroamphetamine.

The correct response is option A: Sodium oxybate.

Sodium oxybate or gamma-hydroxybutyrate is FDA-approved for treating excessive daytime sleepiness and cataplexy in patients with narcolepsy. It had been banned in the United States in 1990 and listed as a Schedule I drug because of its abuse potential and use to facilitate sexual assaults. Because of its value in treating narcolepsy, it is now listed as a Schedule III drug when used medically, and its distribution is under strict control.

Robinson DM, Keating GM. Sodium oxybate: a review of its use in the management of narcolepsy. CNS Drugs. 2007; 21:350–352

Drasbek KR, Christensen J, Jensen K. Gamma-hydroxybutyrate—a drug of abuse. Acta Neurol Scand. 2006; 114:145

---

81 A patient recounts a story about getting angry with a store clerk. The therapist asks a factual question about the circumstance, inspiring rage in the patient, who finds him to be uncaring and seeking to blame her. The therapist says, "I wonder if what you're feeling right now is just like the feeling you had in the store, when you attributed the same uncaring attitude toward the clerk. These kinds of misreadings seem to make you very upset in many different settings." Which of the following most accurately describes this type of intervention?

A. Genetic interpretation.
B. Transference interpretation.
C. Clarification.
D. Observation.
E. Empathic validation.

The correct response is option B: Transference interpretation.

This is a paraphrasing of a vignette example of a transference interpretation that appeared in an article by Gabbard and Horowitz in *The American Journal of Psychiatry*, March 2009. In a transference interpretation, the therapist points out how a patient's early relational pattern, which recurs in many domains of the patient's life, is repeating itself in the "here and now" between therapist and patient. *Clarification* refers to the process of helping a patient specify vague issues. In a genetic interpretation, the therapist draws a link between present occurrences and a patient's early family relationships. When a therapist strives to put himself in the patient's position and states how that must feel, he performs an *empathic validation*. Although the therapist is technically making an observation about the patient, *observation* in psychotherapy is different from interpretation in that it does not explain or link behaviors.

Gabbard GO, Horowitz MJ: Insight, transference interpretation, and therapeutic change in the dynamic psychotherapy of borderline personality disorder. Am J Psychiatry 2009; 166: p 517

Gabbard GO: Long-Term Psychodynamic Psychotherapy: A Basic Text. Washington DC, American Psychiatric Publishing, 2004, pp 59–77

---

82 Consideration of genotyping for human leukocyte antigen allele HLA-B 1502 has been recommended by the FDA prior to starting carbamazepine on patients with which of the following ancestries?

A. European.
B. African.
C. Asian.
D. Hispanic.
E. Native American.

The correct response is option C: Asian.

According to the FDA, "the risk of Stevens Johnson syndrome (SJS)/toxic epidermal necrolysis (TEN) from carbamazepine is significantly increased in patients positive for the HLA-B*1502 allele. This allele is found almost exclusively in patients with ancestry across broad areas of Asia, including South Asian Indians. Owing to wide variability in rates of HLA-B*1502 even within ethnic groups, the difficulty in ascertaining ethnic ancestry, and the likelihood of mixed ancestry, screening for HLA-B*1502 should be performed for most patients of Asian ancestry. Prevalence of HLA-B*1502 has not been studied in many regions of Asia. The following figures must therefore be considered no more than a rough guide in deciding which patients to screen:

- 10%–15% or more of patients may carry the allele in parts of China, Thailand, Malaysia, Indonesia, the Philippines, and Taiwan.
- South Asians, including Indians, appear to have intermediate prevalence of HLA-B 1502, averaging 2%–4% but higher in some groups.
- HLA-B 1502 appears to be present at a low frequency, <1%, in Japan and Korea.

Although testing negative for HLA-B*1502 allele is associated with a lower risk of such reactions, the risk is not reduced to zero."

FDA U.S. Food and Drug Administration: Information for Healthcare Professionals: Dangerous or Even Fatal Skin Reactions - Carbamazepine (marketed as Carbatrol, Equetro, Tegretol, and generics). http://www.fda.gov/Drugs/DrugSafety/PostmarketDrugSafetyInformationforPatientsandProviders/ucm124718.htm

Ferrel PB, Jr. and McLeod HL. Carbamazepine, HLA-B*1502 and risk of Stevens-Johnson syndrome and toxic epidermal necrolysis: US FDA recommendations. Pharmacogenetics 2008; 9:1543–1546

83 An 84-year-old woman with a history of Alzheimer's disease presents to an emergency department after a fall. She had been experiencing difficulty sleeping at night for several months and was increasingly combative and suspicious of her daughter, with whom she lived. In developing a plan of treatment for this patient, which of the following principles is most appropriate to incorporate?

A. Adjust doses of medication slowly with long intervals between dose increments.
B. Prescribe small doses of several different medications rather than using one medication.
C. Use a long-acting injectable medication to aid adherence.
D. Use an initial loading dose of medication to speed response.

The correct response is option A: Adjust doses of medication slowly with long intervals between dose increments.

Individuals with dementia may be more sensitive to adverse effects such as anticholinergic effects, orthostasis, sedation, and Parkinsonism because of alterations in absorption, distribution metabolism, and/or elimination of medications. Consequently, smaller initial doses, smaller increments in dose, and long periods of time between dose changes are recommended. The use of more than one medication, although sometimes unavoidable, may further influence the pharmacokinetics of many medications and obscure causes of adverse effects if they appear. Although long-acting injectable medications can aid adherence, the potential for long-lasting adverse effects would be problematic in an older patient with dementia.

American Psychiatric Association Practice Guideline for the Treatment of Patients with Alzheimer's Disease and Other Dementias, 2nd ed. 2007, p 12. http://psychiatryonline.org/guidelines.aspx

84 A 28-year-old woman with bipolar I disorder is pregnant for the first time. Throughout the pregnancy, she has been maintained on a mood stabilizer. At the time of birth, the baby is noted to have a cardiovascular defect consistent with Ebstein's anomaly. The mood stabilizer the woman was taking was most likely:

A. Carbamazepine.
B. Haloperidol.
C. Lithium.
D. Lorazepam.
E. Valproate.

The correct response is option C: Lithium.

First-trimester exposure to lithium, valproate, or carbamazepine is associated with greater risk of birth defects. With lithium exposure, the relative risk for Ebstein's anomaly, a cardiovascular defect, is 10–20 times greater than the risk in the general population, although the absolute risk is low at about 1–2 per 1,000 births. Exposure to carbamazepine and valproate during the first trimester is associated with neural tube defects and craniofacial abnormalities. High-potency antipsychotic medications are preferred in the treatment of psychotic symptoms during pregnancy because they are less likely to have associated anticholinergic, antihistaminergic, or hypotensive effects. In general, teratogenic effects with benzodiazepines are likely to be small.

American Psychiatric Association Practice Guideline for the Treatment of Patients with Bipolar Disorder, 2nd ed (2002). http://psychiatryonline.org/guidelines.aspx

85 According to simple Mendelian inheritance, if a disease gene is recessive, what is the likelihood of developing the disease if one parent has two dominant genes and the other two recessive genes?

A. 0%.
B. 25%.
C. 50%.
D. 75%.
E. 100%.

The correct response is option A: 0%.

Because the disease will only occur in the absence of a dominant gene, two recessive genes will be necessary for the condition to appear. Therefore, the children will not be at risk for developing the disease, but they will be carriers.

	r	r
R	Rr	Rr
R	Rr	Rr

Sadock BJ, Sadock VA (eds): Kaplan & Sadock's Comprehensive Textbook of Psychiatry, 9th ed. Philadelphia, Lippincott Williams & Wilkins, 2009, pp 301–302

Smoller JW, Sheidley BR, Tsuang MT. Psychiatric Genetics: Applications in Clinical Practice. American Psychiatric Publishing, 1st edition, 2008, p 196

86 Which of the following is the medication most often associated with an increased risk of falls in persons age 80 or older?

A. Antihypertensives.
B. Benzodiazepines.
C. Antidepressants.
D. Histamine H_1 receptor antagonists.
E. Atypical antipsychotics.

The correct response is option B: Benzodiazepines.

In patients 80 years or older, it is estimated that at least one-third of injurious falls (falls associated with hospitalization, fracture, head trauma, or death) are related to the use of benzodiazepines. Approximately 10% of the falls in this age group are fatal.

Pariente A, Dartigues JF, Benichou J, Letenneur L, Moore N, Fourrier-Réglat A. Benzodiazepines and injurious falls in community dwelling elders. Drugs Aging. 2008; 25(1):61–70

87 Patients who are being treated with exposure therapy for anxiety disorders are:

A. Encouraged to think about nonthreatening situations during the treatment.
B. Encouraged to focus on their fears and allow feelings of anxiety to occur.
C. Required to conduct the therapy in real-life or fully realistic situations.
D. Required to develop a protocol and start with the most feared stimulus first.
E. Required to be on an appropriate type and dose of antianxiety medication.

The correct response is option B: Encouraged to focus on their fears and allow feelings of anxiety to occur.

For exposure therapy to be effective, the patient must pay attention fully to the details of the experience and allow the feelings of anxiety and arousal to occur. Exposure is designed to help the patient confront their fears while staying psychologically engaged, allowing the processes involved in fear reduction (habitation and extinction) to occur. Generally, patients start with the least feared situations. Exposure can occur using imagination, role-play, virtual reality, or in real-life situations. Thinking about other things can interfere with the process, and medication is not a required component of the treatment.

Scheier FR, Luterek JA, Heimberg RG, Leonardo E: Social phobia, in Clinical Manual of Anxiety Disorders. Edited by DJ Stein. Washington, DC. American Psychiatric Publishing, 2004, p 77

88 What were the findings of the Treatment for Adolescents with Depression Study (TADS), with regard to efficacy of treatment?

A. Fluoxetine alone was most effective.
B. Cognitive-behavioral therapy (CBT) alone was most effective.
C. Fluoxetine plus cognitive-behavioral therapy was most effective.
D. Interpersonal therapy alone was most effective.
E. Fluoxetine plus interpersonal therapy was most effective.

The correct response is option C: Fluoxetine plus cognitive-behavioral therapy was most effective.

TADS evaluated and compared the efficacy of four treatment approaches: Combined CBT-fluoxetine, fluoxetine alone, CBT alone, and placebo. The results of the study indicated that 71% of adolescents improved with the combined treatment, 60.6% improved with fluoxetine alone, 43.2% improved with CBT alone, whereas 34.8% showed improvement with placebo. Interpersonal therapy was not evaluated in this study.

March JS, Silva S, Petrycki S, Curry J, et al: Treatment for Adolescents with Depression Study (TADS) team. Fluoxetine, cognitive-behavioral therapy, and their combination for adolescents with depression: Treatment for Adolescents with Depression Study (TADS) randomized controlled trial. Journal of the American Medical Association. 2004 Aug 18; 292(7):807–820

AACAP practice parameter for the assessment and treatment of children and adolescents with depressive disorders. J Am Acad Child Adolesc Psychiatry. 2007. FOCUS: Child and Adolescent Psychiatry. Summer 2008; 6(3):387–8

Emslie GJ, Kennard BD, Mayes TL, Nightingale-Teresi J, et al: Fluoxetine versus placebo in preventing relapse of major depression in children and adolescents. FOCUS: Child and Adolescent Psychiatry. Summer 2008; 6(3):356

89 A 76-year-old woman with a long history of generalized anxiety disorder presents to a psychiatrist. She is interested in the possibility of pharmacotherapy for this disorder. She has a history of hypertension, for which she takes amlodipine, but otherwise is in good health. The most accurate advice regarding the use of pharmacotherapy for this patient is that medications are:

A. Generally not effective in treating anxiety in elderly patients.
B. Contraindicated due to the increased side effects in older adults.
C. Less effective than psychotherapy for anxiety in older adults.
D. Not recommended owing to the high potential for drug-drug interactions.
E. A first-line treatment for anxiety in the elderly.

The correct response is option E: A first-line treatment for anxiety in the elderly.

The same treatments that are effective for anxiety in younger persons are also effective in the elderly. Although both pharmacotherapy and behavioral interventions are reasonably effective, the weight of evidence suggests that there are higher average treatment effects with pharmacological interventions. Although side effects, drug interactions, and patient preferences should be taken into account, in most elderly patients pharmacotherapy is likely to be the first-line treatment recommendation for anxiety disorders. With regard to generalized anxiety disorder, Pinquart and Duberstein (2007) evaluated six medication studies and eight behavioral studies.

Pinquart M, Duberstein PR. Treatment of anxiety disorders in older adults: a meta-analytic comparison of behavioral and pharmacological interventions. Am J Geriatr Psychiatry. 2007; 15(8):639–651

90 You are treating a 16-year-old patient for ADHD who has multiple café au lait spots visible on both arms and legs. A diagnosis of neurofibromatosis is made by a neurology consultant. Which one of the following modes of genetic transmission is seen in this illness?

A. Autosomal dominant.
B. Autosomal recessive.
C. Non-Mendelian inheritance.
D. X-linked recessive.
E. X-linked dominant.

The correct response is option A: Autosomal dominant.

Neurofibromatosis type I is characterized by café au lait spots, neurofibromas, and Lisch nodules. It is also associated with ADHD and having an IQ 5–10 points below average. It is inherited on chromosome 17 in an autosomal dominant pattern.

Kaufman DM: Clinical Neurology for Psychiatrists, 5th ed. Philadelphia, WB Saunders Company, 2001, pp 329–333

http://ghr.nlm.nih.gov/handbook/inheritance/inheritancepatterns

Smoller JW, Sheidley BR, Tsuang MT. Psychiatric Genetics: Applications in Clinical Practice. American Psychiatric Publishing, 1st edition, 2008, p 202

91 Which of the following combination treatments has the best evidence for producing a short-term benefit of more rapid stabilization for the acute symptom treatment of panic disorder?

A. CBT and SSRI.
B. Benzodiazepine and SSRI.
C. CBT and benzodiazepine.
D. SSRI and buspirone.

The correct response is option B: Benzodiazepine and SSRI.

According to The American Psychiatric Association Practice Guideline for the Treatment of Patients With Panic Disorder, benzodiazepines may be used along with antidepressants to help control symptoms until the antidepressant takes effect. Studies suggest that the benzodiazepine confers a short-term benefit of stabilization of panic symptoms. However, the advantage of the combination does not continue and individuals receiving SSRI alone catch up to those receiving the combination after the first few weeks of treatment. The benefit of quicker stabilization should be weighed against the possibility of an increased side-effect burden. Studies of medication and psychosocial treatment have not shown a clear and lasting advantage for this combination.

Goddard AW, Brouette T, Almai A, Jetty P, Woods SW, Charney D. Early coadministration of clonazepam with sertraline for panic disorder. Arch Gen Psychiatry. 2001 Jul;58(7):681–6

Pollack MH, Simon NM, Worthington JJ, Doyle AL, Peters P, Toshkov F, Otto MW. Combined paroxetine and clonazepam treatment strategies compared to paroxetine monotherapy for panic disorder. J Psychopharmacol. 2003 Sep;17(3):276–82

92 A 22-year-old man presents repeatedly over a year with concerns that he is suffering from AIDS. He has never been found to be HIV positive, but he is not convinced despite having negative tests. He does not meet the criteria for major depressive disorder, generalized anxiety disorder, or obsessive-compulsive disorder. Which of the following is the most likely diagnosis?

A. Body dysmorphic disorder.
B. Illness anxiety disorder.
C. Conversion disorder.
D. Somatic symptom disorder.
E. Unspecified somatic symptom disorder.

The correct response is option B: Illness anxiety disorder.

Illness anxiety disorder is characterized by 6 months or more of a general preoccupation with fears or the idea of having a serious undiagnosed medical illness. This preoccupation causes significant distress and impairment; it is not accounted for by another psychiatric or medical disorder. The emphasis is on fear of having a disease, and emphasis in somatic symptom disorder is the concern with symptoms. Illness anxiety disorder is equally prevalent among men and women. Conversion disorder usually involves one or more symptoms of altered voluntary motor or sensory function rather than a particular disease.

Sadock BJ and Sadock VA (eds). Kaplan and Sadock's Synopsis of Psychiatry, 10th ed. Philadelphia: Lippincott Williams and Wilkins; 2007. p 643

American Psychiatric Association: Diagnostic and Statistical Manual of Mental Disorders, 5th Edition. Arlington, VA, American Psychiatric Association, 2013, pp 309–327

---

93 Which of the following neurotransmitters has the largest body of evidence associating it with the reinforcing effects of various types of drugs of abuse?

A. Acetylcholine.
B. Dopamine.
C. GABA.
D. Glutamate.
E. Serotonin.

The correct response is option B: Dopamine.

Although all of the answer choices have been associated in one way or another with the reinforcing effects of drugs, the most consistently associated neurotransmitter has been dopamine. The concentrations of dopamine are increased in the limbic regions by drugs of abuse. It is thought that the reinforcing effects of drugs of abuse are due to their ability to exceed the magnitude and duration of the increases in dopamine in the nucleus accumbens when compared to natural reinforcers like sleep and sex.

Kalivas PW, Volkow ND: The neural basis of addiction: a pathology of motivation and choice. Am J Psychiatry 2005; 162:1403–1413. Reprinted in FOCUS: Substance Abuse, Spring 2007; 2:208–219

Pierce RC, Kumaresan V: The mesolimbic dopamine system: the final common pathway for the reinforcing effect of drugs of abuse? Neuroscience & Biobehavioral Reviews 2006; 30:215–38

Volkow ND, Li TK: Drug addiction: the neurobiology of behaviour gone awry. Nature Reviews Neuroscience 2004; 5:963–70

---

94 Which of the following is the preferred method to confirm a clinical diagnosis of narcolepsy?

A. Functional magnetic resonance imaging (fMRI).
B. Apnea monitoring.
C. Multiple sleep latency test (MSLT).
D. Human leukocyte antigen (HLA) testing.
E. Cerebrospinal fluid (CSF) hypocretin levels.

The correct response is option C: Multiple sleep latency test (MSLT).

The MSLT, which involves measuring REM sleep latency, consists of four or five 20-minute naps scheduled about 2 hours apart. It is usually performed after an overnight sleep study. HLA testing lacks diagnostic specificity, and CSF hypocretin levels require a lumbar puncture. Apnea monitoring is essential for diagnosing sleep apnea.

Dauvilliers Y, Arnulf I, Mignot E. Narcolepsy with cataplexy. Lancet. 2007; 369:499–511

Moore DP. Textbook of Clinical Neuropsychiatry, 2nd ed. London, Hodder Arnold, 2008. pp 575–577

95 Which of the following psychotherapeutic interventions represents the best approach for a patient with germ obsessions who washes his hands every time he touches something he considers dirty?

A. Having the patient place his hands in a container of mud.
B. Having the patient snap his wrist with a rubber band when he washes his hands.
C. Pointing out to the patient that the germ phobia is an example of distorted thinking.
D. Having the patient touch a dirty object, then not allowing him to wash his hands.
E. Providing the patient with coping cards to remind him that the hand washing is unnecessary.

The correct response is option D: Having the patient touch a dirty object, then not allowing him to wash his hands.

This is an example of exposure and response prevention (ERP). Wrist-snapping represents aversive conditioning. Placing the patient's hands in mud represents flooding. The coping cards and distorted thinking are tenets of CBT. While these may be helpful in some instances, ERP is the best form of therapy for OCD.

Sadock BJ, Sadock VA: Kaplan & Sadock's Synopsis of Psychiatry: Behavioral Sciences/Clinical Psychiatry, 10th ed. Philadelphia, Lippincott Williams & Wilkins, 2007, p 611

96 A military veteran is diagnosed with PTSD after his wife encourages him to seek treatment because of problems adjusting to civilian life. It is clear that survivor guilt is a major source of distress. Which of the following is the best intervention for this issue?

A. Vocational counseling.
B. Couples therapy.
C. Individual psychotherapy.
D. Fluoxetine.
E. Risperidone.

The correct response is option C: Individual psychotherapy.

Individuals with PTSD often have multiple problems that require different interventions. Interpersonal withdrawal, survivor guilt, or shame may be more responsive to psychosocial interventions than medication. The other options may be helpful for other aspects of the patient's functioning.

American Psychiatric Association Practice Guideline for the Treatment of Patients with Acute Stress Disorder and Posttraumatic Stress Disorder. Am J Psychiatry. 2004; 161(11):37. http://psychiatryonline.org/guidelines.aspx
Gabbard GO (ed): Treatments of Psychiatric Disorders 4th ed. American Psychiatric Publishing, Washington, DC. 2007; pp 520–525

97 Which of the following cultural groups is most likely to want to be informed of a terminal prognosis?

A. Mexican Americans.
B. Korean Americans.
C. African Americans.
D. Japanese Americans.
E. Navajo Americans.

The correct response is option C: African Americans.

Blackhall et al. (1995) studied cultural differences in attitudes toward disclosing information about terminal illness. African Americans (and European Americans) were found to be more likely to want this disclosure than Mexican or Korean Americans. Japanese tend to expect little specific information from their physicians. On the other hand, Navajos believe that language can "shape reality and control events." Therefore being given a negative prognosis is felt to be dangerous physically and emotionally as well as disrespectful.

Breitbart W, Lintz K. Psychiatric Issues in the care of dying patients. Wise MG, Rundell JR (eds): Textbook of Consultation-Liaison Psychiatry, 2nd ed. Washington, DC, American Psychiatric Publishing, 2002, pp 775–776
Blackhall LJ, Murphy ST, Frank G, et al: Ethnicity and attitudes toward patient autonomy. JAMA 1995, 278:820–825
Levenson JL (ed): Textbook of Psychosomatic Medicine. Arlington, VA, American Psychiatric Publishing, 2005, p 996

98 When diagnosing major depressive disorder in young children, which of the following signs or symptoms is MORE likely to be present than would be expected in an adolescent or adult?

A. Diurnal variation in mood.
B. Hypersomnia.
C. Melancholia.
D. Poor self-esteem.
E. Somatic complaints.

The correct response is option E: Somatic complaints.

Although the essential features of major depressive disorder are similar in children, adolescents, and adults, there are noticeable differences in phenomenology. Younger children, unable to express emotions as adequately as adolescents and adults, tend to present with more somatic complaints, psychomotor agitation, and, at times, mood-congruent hallucinations. The most common somatic complaints are headaches and abdominal pain/discomfort. With age, these symptoms begin to decrease, but self-esteem seems to worsen. By adolescence, somatic complaints and depressed appearance decrease in frequency and are commonly replaced by symptoms of anhedonia, diurnal variation, hopelessness, psychomotor retardation, and delusions.

Dulcan MK and Wiener JM. Essentials of Child and Adolescent Psychiatry, Arlington, VA, American Psychiatric Publishing, 2006. pp 268–269

99 A mutation on which of the following chromosomes has been associated with early-onset Alzheimer's dementia?

A. Chromosome 2.
B. Chromosome 19.
C. Chromosome 21.
D. Y chromosome.
E. X chromosome.

The correct response is option C: Chromosome 21.

Many individuals with Down syndrome develop early-onset Alzheimer's dementia. Therefore, chromosome 21 has been linked to this illness. Other linked chromosomes are 1 and 14. Chromosome 19 is linked to late-onset Alzheimer's dementia. Alzheimer's is not sex-linked.

Alzheimer's Disease Genetics fact Sheet from U.S. National Institutes of Health National Institute on Aging [Retrieved 8/16/09] http://www. nia.nih.gov/Alzheimers/Publications/geneticsfs.htm

Smoller JW, Sheidley BR, Tsuang MT. Psychiatric Genetics: Applications in Clinical Practice. American Psychiatric Publishing, 1st edition, 2008, p 181

100 A 16-year-old girl is brought by her parents for an evaluation as part of the admission process for a weight reduction program. The adolescent agrees that she is overweight and that she would like to lose weight. Which of the following would be MOST indicative that she will be successful in the program?

A. BMI <30.
B. No family history of eating disorders.
C. Mother successfully lost weight.
D. She is willing to take medication.
E. She is willing to change her eating habits.

The correct response is option E: She is willing to change her eating habits.

To be able to participate successfully in a weight reduction and management program, adolescents must be willing to change their lifestyle habits.

Zametkin AJ, Zoon CK, Klein HW, Munson S. Psychiatric aspects of child and adolescent obesity: a review of the past 10 years. J Am Acad Child Adolesc Psychiatry 2004; Reprinted in FOCUS. Fall 2004; 2 (4):634

101 A 25-year-old woman complains about shortness of breath, chest pain, and diaphoresis. She has had multiple attacks in the past 3 weeks. Her medical workup is negative. Which of the following medications is the best choice considering efficacy and side-effect profile?

A. Propranolol.
B. Desipramine.
C. Bupropion.
D. Sertraline.
E. Alprazolam.

The correct response is option D: Sertraline.

The APA Practice Guideline for Panic Disorder suggests the SSRIs as the most useful agents currently because of the data supporting their effectiveness and favorable side-effect profile. The TCAs (desipramine) have been shown to be effective, but the side-effect profile makes them less well tolerated (e.g., anticholinergic, sleep disturbance, sweating, hypotension, weight gain, etc.). There is no good evidence that either propranolol or bupropion are effective for panic disorder. Finally, alprazolam was a major choice for treatment some time ago, but its side-effect profile including tolerance, difficulty in discontinuing drug without rebounds, sedation, and other common side effects of the benzodiazepines caused it to be replaced by other agents.

American Psychiatric Association Practice Guideline for the Treatment of Patients With Panic Disorder, 2nd ed (2008). http://psychiatryonline.org/guidelines.aspx

102 The "parent of origin" effect is defined as transmission of a risk for disease based on whether an autosome has been transmitted by the mother or father. As one example of this phenomenon in psychiatric genetics, duplications of chromosome 15q inherited from the mother, but not the father, have been found to account for a small but significant proportion of cases of which of the following disorders?

A. Schizophrenia.
B. Bipolar disorder.
C. Obsessive-compulsive disorder.
D. Alcohol dependence.
E. Autism.

The correct response is option E: Autism.

Duplications of chromosome 15q inherited from the mother (but not from the father) have been associated with cases of autism. Duplicated genetic material may lead to normal development when originating with the father, but often leads to developmental abnormalities when originating with the mother. Each of the recent CNV studies of ASD has provided strong support for contribution of chromosome 15q11-13 duplication to ASD risk. The rate of chromosome 15q11-13 duplication is 1% in ASD.

Mason CE, State MW, Moldin SO. Genome, Transcriptome, and Proteome: Charting a New Course to Understanding the Molecular Neurobiology of Mental Disorders. Chapter 1.11. in Sadock BJ, Sadock VA. Ruiz P (eds): Kaplan and Sadock's Comprehensive Textbook of Psychiatry, 9th ed. Philadelphia, Lippincott Williams & Wilkins, 2009, pp 147–161
Campbell DB. Advances and challenges in the genetics of autism. FOCUS Summer 2010;8(3):339–349

103 A 14-year-old girl presents with significant weight loss. She reports that about 1 year ago she became concerned that she was overweight and began self-inducing vomiting. Since then, she has continued to use purgatives in addition to misusing laxatives, diuretics, and enemas as a means of weight control after binging. She is intensely afraid of becoming fat. She is in the 65th percentile for weight based on height, appears cachetic, but insists she is obese. She has not experienced menses for 6 months. Which of the following symptoms will MOST likely be elicited from the patient?

A. A need for orderliness and control.
B. Competitiveness.
C. Obsessional thinking.
D. Perfectionism.
E. Comorbid impulsivity.

The correct response is option E: Comorbid impulsivity.

Anorexia nervosa typically has its onset in an adolescent female who perceives herself to be overweight. The cardinal symptoms are refusal to maintain body weight at or above a minimally normal weight for age and height; intense fear of gaining weight; and denial of the seriousness of the current low body weight. DSM-5 distinguished between two subtypes—restricting and binge eating/purging. The binge eating/purging type is characterized by regularly engaging in binge-eating or purging behavior such as self-induced vomiting or the misuse of laxatives, diuretics, or enemas. When compared with patients with restricting anorexia, those with binge eating/purging type are more likely to have comorbid impulsivity, including substance use disorder, personality disorders, mood lability, and suicidality.

Dulcan MK, Weiner JM. Essentials of Child and Adolescent Psychiatry. Arlington (VA): American Psychiatric Publishing, 2006. pp 527–528

Hales RE, Yudofsky SC, Gabbard GO (eds): The American Psychiatric Publishing Textbook of Psychiatry, 5th ed. Arlington, VA, American Psychiatric Publishing, 2008, p 974

American Psychiatric Association: Diagnostic and Statistical Manual of Mental Disorders, 5th Edition. Arlington, VA, American Psychiatric Association, 2013, p 341

---

104 Cognitive deficits in schizophrenia have been associated with a decrease in $GABA_A$ receptors in which of the following brain areas?

A. Lateral amygdala.
B. Medial amygdala.
C. Dorsolateral prefrontal cortex.
D. Medial prefrontal cortex.
E. Nucleus accumbens.

The correct response is option C: Dorsolateral prefrontal cortex.

Several lines of evidence have linked cognitive impairments in schizophrenia with altered levels of $GABA_A$ receptors in the dorsolateral prefrontal cortex. Whereas the prefrontal cortex in general has been associated with cognitive function, it is specifically the dorsolateral prefrontal cortex that has been associated with cognitive deficits in schizophrenia. The amygdala is primarily involved in regulating emotional behavior and the nucleus accumbens with reward.

Lewis DA, Moghaddam B. Cognitive dysfunction in schizophrenia: convergence of)'-aminobutyric acid and glutamate alterations. Arch Neurol 2006; 63:1372–6

---

105 A 19-year-old man presents for an outpatient evaluation of increasing concerns about germs and contamination that are now resulting in several hours per day of hand washing and cleaning rituals to relieve anxiety. He is started on sertraline, the dose of which is increased 50 mg every other day until reaching 200 mg daily. After 1 week of treatment at this dose, he has not experienced any relief of the symptoms. However, the medication is well tolerated without significant side effects. In developing further plan of treatment, which of the following is the appropriate total length of time to continue sertraline before changing to another pharmacologic agent?

A. 2 weeks.
B. 4 weeks.
C. 6 weeks.
D. 8 weeks.
E. 10 weeks.

The correct response is option E: 10 weeks.

At least 10 and perhaps 12 weeks of pharmacological treatment is needed before one can conclude that an SSRI has failed in relieving symptoms of OCD. Equally important is an adequate dose, usually on the high end of the dosing spectrum. The SSRI chosen, as with other disorders, should be a good fit for a particular patient in terms of its side-effect profile. Many SSRIs have FDA approval for OCD. The first challenge in treating with medication is working with the patient to maintain medication adherence.

Koran LM. Obsessive-compulsive disorder: an update for clinicians. FOCUS: OCD; Summer 2007; 3:299–313

Stein DJ, Hollander E, Rothbaum BO (eds): Textbook of Anxiety Disorders, 2nd ed. Arlington, VA, American Psychiatric Publishing, 2010, p 314

---

106 A psychiatric consult is requested for a patient who has burns over 60% of his body. The patient has begun refusing dressing changes despite pretreatment with morphine. Pain control is adequate except during dressing changes. Upon examination, the patient reports that the pain is too severe to tolerate, and he does not feel that the morphine is adequately controlling his pain. The psychiatrist should recommend which of the following agents as an additional medication prior to dressing changes?

A. Long-acting morphine.
B. Methadone.
C. Meperidine.
D. Fentanyl.
E. Codeine.

The correct response is option D: Fentanyl.

This patient is undermedicated during dressing changes and requires better analgesic control. Fentanyl is the recommended agent for managing the pain associated with dressing changes because of its rapid onset and short duration of action. The other medications have a less favorable onset/duration of action profile than fentanyl.

Wise MG, Rundell JR (eds): The American Psychiatric Publishing Textbook of Consultation-Liaison Psychiatry, 2nd ed. Washington, DC, American Psychiatric Publishing, 2002, p 612

American Psychiatric Publishing Textbook of Psychosomatic Medicine. Levenson JL (ed) 2005, p 660

---

107 A 36-year-old moderately obese man is seen for evaluation of depressed mood, difficulty falling asleep, poor appetite, and diminished concentration at work, all of which have been worsening over the past few weeks. When treatment options are discussed, he reports particular concerns about sexual side effects. Considering the patient's concerns, which one of the following medications would be most appropriate to suggest as an initial treatment?

A. Bupropion.
B. Fluoxetine.
C. Mirtazapine.
D. Nortriptyline.
E. Venlafaxine.

The correct response is option A: Bupropion.

In direct comparative studies that specifically evaluated sexual functioning, bupropion was significantly less likely to be problematic than SSRIs, TCAs, or SNRIs. Mirtazapine does not cause significant problems with sexual side effects but may cause significant weight gain (as can nortriptyline). Thus bupropion would be the medication of choice.

Clayton AH, Croft HA, Horrigan JP, Wightman DS, et al: Bupropion extended release compared with Escitalopram: effects on sexual functioning and antidepressant efficacy in 2 randomized, double-blind, placebo-controlled studies. J Clin Psychiatry 2006; 67:736–746

Jefferson JW: Bupropion extended-release for depressive disorders. Expert Rev Neurother 2008; 8:715–722

---

108 Which of the following disorders has the most evidence supporting familial aggregation of the disorder?

A. Posttraumatic stress disorder.
B. Adjustment disorder, mixed features.
C. Panic disorder.
D. Social phobia.
E. Specific phobia.

The correct response is option C: Panic disorder.

Among these disorders, the strongest aggregate evidence for familial aggregation is for panic disorder. Panic disorder, generalized anxiety disorder, phobias, and OCD all have significant familial aggregation. More research has been done on the genetics of panic disorder compared to other anxiety disorders.

Merikangas KR, Low NC. Genetic epidemiology of anxiety disorders. Handb Exp Pharmacol. 2005; (169):163–79

Hettema JM, Neale MC & Kendler KS. A review and meta-analysis of the genetic epidemiology of anxiety disorders. Am J Psychiatry 2001; 158:1568–1578

---

109 Which of the following medical complications is most likely to be seen in a patient with bulimia nervosa?

A. Decreased serum amylase.
B. Hyperchloremia.
C. Metabolic acidosis.
D. Hypokalemia.
E. Hyperthyroxinemia.

The correct response is option D: Hypokalemia.

Self-induced vomiting in patients with bulimia nervosa can result in metabolic alkalosis, hypochloremia, hypokalemia, increased serum amylase, and cardiac arrhythmias. Dangers of hypokalemia include weakness, lethargy, and possible cardiac arrhythmias.

Hales RE, Yudofsky SC, Gabbard GO (eds): The American Psychiatric Publishing Textbook of Psychiatry, 5th ed. Washington, DC, American Psychiatric Publishing, 2008. pp 983–985

Mehler PS. Bulimia nervosa. N Engl J Med 2003; 349:876–877

---

110 Evidence to date from OCD genetic studies indicates that its inheritance is best characterized by which pattern?

A. Automsomal dominant.
B. Autosomal recessive.
C. Sex-linked recessive.
D. Complex.
E. Mendelian.

The correct response is option D: Complex.

OCD is a complex genetic disorder that seems to also be strongly influenced by environmental and non-genetic biologic processes. There is emerging evidence that complex disorders may result from both rare genes of major effect and a combination of common genes of lesser effect. Studies of OCD report increased prevalence of this disorder among relatives. Twin studies have confirmed that a genetic component underlies the illness. Genome-wide significant findings have yet to be identified. Segration analyses have clarified that transmission does not occur in a simple Mendelian fashion.

Stewart SE, Pauls DL: The genetics of obsessive-compulsive disorder. FOCUS Summer 2010;8(3):350–357

---

111 A 72-year-old woman is referred to a psychiatrist because the family has noticed increasing apathy. In evaluating the patient, which of the following would be the most useful first step for revealing the likely underlying pathology?

A. An empirical trial of an antidepressant.
B. An MRI of the brain.
C. History and a full mental status examination.
D. Thyroid function testing.
E. Neuropsychological evaluation.

The correct response is option C: History and a full mental status examination.

Apathy is common in the elderly, and recent research suggests that it is distinct from depression and should not be treated automatically as a variant of major depression. Both clinical and neurobiological research suggests that apathy in the elderly is most often associated with neurocognitive disorders and may be a harbinger of progressive cognitive decline. Laboratory tests such as an MRI, thyroid function, and urine drug testing are most likely to play a confirmatory role when the history and examination suggest a specific pathology. MRI and similar neuroanatomical evaluations have shown that specific anatomical areas may underlie the pathology of apathy; however, these findings represent relative differences seen in population comparisons and are not sensitive enough to be considered a diagnostic tool.

Lyketsos C. Apathy and agitation: challenges and future directions. Am J Geriatr Psychiatry. 2007; 15(5):361–364

---

112 Which of the following is believed to be the chief factor in predicting outcome of psychodynamic psychotherapy?

A. Transference.
B. Countertransference.
C. Therapeutic alliance.
D. Resistance.
E. On-time payments.

The correct response is option C: Therapeutic alliance.

Although most of the above-mentioned choices are significant aspects of psychotherapy, therapeutic alliance is a strong predictor of outcome in individual psychotherapy across diverse treatment orientations and modalities. The strength of the therapeutic relationship is correlated with outcome across schools of psychotherapy.

Sadock BJ, Sadock VA. Kaplan and Sadock's Synopsis of Psychiatry: Behavioral Sciences/Clinical Psychiatry. Lippincott Williams & Wilkins; 10th edition, 2007, p 495

Gabbard GO (ed): Textbook of Psychotherapeutic Treatments. Arlington, VA: American Psychiatric Publishing, 2009, p 714

---

113 An adolescent girl becomes anxious and "panicky" at the thought of spiders. She cannot join her high school classmates for lunch outside because of the fear that she "will run into a spider." The most appropriate diagnosis is:

A. Agoraphobia.
B. Acute stress disorder.
C. Generalized anxiety disorder.
D. Specific phobia.
E. Social phobia.

The correct response is option D: Specific phobia.

Specific phobias are marked and persistent fears that are excessive or unreasonable, cued by the presence of anticipation of a specific object (e.g., animals) or situation (e.g., heights, flying). Social phobias concern the avoidance of social situations, and agoraphobia is characterized by anxiety about being in places or situations from which escape might be difficult. In this case, the anxiety is specifically related to a fear of spiders.

American Psychiatric Association: Diagnostic and Statistical Manual of Mental Disorders, 5th Edition. Arlington, VA, American Psychiatric Association, 2013, pp 197–202

---

114 A 31-year-old female describes dramatic fluctuations in mood and self-esteem. Which one of the following features would be most helpful in distinguishing bipolar II disorder from borderline personality disorder during a period of elevated mood?

A. Suicidal ideation with depressed mood.
B. Psychosis while mood is elevated or irritable.
C. Impulsivity while mood is elevated or irritable.
D. A history of continued functioning through mood fluctuations.
E. Mood fluctuations are observed by others.

The correct response is option B: Psychosis while mood is elevated or irritable.

In a hypomanic episode, by definition, psychosis is never present, whereas borderline patients may experience transient paranoia or dissociation when under stress. Personality disorders such as borderline personality disorder may have symptom overlap with bipolar disorders. In bipolar disorders, symptoms must represent a distinct episode, and the noticeable increase over baseline required for the diagnosis of bipolar disorder must be present.

American Psychiatric Association: Diagnostic and Statistical Manual of Mental Disorders, 5th Edition. Arlington, VA, American Psychiatric Association, 2013, pp 197, 202, 217

---

115 Which of the following psychiatric conditions is most commonly associated with self-neglect in the geriatric population?

A. Depression.
B. Generalized anxiety disorder.
C. Panic disorder.
D. Schizophrenia.
E. Personality disorder.

The correct response is option A: Depression.

Depression is a predictor of self-neglect. It has been shown to be as common as 62% in elders who self-neglect in one case-controlled study of older persons referred for self-neglect (compared with 12% in those referred for other reasons). Elders who self-neglect are frequently frail, live in squalor, have untreated medical conditions, and frequently refuse medical interventions. Neurocognitive disorders are also common in self-neglectors.

Abrams RC, Lachs M, McAvay G, Keohane DJ, Bruce ML. Predictors of self-neglect in community-dwelling elders. Am J Psychiatry. 2002 Oct; 159(10):1724–30
Dyer CB, Pavlik VN, Murphy KP, Hyman DJ. The high prevalence of depression and dementia in elder abuse or neglect. J Am Geriatr Soc. 2000 Feb; 48(2):205–8

---

116 According to the AMA Code of Medical Ethics, which of the following educationally related gifts from a pharmaceutical company is ethically acceptable?

A. Money to help defray hotel costs during a CME event.
B. Scholarships awarded to individual residents to attend educational conferences.
C. Reimbursement of travel for a guest faculty speaker.
D. Money to compensate a psychiatrist for time spent at a CME event.

The correct response is option C: Reimbursement of travel for a guest faculty speaker.

Scholarships awarded to students cannot be awarded to individuals, only to institutions. Gifts should serve an educational purpose and cannot be used to compensate a clinician for time or cost spent attending a CME event. Faculty speakers can be compensated financially by pharmaceutical companies.

Wahl DS, Milone RD et al: Ethics Primer of the American Psychiatric Association, Washington, DC, American Psychiatric Publishing, 2001; 48
Jibson MD; Interactions between physicians and industry: FOCUS Fall 2007

117 Which of the following statements best describes the association between PTSD and the subsequent emergence of drug use problems?

A. Young adults with PTSD due to earlier lifetime traumas, with no prior drug use disorders, are about five times more likely to develop drug-related problems subsequently compared with traumatized young adults without PTSD.
B. Experiencing significant trauma without the presence of PTSD is sufficient to subsequently increase the prevalence of drug use disorders substantially.
C. After controlling for factors such as sex, age, and ethnicity, PTSD confers no additional increased risk of subsequent drug use disorders.
D. After controlling for factors such as childhood conduct problems and risk taking, PTSD confers no additional increased risk of subsequent drug use disorders.
E. After controlling for factors such as family socioeconomic status (SES) and years of education, PTSD confers no additional increased risk of subsequent drug use disorders.

The correct response is option A: Young adults with PTSD due to earlier lifetime traumas, with no prior drug use disorders, are about five times more likely to develop drug-related problems subsequently compared with traumatized young adults without PTSD.

A large, longitudinal prospective study has shown that in young adults who have no features of drug use disorder, the presence of PTSD following lifetime history of significant trauma increases the relative risk of subsequent drug use and abuse problems nearly 5 times (relative risk 4.9), and this increased risk remains substantial even after controlling for a host of early factors that in themselves also increase the risk for adult drug use including sex, age, ethnicity, childhood conduct problems, risk taking, family SES, and years of education.

Reed PL, Anthony JC, Breslau N. Incidence of drug problems in young adults exposed to trauma and posttraumatic stress disorder: do early life experiences and predispositions matter? Arch Gen Psychiatry. 2007; 64(12):1435–1442

118 Borderline personality disorder is marked by pervasive instability of self-image, emotions, and impulsivity. Which of the following is a DSM diagnostic criteria for this diagnosis?

A. Consistent irresponsibility.
B. Lack of remorse after injuring others.
C. Requiring excessive admiration.
D. Sense of entitlement.
E. Unstable sense of self.

The correct response is option E: Unstable sense of self.

Although patients with borderline personality disorder may display or possess any of the other features listed, unstable sense of self is the only one that is a diagnostic criterion for this diagnosis. Consistent irresponsibility as well as lack of remorse after injuring others are criteria for antisocial personality disorder; entitlement and requiring admiration are criteria for narcissistic personality disorder.

American Psychiatric Association: Diagnostic and Statistical Manual of Mental Disorders, 5th Edition. Arlington, VA, American Psychiatric Association, 2013, p 663

119 Which of the following should be the initial treatment of a patient with illness anxiety?

A. Cognitive-behavioral therapy.
B. Treatment of incidental physical exam findings.
C. Scheduling regular physical examinations.
D. Discussing the false nature of the illness pharmacotherapy with SSRIs.

The correct response is option C: Scheduling regular physical examinations.

As with somatic symptom disorder, in which the preoccupation is on symptoms, the first-line treatment for illness anxiety disorder is reassurance to diminish the preoccupation with fear of having a disease. This can be accomplished by scheduling regular medical appointments with a clear goal. Cognitive therapy, as well as other forms of psychotherapy, may be helpful. Pharmacotherapy is helpful in treating any underlying drug-responsive conditions. Discussing the false nature of the illness is not helpful. Treatment of physical complaints should be done when objective evidence calls for it.

Hales RE, Yudofsky SC, Gabbard GO (eds): The American Psychiatric Publishing Textbook of Psychiatry, 5th ed. Washington, DC, American Psychiatric Publishing, 2008, p 632

American Psychiatric Association: Diagnostic and Statistical Manual of Mental Disorders, 5th Edition. Arlington, VA, American Psychiatric Association, 2013, pp 309–313

---

120 A 33-year-old man with schizophrenia and alcohol dependence acknowledges that when he drinks beer the police tend to arrest him and bring him to the psychiatric hospital. He agrees to "take medicine to help [him] not drink so much." Owing to issues of noncompliance, his current medication is a long-acting injectable antipsychotic. He lives on his own and keeps his clinic appointments but has had difficulties adhering to oral medication regimens. The best medication to augment the treatment of his alcohol dependence would be:

A. Acamprosate.
B. Clozapine.
C. Disulfiram.
D. Naltrexone.
E. Ondansetron.

The correct response is option D: Naltrexone.

Both acamprosate and disulfiram are available only as oral medications and so are not ideal for a patient with medication adherence problems. Although there are some data suggesting that clozapine may be useful in treating symptoms of both schizophrenia and substance use disorders, it too is available as an oral medication only. Ondansetron has been insufficiently studied in this patient population to recommend its use here. Naltrexone is available as a long-acting injection (Vivitrol), so may be preferable in this situation.

Dermatis H, Galanter M. Clinical advances in pharmacological and integrated treatment approaches for alcohol and drug use disorders. FOCUS: Substance Abuse Spring 2007:2:142

American Psychiatric Association Practice Guideline for the Treatment of Patients with Substance Use Disorders, 2nd Edition, (2006). http://psychiatryonline.com/pracGuide/pracGuideHome. aspx.

---

121 Avoidant personality disorder is marked by social inhibition, sense of inadequacy, and hypersensitivity. Which of the following is a DSM criterion for this disorder?

A. Requiring excessive admiration.
B. Difficulty making everyday decisions.
C. Excessive devotion to work to the exclusion of friendships.
D. Preoccupation with being socially criticized.
E. Reluctance to delegate tasks or to work with others.

The correct response is option D: Preoccupation with being socially criticized.

A patient with avoidant personality disorder may manifest any or all of the other features listed, but only D is a criterion for this diagnosis. Difficulty expressing disagreement and making everyday decisions is diagnostic for dependent personality disorder. Excessive devotion to work and reluctance to delegate is diagnostic criteria for obsessive compulsive personality disorder and requiring excessive admiration is a criteria for narcissistic personality disorder.

American Psychiatric Association: Diagnostic and Statistical Manual of Mental Disorders, 5th Edition. Arlington, VA, American Psychiatric Association, 2013, pp 672–678

122 Which of the following statements gives the most appropriate guidance for patients and their families regarding driving by patients with neurocognitive disorders?

A. Families have no responsibility for getting involved in driving decisions of patients with mild cognitive impairment.
B. All patients with mild cognitive impairment should be reported to their state motor vehicle departments for mandatory tracking.
C. Clinicians should advise all patients with mild cognitive impairment to stop driving and to turn in their driver's licenses.
D. Mildly impaired patients should be advised to stop driving at night.
E. Patients and families should be informed that even mild neurocognitive disorders increase the risk of vehicular accidents.

The correct response is option E: Patients and families should be informed that even mild neurocognitive disorders increase the risk of vehicular accidents.

The guidance from the APA's Practice Guideline for the Treatment of Patients With Alzheimer's Disease and Other Dementias points out that even mild neurocognitive disorder is associated with increased vehicular accidents. Accordingly, mildly impaired patients should be advised to limit their driving to safe situations or to stop driving (there is no imperative and no mandatory reporting law for mildly impaired patients). Families should be informed and involved, because the implementation of the recommendations often falls to them.

American Psychiatric Association Practice Guideline for the Treatment of Patients with Alzheimer's Disease and Other Dementias, 2nd ed. 2007 p 11. http://psychiatryonline.org/guidelines.aspx

123 An 8-year-old boy presents with a 1-month history of stomachaches and headaches every morning just before going to school. When interviewed, he reports having persistent nightmares of being kidnapped and worries about his father having an accident. The most likely diagnosis is:

A. Normal childhood.
B. Agoraphobia.
C. Separation anxiety.
D. Generalized anxiety disorder.
E. Panic disorder.

The correct response is option C: Separation anxiety.

Separation anxiety disorder is excessive anxiety concerning separation from the home or from those to whom the person is attached. When separated from major attachment figures, these individuals are often preoccupied with fears that accident or illnesses will befall them or their attachment figures. It can be differentiated from generalized anxiety disorder by the fact that the anxiety is about separation and not generalized.

American Psychiatric Association: Diagnostic and Statistical Manual of Mental Disorders, 5th Edition. Arlington, VA, American Psychiatric Association, 2013, pp 190–191

Dulcan MK, Weiner JM. Essentials of Child and Adolescent Psychiatry. Arlington (VA): American Psychiatric Publishing, 2006. p 558

124 A 65-year-old man has metastatic head-and-neck cancer that leaves him with a ptosis, facial nerve palsy, and an inability to eat solid foods. He complains of feeling hopeless, that life has lost all meaning, and that he wants to die immediately. He does not meet criteria for major depression. The best descriptor for this triad of symptoms is:

A. Anticipatory grief.
B. Demoralization.
C. Mourning.
D. Denial.
E. Bargaining.

The correct response is option B: Demoralization.

Anticipatory grief precedes death and results from its expectation. Mourning is the process of adaptation to death. Kissane and colleagues described the triad of hopelessness, loss of meaning in life, and desire for death as the demoralization syndrome.

Breitbart W, Gibson C, Chochinov HM. Palliative care, in American Psychiatric Publishing Textbook of Psychosomatic Medicine, Edited by Levenson JA. Arlington, VA, 2005 pp 993–998

Kissane DW. The contribution of demoralization to end of life decision-making. Hastings Cent Rep. 2004 Jul-Aug; 34(4):21–31

Clarke DM, Kissane DW. Demoralization: its phenomenology and importance. Australian & New Zealand Journal of Psychiatry 2002–12; 36:6 733(10) pp 733–742

---

125 A 73-year-old woman was prescribed 10 mg/day of paroxetine for anxiety 1 week ago. She now presents to the physician's office with confusion. Laboratory workup reveals low serum sodium and low plasma osmolarity. Her urine sodium and osmolarity are high. The physician should consider a diagnosis of:

A. Hypothyroidism.
B. Syndrome of Inappropriate Antidiuretic Hormone (SIADH).
C. Hyperparathyroidism.
D. Renal failure.
E. Dehydration.

The correct response is option B: Syndrome of Inappropriate Antidiuretic Hormone (SIADH).

Hyponatremia and SIADH have been associated with SSRI use in elderly patients. The incidence of SIADH does not appear to be dose-dependent. Most cases of SIADH occur within the first 2 weeks of SSRI treatment, but they could occur at any time. Risk factors for elderly patients could include low body mass index and lower baseline sodium (138 mEq/L).

Jacobson SA, Pies RW and Katz IR. Clinical Manual of Geriatric Psychopharmacology. Arlington, VA, American Psychiatric Publishing, 2007. pp 191–192

---

126 A 37-year-old male software designer is brought to the psychiatrist's office by his brother, who reports that the patient has become increasingly suspicious over the last year. Last week, a shopping mall security guard observed him recording license plate numbers. The guard inquired, the patient explained that he was doing statistical research on license plates, and there was no further incident. He told his brother later that he thought he had noticed these cars parked in front of his home, and they might be part of scoping the neighborhood in advance of a crime. The brother is now concerned that it is only a matter of time for the patient to get into his first legal skirmish as a result of this kind of behavior. The patient reports that since his teens, he has needed to be very observant of others to protect himself. He says he has never been a victim of assault or theft only because of his constant vigilance. He experienced several days of auditory hallucinations when he was about 20 years old; "voices" were making deprecatory comments, but he cannot recall further details. These symptoms remitted entirely, and he reports no other psychotic symptoms.

He has worked at the same software company for 10 years, and although he has been promoted several times, most recently 3 months ago, he thinks he was slighted by his supervisor who gave a better position to a colleague. He is satisfied with his single status. Which ONE of the following disorders is the most likely diagnosis?

A. Paranoid personality disorder.
B. Delusional disorder.
C. Schizoid personality disorder.
D. Schizophrenia, paranoid type.
E. Schizotypal personality disorder.

The correct response is option A: Paranoid personality disorder.

The patient's suspiciousness and related behavior places paranoid personality disorder high on the differential diagnosis. The other Cluster A personality disorders are less likely but still on the differential diagnosis. His brief psychotic symptoms 20 years ago do not meet criteria for schizophrenia or delusional disorder, which are characterized by a period of persistent psychotic symptoms, and thus delusional disorder is ruled out.

American Psychiatric Association: Diagnostic and Statistical Manual of Mental Disorders, 5th Edition. Arlington, VA, American Psychiatric Association, 2013, p 652

---

127 A 6-year-old girl is referred by her teacher because of "acting out" behaviors at school, including inappropriate touching of peers and insistence on sitting on adults' laps. During the session, she tells the psychiatrist that her father touches her "secret place." The father explains that he bathes the girl at night and is simply making sure she is clean everywhere. Which of the following is the most appropriate action for the psychiatrist?

A. Advise the father not to give baths and see if the behavior resolves.
B. Tell the teacher to call child protective services.
C. Relay the findings to the teacher and tell her child protective services will not be necessary.
D. Try to gather more history to see if this constitutes sexual abuse.
E. Make a call to child protective services.

The correct response is option E: Make a call to child protective services.

The threshold for reporting is a *suspicion* of child abuse. The determination of abuse is not up to the individual doctor. Revealing findings to the teacher without consent from the parents is a confidentiality violation.

Wahl DS, Milone RD et al: Ethics Primer of the American Psychiatric Association, Washington, DC, American Psychiatric Publishing, 2001; 17–18

---

128 Patients with acute stress disorder have been shown in controlled trials to be least likely to subsequently develop posttraumatic stress disorder when treated with:

A. Cognitive-restructuring therapy.
B. Exposure therapy.
C. Systematic debriefing.
D. Couples therapy.
E. Internet-based CBT.

The correct response is option B: Exposure therapy.

A controlled trial of 90 civilian patients with acute stress disorder following trauma treated with six 90-minute weekly sessions of imaginal and in vivo exposure therapy, cognitive-restructuring therapy, or assignment to a wait list control showed that exposure therapy was clearly superior to cognitive restructuring, which was, in turn, superior to wait list control in preventing the subsequent appearance of PTSD. Whereas at 6 months, 77% of those in the wait list group developed PTSD, only 63% of those receiving cognitive restructuring and 33% of those receiving exposure therapy developed PTSD.

Bryant RA, Mastrodomenico J, Felmingham KL, Hopwood S, Kenny L, Kandris E, Cahill C, Creamer M. Treatment of acute stress disorder: a randomized controlled trial. Arch Gen Psychiatry. 2008; 65(6):659–667

---

129 According to the results of the Clinical Antipsychotic Trials of Intervention Effectiveness (CATIE) study, approximately what percentage of patients had continued on their initial antipsychotic medications by 18 months?

A. 10%.
B. 25%.
C. 50%.
D. 75%.
E. 90%.

The correct response is option B: 25%.

The most prominent finding of the CATIE study is the high all-cause discontinuation rate (74%) for all the antipsychotic medications. This implies that 74% of the patients discontinued the medication, before 18 months of being started on it. The causes for discontinuation included lack of tolerability, lack of efficacy, clinician decision (due to safety concerns), and patient decision (electing to terminate). Among the atypical antipsychotics, the time to discontinuation was significantly longer for patients treated with olanzapine when compared to patients on risperidone and quetiapine.

Lieberman JA, Stroup TS, McEvoy JP, Swartz MS, et al: Effectiveness of antipsychotic drugs in patients with chronic schizophrenia. N Engl J Med. 2005; 353(12):1209–23

Nasrallah HA. The roles of efficacy, safety, and tolerability in antipsychotic effectiveness: practical implications of the CATIE schizophrenia trial. J Clin Psychiatry. 2007; 68 Suppl 1:5–11

---

130 Temperament traits of Harm Avoidance, Novelty Seeking, Reward Dependence, and Persistence are defined as heritable differences underlying automatic responses to danger, novelty, social approval, and intermittent reward, respectively. Which of the following statements about the temperament traits in the general population is MOST accurate?

A. The phenotypic expression of these traits is primarily due to the experiences of the individual.
B. They are normally distributed quantitative traits.
C. They are modifiable based on the goodness of fit with the parent.
D. They are inconsistently manifested in different cultures.
E. They are similar to fluid intelligence in that they show demonstrable changes with aging.

The correct response is option B: They are normally distributed quantitative traits.

Each of the four major dimensions is normally distributed quantitative trait, moderately heritable, observable in early childhood, relatively stable in time, and moderately predictive of adolescent and adult behavior. The four dimensions have been repeatedly shown to be universal across different cultures, ethnic groups, and political systems.

Sadock BJ, Sadock VA (eds): Kaplan and Sadock's Comprehensive Textbook of Psychiatry, 9th ed. Philadelphia, Lippincott Williams & Wilkins, 2009, p 2199

Angres DH. The Temperament and Character Inventory in addiction treatment. Focus 2010 8: 192

---

131 A 37-year-old single man's sex life centers on donning women's lingerie before engaging in sexual activities with willing female partners. He considers himself heterosexual and has never had any interest in having sex with men. He is distressed about his sexual behavior and is now seeking treatment. Which of the following best describes his behavior?

A. Transvestic disorder.
B. Gender dysphoria.
C. Frotteurism.
D. Exhibitionism.

The correct response is option A: Transvestic disorder.

The behaviors are consistent with transvestic disorder. He is a heterosexual male who experiences intense sexual urges while cross-dressing. Furthermore, the behavior causes distress for him.

American Psychiatric Association: Diagnostic and Statistical Manual of Mental Disorders, 5th Edition. Arlington, VA, American Psychiatric Association, 2013, p 702–703

132 A 28-year-old woman presents to the clinic concerned about having ADHD. She has noticed that for the last 3 days she has been "hyper." She stays up until 4 A.M. to rehearse her presentations and awakens easily at 7 A.M. She also now works as late as 9 P.M., whereas she would usually stop at 6 P.M. She finds herself easily distracted and strays from her routine presentation. She experiences these symptoms about three times a year. Talking with her husband reveals that these periods are always followed by a deep depression during which she will rarely get out of bed, does not eat, and will not see clients for about 2 weeks. Her presentation is most consistent with:

A. Cyclothymia.
B. Bipolar I disorder.
C. Bipolar II disorder.
D. ADHD–inattentive type.
E. ADHD–hyperactive/impulsive type.

The correct response is option C: Bipolar II disorder.

The patient's hyperactivity and distractibility are confined to times in which she expresses the other manic symptoms, making ADHD unlikely. Her depressive phases are too severe to classify her as cyclothymic. The mania in bipolar I disorder is associated with *significant* social or occupational dysfunction or hospitalization. The patient in this scenario is impaired but not significantly so.

Sadock BJ, Sadock VA, Ruiz P (eds): Kaplan & Sadock's Comprehensive Textbook of Psychiatry, 9th ed. Philadelphia, Lippincott Williams & Wilkins, 2009, pp 1719–20

American Psychiatric Association Practice Guideline for the Treatment of Patients with Bipolar Disorder, 2nd Edition (2002). http://psychiatryonline.org/guidelines.aspx

133 A 19-year-old woman with anorexia presents with shortness of breath and symptoms consistent with heart failure. She admits to using large amounts of ipecac. Which of the following test results would be most consistent with ipecac-induced toxicity?

A. Decrease in the serum CK value.
B. Decrease in lactate dehydrogenase.
C. Shortening of the QTc interval.
D. Enlarged heart.
E. Bradycardia.

The correct response is option D: Enlarged heart.

Ipecac abuse is associated most predominantly with a myopathy that involves "Z-band streaming." This can result in increased CPK and lactate dehydrogenase and cardiac abnormalities including tachycardia, QTc prolongation, an enlarged heart on echocardiogram, and reduced ejection fraction. The cardiovascular changes usually reverse when the ipecac is stopped. Direct testing for ipecac alkaloids can be done in urine, serum, or tissue samples and are present for several weeks after use.

Silber TJ: Ipecac syrup abuse, morbidity, and mortality: isn't it time to repeal its over-the-counter status? J Adolescent Health 2005; 37(3):256–260

134 An assessment of a 25-year-old woman as a candidate for psychotherapy reveals that she is able to delay gratification in order to attain personal goals but remains egocentric and defensive. She is noted to have frequent distress when attachments and desires are frustrated. She functions well under good conditions but frequently experiences problems under stress. On the basis of the *stages in the development of self-awareness and well-being,* this woman is MOST likely at what stage?

A. Stage 0: unaware.
B. Stage 1: average adult cognition.
C. Stage 2: metacognition.
D. Stage 3: contemplation.

The correct response is option B: Stage 1: average adult cognition.

A full assessment of personality requires consideration of a person's level of self-awareness and well-being. There are four stages of self-awareness along the path to well-being. Stage 0 (unaware) is characterized by immaturity, seeking immediate gratification and a "child-like" ego state. Stage 1 (average adult cognition) includes individuals who are purposeful but egocentric; they are able to delay gratification but have frequent negative emotions such as anxiety, anger, and disgust. In Stage 2 (metacognition), individuals are mature and allocentric; they are aware of their own subconscious thinking; are calm and patient; and so are able to supervise conflicts and relationships. Stage 3 (contemplation) is the highest stage. These people are calm and wise; demonstrate impartial awareness; are creative and loving; are able to access what was previously unconscious as needed without effort or distress.

Sadock BJ, Sadock VA (eds): Kaplan and Sadock's Comprehensive Textbook of Psychiatry, 9th ed. Philadelphia, Lippincott Williams & Wilkins, 2009, pp 2233

---

135 Which of the following techniques or therapies has been shown, in a randomized controlled trial, to be most helpful in the treatment of acute stress disorder?

A. Cognitive restructuring.
B. Individual psychological debriefing.
C. Exposure-based therapy.
D. Eye movement desensitization and reprocessing (EMDR).
E. Group debriefing.

The correct response is option C: Exposure-based therapy.

The cognitive-behavioral therapy technique of exposure-based therapy has been found to be superior to cognitive restructuring. Debriefing, either individually or in group, has not been found to be effective. EMDR has not been tested for the treatment of acute stress disorder.

Gabbard, GO. Treatment of Psychiatric Disorders, 4th ed. Washington, DC, American Psychiatric Press, 2007, pp 519–522

American Psychiatric Association Practice Guideline for the Treatment of Patients with Acute Stress Disorder and Posttraumatic Stress Disorder. 2004; pp 61–62. http://psychiatryonline.org/guidelines.aspx

Bryant RA, Mastrodomenico J, Felmingham KL, Hopwood S, et al: Treatment of acute stress disorder: a randomized controlled trial. Arch Gen Psychiatry. 2008; 65(6):659–667

---

136 Which of the following medications should be the first-line treatment for generalized anxiety disorder?

A. Diazepam.
B. Lorazepam.
C. Buspirone.
D. Paroxetine.
E. Hydroxyzine.

The correct response is option D: Paroxetine.

Efficacy and the favorable side-effect profile make SSRIs (paroxetine) the current first-line choice. Long-acting benzodiazepines (diazepam) are also effective, but concern about dependence and cognitive problems make them a second-line choice. Short-acting benzodiazepines (lorazepam) pose even greater risk for dependence. Buspirone has a longer wait until active. Although it has a favorable side-effect profile, some consider it less effective than other drugs. Hydroxyzine, a histamine receptor antagonist, was found to be effective with no problem of dependence. Its major side effect is sedation. It does not appear to be very widely used.

Stein DJ, Hollander E, Rothbaum BO (eds): Textbook of Anxiety Disorders, 2nd ed. Arlington, VA, American Psychiatric Publishing, 2010, pp 193–213

Hales RE, Yudofsky SC, and Gabbard GO (eds). American Psychiatric Textbook of Psychiatry, 5th ed. Arlington, VA, American Psychiatric Publishing, 2008, pp 534–35

137 After performing a thorough history and physical, a psychiatrist suspects that the patient has bipolar I disorder, rapid cycling. Which of the following tests should be ordered to rule out an underlying medical etiology?

A. CSF 5-HIAA.
B. 24-hour urine.
C. Thyroid function tests.
D. Liver function tests.
E. Dexamethasone suppression test.

The correct response is option C: Thyroid function tests.

The initial intervention in patients who experience rapid cycling is to identify and treat medical conditions such as hypothyroidism. Autoimmune thyroid disease as manifested in positive TPO antibodies, with or without frank hypothyroidism, may contribute to rapid cycling. Low levels of 5-HIAA are associated with increased impulsivity. Twenty-four-hour urine collections are most associated with pheochromocytomas. Liver function tests (liver-associated enzymes) are often part of the monitoring requirements for mood stabilizers. Although a dexamethasone suppression test has had some studies linking it to bipolar disorder, it is rarely used.

Oomen HA, Schipperijn AJ, Drexhage HA. The prevalence of affective disorders and in particular rapid-cycling bipolar disorder in patients with abnormal thyroid function tests. Clin Endocrinol. 1996; 45:215–223
American Psychiatric Association Practice Guideline for the Treatment of Patients with Bipolar Disorder, 2nd Edition (2002). http://psychiatryonline.org/guidelines.aspx

138 The symptom domain most strongly correlated with functional impairment in schizophrenia is:

A. Positive symptoms.
B. Negative symptoms.
C. Cognitive impairment.
D. Mood disturbance.

The correct response is option C: Cognitive impairment.

Among the four symptom domains of schizophrenia—positive symptoms (hallucinations, delusions); negative symptoms (blunted affect, alogia, anhedonia, social isolation, lack of motivation); cognitive impairment; and mood disturbance—cognitive dysfunction has the highest correlation with functional impairment. Improvements in cognition are highly correlated with better quality of life.

Marder SR. Neurocognition as a treatment target in schizophrenia. FOCUS: Schizophrenia. Spring 2008; 6(2):180–183

139 A 37-year-old woman, in dynamic psychotherapy for borderline personality disorder, has been expressing an unrealistic overvaluation of the therapist. After many months of this expressed high regard, she suddenly becomes enraged after the therapist fails to return her call and now declares the therapist to be "the worst ever." Which of the following would be the most appropriate way to handle the patient's new reaction?

A. Avoid directly responding and instead encourage the patient to further express her emotions.
B. Apologize for the missed call and then suggest they move on with the current work.
C. Acknowledge the failing and then question how the patient's opinion could change so dramatically.
D. Propose that they clarify an appropriate call-back policy to avoid future mishaps.
E. Suggest to the patient that such inevitable mistakes are an important part of the therapy.

The correct response is option C: Acknowledge the failing and then question how the patient's opinion could change so dramatically.

One of the primary goals of dynamic psychotherapy is to increase a patient's insight into the workings of his or her own mind. Patients with borderline personality disorders have chaotic relationships with oscillations between idealization and devaluation. Although a therapist should honestly acknowledge mistakes, the patient's seeming overreaction to this mistake provides an opportunity to explore the patient's defensive style and help the patient see how these reactions likely affect other areas of the patient's life.

Cabaniss D. Personality disorders. FOCUS 2005; 3:383–384

---

140 Which of the following is the most accurate information to give families regarding the risk of using antipsychotics to treat agitation in elderly patients with moderate dementia of the Alzheimer's type?

A. There is an increased risk of mortality but only for the antipsychotics risperidone and olanzapine.
B. Increased mortality in the elderly has been associated with both atypical and conventional antipsychotics.
C. Although suggested by earlier studies, subsequent studies have not found a significant risk of mortality with atypical antipsychotics.
D. The risk is unknown, as inadequate data exist to make any conclusive statements.
E. Although newer antipsychotics may have a risk, typical antipsychotics appear to be safe.

The correct response is option B: Increased mortality in the elderly has been associated with both atypical and conventional antipsychotics.

Recently published studies suggest that both conventional and atypical antipsychotic medications are associated with increased risk of death in elderly patients, leading the FDA to require manufacturers to add a black box warning to this effect. In a prior FDA-conducted meta-analysis of 17 placebo-controlled studies concerning atypical antipsychotics over the course of the 10-week trials, 4.5% of those taking active medications died compared to 2.6% of those taking placebo.

Gill SS, Bronskill SE, Normand SL, Anderson GM, et al: Antipsychotic drug use and mortality in older adults with dementia. Ann Intern Med. 2007; 146(11):777–786
Schneeweiss S, Setoguchi S, Brookhart A, Dormuth C, Wang PS. Risk of death associated with the use of conventional versus atypical antipsychotic drugs among elderly patients. CMAJ. 2007; 176(5):627–632
Kuehn BM. FDA: Antipsychotics risky for elderly. JAMA. 2008; 300(4):379–380
Cheong JA: Ask the expert: Geriatric Psychiatry. FOCUS. 2009; 7:36–37

---

141 The use of stimulants to treat ADHD is relatively contraindicated if the child has which of the following comorbid conditions?

A. Tic disorder.
B. Preexisting cardiovascular disease.
C. Seizure disorder.
D. Anxiety disorder.
E. Bipolar disorder.

The correct response is option B: Preexisting cardiovascular disease.

The FDA indicates that stimulants should not be used when individuals have a number of comorbid conditions. However, studies and the literature indicate that none of the options except B (preexisting cardiovascular disease) appear to be significantly exacerbated by the use of stimulants. The American Heart Association has recommended that all children receiving stimulant medications receive an EKG prior to initiating treatment.

AACAP Practice parameter of the use of stimulant medications in the treatment of children, adolescents, and adults. J Am Acad Child Adolesc Psychiatry. 2007. Reprinted in FOCUS: Child and Adolescent Psychiatry. Fall 2004; 2(4):644–645

Practice parameter for the assessment and treatment of children and adolescents with ADHD. J Am Acad Child Adolesc Psychiatry. 2007; 46:911–912. Reprinted in FOCUS: Child and Adolescent Psychiatry. Summer 2008; (3) pp 401–426

Winterstein AG, Gerhard T, Shuster J, Johnson M, Zito JM, Saidi A. Cardiac safety of central nervous system stimulants in children and adolescents with attention-deficit/hyperactivity disorder. Pediatrics. Dec 2007; 120(6): e1494–501

Cardiovascular monitoring of children and adolescents with heart disease receiving stimulant drugs: a scientific statement from the American Heart Association Council on Cardiovascular Disease in the Young Congenital Cardiac Defects Committee and the Council on Cardiovascular Nursing. Circulation. 2008 May 6; 117(18) pp 2407–23

---

142 A patient describes a dinner party at which he felt increasing anxiety and a sense that people were avoiding him. He discussed this with his wife and she became irritated with him, noting that it would help if he could look people in the eye and not wear the same worn-out suit jacket to every party. He tried to explain that this was his lucky jacket and it protected them both from car accidents, but she just shook her head. On the basis of this, which of the following personality disorders is most likely?

A. Schizoid.
B. Schizotypal.
C. Antisocial.
D. Borderline.
E. Narcissistic.

The correct response is option B: Schizotypal.

Schizotypal personality disorder is a pervasive pattern of social and interpersonal deficits marked by acute discomfort with, and reduced capacity for, close relationships, as well as cognitive distortions of behavior. This may include odd social behaviors, loose, vague, or idiosyncratic speech, paranoia in social situations, and magical thinking.

American Psychiatric Association: Diagnostic and Statistical Manual of Mental Disorders, 5th Edition. Arlington, VA, American Psychiatric Association, 2013, p 655

---

143 What is the leading cause of disability in the world for persons 15–44 years of age?

A. Bipolar disorder.
B. Schizophrenia.
C. Self-inflicted injuries.
D. Unipolar major depression.
E. Alcohol use.

The correct response is option D: Unipolar major depression.

When ranked according to the percent total disability-adjusted life year, the global burden of disease is greatest for major depression. All of the other listed mental illnesses are also ranked in the top ten leading causes of disability.

Murray CJL, Lopez AD: The Global Burden Of Disease: A Comprehensive Assessment Of Mortality And Disability From Diseases, Injuries, and Risk Factors in 1990 and Projected to 2020. Cambridge, MA, Harvard University Press, 1996 (Table 5.4)

Hales RE, Yudofsky SC, Gabbard GO (eds): The American Psychiatric Textbook of Psychiatry, 5th ed. Arlington, VA, American Psychiatric Publishing, 2008. pp 472

---

144 A busy 33-year-old female executive decides that she will end 10 years of smoking. She tried once before but was unsuccessful. She travels several times a month and agrees to use a nicotine inhaler, along with brief telephone counseling appointments. When is she most likely to relapse?

A. On the quit date.
B. During the first few days of the quit date.
C. 1 week after the quit date.
D. 2 weeks after the quit date.

The correct response is option B: During the first few days of the quit date.

Most patients relapse within a couple of days of stopping smoking. It is therefore important for the psychiatrist or the psychiatrist's staff to contact the patient right after the quit date for support.

American Psychiatric Association Practice Guideline for the Treatment of Patients with Substance Use Disorders, 2nd Edition (2006), p 362–364. http://psychiatryonline.org/guidelines.aspx

145 Clinical efficacy of typical (first-generation) antipsychotic medications is highly correlated with binding to which of the following receptors?

A. Dopamine, D_1.
B. Dopamine, D_2.
C. Serotonin, 5-HT_{2a}.
D. Muscarinic, M_4.
E. Adrenoceptors, α_2.

The correct response is option B: Dopamine, D_2.

Clinical efficacy of typical antipsychotic medications is highly correlated with binding to dopaminergic D_2 receptors. The dose of a typical antipsychotic that is likely to be effective is the dose that occupies an appropriate number of D_2 receptors. For dopamine receptor antagonists, this implies approximately 60%–70% of receptors.

Kane JM, Stroup TS, Marder SR. Schizophrenia: Pharmacological Treatment, in Kaplan & Sadock's Comprehensive Textbook of Psychiatry, 9th ed. Edited by Sadock BJ, Sadock VA, Ruiz P. Philadelphia, Lippincott Williams & Wilkins, 2009, pp 1547–56

Miyamoto S, Duncan GE, Marx CE, Lieberman JA. Treatments for schizophrenia: a critical review of pharmacology and mechanisms of action of antipsychotic medications. Mol Psychiatry. 2005, Jan; 10(1):79–104

146 Which of the following is a single-locus (monogenic) disorder?

A. Alzheimer's disease.
B. Bipolar disorder.
C. Autism.
D. Huntington's disease.
E. Obsessive-compulsive disorder.

The correct response is option D: Huntington's disease.

Huntington's disease is a neurodegenerative genetic disorder caused by a single gene mutation (the Huntington gene) producing a trinucleotide repeat on chromosome 4. Its transmission follows simple Mendelian inheritance. The other options are polygenic disorders with more complex inheritance patterns.

Smoller JW, Sheidley BR, Tsuang MT. Psychiatric Genetics: Applications in Clinical Practice. American Psychiatric Publishing, 1st edition, 2008, p 48

Sadock BJ, Sadock VA (eds): Kaplan & Sadock's Comprehensive Textbook of Psychiatry, 9th ed. Philadelphia, Lippincott Williams & Wilkins, 2009, pp 299–333

147 The absence of which of the following features differentiates social communication disorder from autism spectrum disorder in DSM-5?

A. Deficits of nonverbal communicative behaviors.
B. Deficits in developing relationships appropriate to the developmental level.
C. Deficits in social-emotional reciprocity.
D. Symptoms present in the early developmental period.
E. Restrictive and repetitive behavior, interests, or activities.

The correct response is option E: Restrictive and repetitive behavior, interests, or activities.

Autism spectrum disorder (ASD) is a new DSM-5 name that reflects a scientific consensus that four previously separate disorders are actually a single condition with different levels of symptom severity in two core domains. ASD now encompasses the previous DSM-IV autistic disorder (autism), Asperger's disorder, childhood disintegrative disorder, and pervasive developmental disorder not otherwise specified. ASD is characterized by 1) deficits in social communication and social interaction and 2) restricted repetitive behaviors, interests, or activities (RRBs). Because both components are required for diagnosis of ASD, social communication disorder is diagnosed if no RRBs are present.

American Psychiatric Association: Diagnostic and Statistical Manual of Mental Disorders, 5th Edition. Arlington, VA, American Psychiatric Association, 2013; Highlights of changes from DSM-IV to DSM-5, p 809

148 Medications from which one of the following classes have the greatest potential for worsening symptoms of borderline personality disorder?

A. Selective serotonin reuptake inhibitors.
B. Monoamine oxidase inhibitors.
C. Anticonvulsants.
D. Atypical antipsychotics.
E. Benzodiazepines.

The correct response is option E: Benzodiazepines.

Patients with borderline personality disorder may exhibit disinhibition with benzodiazepines. All of the other classes of drugs listed may be helpful in treating specific symptoms of this disorder.

Sadock BJ, Sadock VA: Kaplan and Sadock's Synopsis of Psychiatry, 10th ed. Philadelphia, Lippincott Williams & Wilkins, 2007, p 801

149 In order to be given the diagnosis of mild neurocognitive disorder (NCD), a patient must have:

A. A memory impairment.
B. A cognitive decline in at least one domain.
C. Cognitive complaints in multiple domains.
D. Compromised general cognitive function.
E. Cognitive and memory complaints meeting criteria for mild dementia.

The correct response is option B: A cognitive decline in at least one domain.

Core to the diagnosis of mild NCD is a cognitive decline in at least one domain of the cognitive domains of memory, attention, language, executive function, perceptual motor, or social cognition. The distinction between major and mild NCD exists along a continuum. Typically, the associated features will be specific to the etiological subtype.

Palmer K, Bäckman L, Winblad B, Fratiglioni L. Mild cognitive impairment in the general population: occurrence and progression to Alzheimer disease. Am J Geriatr Psychiatry. 2008; 16(7):603–611

Chertkow H, Massoud F, Nasreddine Z, Belleville S, et al: Diagnosis and treatment of dementia:3. Mild cognitive impairment and cognitive impairment without dementia. CMAJ. 2008 May 6; 178(10):1273–85

American Psychiatric Association: Diagnostic and Statistical Manual of Mental Disorders, 5th Edition. Arlington, VA, American Psychiatric Association, 2013, pp 605–611

150 A 42-year-old patient requests treatment for anxiety and interpersonal difficulties. The patient reports feelings of social inadequacy and sensitivity to rejection for the past 20 years. The patient does not attend social events or interact with others as a result of this anxiety, worries excessively about being criticized by others, and feels inferior to others. This has caused occupational problems since the patient is only able to function in jobs that have virtually no social interaction. The patient is unhappy that he has no friends and has never been romantically involved. Which of the following is the most likely diagnosis?

A. Schizoid personality disorder.
B. Generalized anxiety disorder.
C. Avoidant personality disorder.
D. Social anxiety disorder.
E. Obsessive-compulsive disorder.

The correct response is option C: Avoidant personality disorder.

This patient meets the DSM-5 criteria for avoidant personality disorder. The differential diagnosis would include social anxiety disorder. There is a great deal of overlap between these disorders. However, avoidant personality disorder generally involves avoidance of situations and relationships with the potential for rejection or disappointment, whereas social anxiety disorder is characterized by specific fears related to social performance. The differential diagnosis also includes schizoid personality disorder. However, this patient is concerned about not having friends and romantic experiences, and a patient with schizoid personality disorder is likely not to desire these kinds of relationships.

Hales RE, Yudofsky SC, Gabbard GO (eds): The American Psychiatric Publishing Textbook of Psychiatry, 5th ed. American Psychiatric Publishing, Washington, DC. 2008. pp 846–847

American Psychiatric Association: Diagnostic and Statistical Manual of Mental Disorders, 5th Edition. Arlington, VA, American Psychiatric Association, 2013, pp 672–675

151 The parents of a 10-year-old boy who has had both motor and vocal tics for over a year are wondering whether he will remain symptomatic as an adult. Which of the following statements MOST accurately describes the probable outcome of children with these symptoms?

A. By age 18, 50% of children are not symptomatic.
B. Symptoms continue to increase in adolescence and adulthood.
C. The motor tics resolve but the vocal tics persist.
D. The tics decrease in adolescence but then increase again in adulthood.

The correct response is option A: By age 18, 50% of children are not symptomatic.

Tourette's disorder includes the presence of both vocal tics and multiple motor tics. Transient tic disorder also has both motor and verbal tics, but if the symptoms last more than one 1 year, the diagnosis is converted to Tourette's disorder. Therefore, this child meets the DSM-5 criteria for the definition of Tourette's disorder. Although Tourette's disorder is described as a lifelong disease, prevalence is 10 times higher among children than adults, and longitudinal studies show that symptoms decrease or fully remit in 50% of affected individuals by age 18 years, demonstrating a more benign and less chronic outcome for many individuals.

Swain JE, Scahill L, Lombroso PL, King RA, Leckman JL. Tourette syndrome and tic disorders: a decade of progress. J Am Acad Child Adolesc Psychiatry. 2007; 46:948

Bloch MH, Peterson BS, Scahill L, Otka J, et al: Adulthood outcome of tic and obsessive-compulsive symptom severity in children with Tourette syndrome. Arch Pediatr Adolesc Med. 2006 Jan; 160(1):65–9

Leckman JF, Zhang H, Vitale A, Lahnin F, et al: Course of tic severity in tourette syndrome:the first two decades. Pediatrics. 1998 July; 102(1):14–19

152 Increased risk of developing diabetes mellitus and dyslipidemia have most commonly been linked to:

A. Perphenazine.
B. Quetiapine.
C. Risperidone.
D. Ziprasidone.
E. Olanzapine.

The correct response is option E: Olanzapine.

Olanzapine and clozapine are associated with increased risks of developing diabetes mellitus and dyslipidemia. A recent comparative antipsychotic trial in schizophrenia suggested significantly greater weight gain for olanzapine than for the other antipsychotics—perphenazine, quetiapine, risperidone, and ziprasidone. Clozapine and olanzapine are associated with the most weight gain, risperidone and quetiapine with moderate weight gain, and ziprasidone and aripiprazole with minimal weight change.

Newcomer JW: Second-generation (atypical) antipsychotics and metabolic effects: a comprehensive literature review. CNS Drugs 2005; 19(suppl 1):1–93

Lieberman JA, Stroup TS, McEvoy JP, Swartz MS, et al: Effectiveness of antipsychotic drugs in patients with chronic schizophrenia. N Engl J Med 2005; 353:1209–1223

Hirschfeld RMA: "Guideline Watch: Practice Guideline for the Treatment of Patients with Bipolar Disorder, 2nd Edition" APA Practice Guidelines November 2005. Reprinted in FOCUS: Bipolar Disorder Winter 2007; 1:36

153 Patients in a study were asked to exert behavioral inhibition when confronted with negative stimuli. fMRI investigations demonstrated decreased activation of the subgenual anterior cingulate cortex and the posterior medial orbitofrontal cortex and increased activity in the left and right extended amygdala and ventral striatum relative to controls. These fMRI findings were associated with which of the following diagnoses?

A. Narcissistic personality disorder.
B. Attention-deficit/hyperactivity disorder.
C. Paranoid personality disorder.
D. Borderline personality disorder.
E. Schizophrenia.

The correct response is option D: Borderline personality disorder.

Previous neuropsychological studies have suggested that impulsivity and negative affectivity may be related to orbitofrontal dysfunction. The study was organized to examine the hypothesis that patients with borderline personality disorder who are experiencing negative emotional states would show deficient inhibitory function of the prefrontal cortex. When confronted with negative stimuli and asked to exert behavioral inhibition, relative to control subjects, patients with borderline personality disorder showed decreased activation of the subgenual anterior cingulate cortex and the posterior medial orbitofrontal cortex and increased activity in the left and right extended amygdala and ventral striatum.

Silbersweig D, Clarkin JF, Goldstein M, Kernberg OF, et al: Failure of frontolimbic inhibitory function in the context of negative emotion in borderline personality disorder. Am J Psychiatry, December 2007; 164:1832–1841

---

154 Binge-eating disorder is characterized by:

A. Feelings of being unable to control one's intake of food.
B. Consumption of a large amount of food over a 24-hour period.
C. Purging after eating a large amount of food.
D. Increasing amounts of exercise.
E. Progressive weight loss.

The correct response is option A: Feelings of being unable to control one's intake of food.

Binge-eating disorder occurs in patients without compensatory behaviors such as purging, fasting, or excessive exercise. These patients consume a large quantity of food in a discrete period of time (e.g., within any 2-hour period) while feeling unable to control their intake. Binge-eating is associated with significant psychiatric comorbidity, including mood, anxiety, and substance use disorders.

American Psychiatric Association: Diagnostic and Statistical Manual of Mental Disorders, 5th Edition. Arlington, VA, American Psychiatric Association, 2013, pp 350–353

---

155 A patient who has been diagnosed with PTSD reports nightmares and sleep disruption. Which one of the following medications has been shown to be effective for the treatment of trauma-related nightmares and sleep disruption in patients with PTSD?

A. Topiramate.
B. Sertraline.
C. Prazosin.
D. Gabapentin.
E. Propranolol.

The correct response is option C: Prazosin.

According to the March 2009 PTSD Guideline Watch of the APA, prazosin is the pharmacotherapy for sleep problems related to PTSD that is supported by the greatest number of peer-reviewed studies. SSRIs are not effective in treating PTSD-related nightmares. Anticonvulsants have not been shown to be efficacious for PTSD symptoms. Although propranolol has some efficacy in reducing symptoms of posttraumatic physiologic arousal, recent studies failed to demonstrate a significant separation from placebo for PTSD symptoms in general.

Benedek DM, Friedman MJ, Zatzick D, Ursano RJ: Guideline Watch (March 2009): Practice Guideline for the Treatment of Patients With Acute Stress Disorder and Posttraumatic Stress Disorder; Focus 2009; 7:204–213. http://psychiatryonline.org/guidelines.aspx

---

156 A 3-day-postpartum mother with no prior psychiatric diagnosis is concerned about feeling depressed. She endorses a decrease in energy, difficulty sleeping despite being tired, decreased appetite, and frequent mood swings saying, "One minute I'm fine, the next minute I'm crying." Which of the following is the most appropriate treatment?

A. Psychoeducation.
B. Cognitive-behavioral therapy.
C. Pharmacotherapy.
D. Hospitalization.
E. Psychodynamic psychotherapy.

The correct response is option A: Psychoeducation.

The mother is most likely experiencing postpartum blues or baby blues. The symptoms of postpartum blues mimic depression and usually peak by day 5 and resolve by day 10 postpartum. By definition, postpartum blues is transient. In addition to psychoeducation and validation of her experience, she should also be monitored for signs and symptoms of a progression into a full postpartum depression or anxiety disorder.

Sadock BJ, Sadock VA, Ruiz P (eds): Kaplan & Sadock's Comprehensive Textbook of Psychiatry, 9th ed. Philadelphia, Lippincott Williams & Wilkins, 2009, p 2553

Payne JL. Antidepressant use in the postpartum period: practical considerations Am J Psychiatry. 2007 Sep; 164(9):1329–32

---

157 A 44-year-old woman presents with a general history of alcohol abuse and significant depressive and anxiety symptoms over 20 years. It is unclear whether the substance use was in response to the affective symptoms or if the affective symptoms were substance-induced. Which of the following procedures would help make this determination?

A. Administer the MacAndrew Alcoholism Scale–Revised (MAC-R).
B. Conduct a detailed mental status exam, focusing on form of thought.
C. Draw a timeline of all substances used and all psychiatric symptoms.
D. Measure the percent carbohydrate-deficient transferrin.
E. Obtain serial urine toxicology tests.

The correct response is option C: Draw a timeline of all substances used and all psychiatric symptoms.

Plotting a life timeline of both substance use and psychiatric symptoms can help delineate the respective courses of substance-related and psychiatric symptomatology and any relationships between the two. The MacAndrew scale may help distinguish patients with substance use problems from those without, but it is less reliable among psychiatric populations. The other options would provide information about more recent use or psychiatric status and so are unlikely to provide the desired historical clarification.

Practice Guideline for the Treatment of Patients with Substance Use Disorders, 2nd Edition. Arlington, VA, American Psychiatric Association, 2006, Section II.B., General Treatment Principles, Assessment. http://psychiatryonline.org/guidelines.aspx

---

158 A depressed 62-year-old man being treated with an SSRI is admitted to the hospital with motoric immobility, posturing, grimacing, echolalia, and echopraxia. Intravenous administration of lorazepam and amobarbital leads to no relief. Which of the following treatments should be considered?

A. Add a second antidepressant.
B. Begin a mood stabilizer.
C. Initiate electroconvulsive therapy.
D. Add dantrolene.
E. Administer intravenous haloperidol.

The correct response is option C: Initiate electroconvulsive therapy.

Catatonic features may occur in the context of mood disorders and are characterized by at least two of the following manifestations: motoric immobility, as evidence by catalepsy or stupor; extreme agitation; extreme negativism; peculiarities of voluntary movement, as evidenced by posturing, stereotyped movements, mannerisms, or grimacing; and echolalia or echopraxia. When catatonia dominates the presentation, urgent biological treatment is indicated. Immediate relief may be obtained by intravenous benzodiazepines. Concurrent antidepressant mediation treatment should be considered. However, when relief is not immediately obtained, the urgent provision of electroconvulsive therapy is indicated.

American Psychiatric Association Practice Guideline for the Treatment of Patients With Major Depressive Disorder, 3rd ed (2010). http://psychiatryonline.org/guidelines.aspx

---

159 Which of the following antidepressants is the best choice for a patient who wants to avoid orgasm dysfunction as a side effect?

A. Bupropion.
B. Sertraline.
C. Venlafaxine.
D. Escitalopram.
E. Fluoxetine.

The correct response is option A: Bupropion.

In double-blind studies that specifically assessed sexual function, bupropion has been shown to have a more favorable sexual side-effect profile than any of the other options.

Clayton AH, Croft HA, Horrigan JP, Wightman DS, et al: Bupropion extended release compared with escitalopram: effects on sexual functioning and antidepressant efficacy in 2 randomized, double-blind, placebo-controlled studies. J Clin Psychiatry. 2006; 67:736–746

Modell JG, Katholi CR, Modell JD, DePalma RL. Comparative sexual side effects of bupropion, fluoxetine, paroxetine, and sertraline. Clin Pharmacol Ther. 1997; 61:476–487

Thase ME, Clayton AH, Haight BR, Thompson AH, et al: A double-blind comparison between bupropion XL and venlafaxine XR. J Clin Psychopharmacol. 2006; 26:482–488

---

160 A 20-year-old female college student presents to the counseling center with concerns about her alcohol use. She describes two occasions in the past year when she attended parties and had "way too much to drink." Following these occasions she feels "lousy," postpones studying, and then must stay up late to study for tests. When she's gone to most other parties, she's had four or five drinks with no ill effects. There are no other substance-related symptoms. She expresses some concern about her drinking and asks for recommendations. The best intervention at this point would be to:

A. Provide a brief intervention.
B. Prescribe disulfiram.
C. Recommend attending Alcoholics Anonymous.
D. Prescribe naltrexone.
E. Prescribe acamprosate.

The correct response is option A: Provide a brief intervention.

Brief intervention is the term used to describe a therapy delivered over one to three sessions, sometimes with telephone follow-up, that provides assessment of substance use, advice on reducing or stopping use and motivational feedback. Its efficacy has been demonstrated in a variety of treatment settings, including the primary care physician's office.

Prescribing medication or recommending attending Alcoholics Anonymous would be more appropriate for someone with a diagnosis of alcohol dependence rather than misuse. The patient is a heavy drinker and is at risk for developing a substance use disorder as well as other complications related to heavy alcohol use, so intervention is indicated.

American Psychiatric Association Practice Guideline for the Treatment of Patients with Substance Use Disorders, 2nd Edition (2006). http://psychiatryonline.org/guidelines.aspx

161 Which of the following medications has the greatest body of evidence supporting its use as a monotherapy for acute bipolar depression?

A. Bupropion.
B. Lamotrigine.
C. Valproate.
D. Olanzapine.
E. Quetiapine.

The correct response is option E: Quetiapine.

Quetiapine is FDA-approved as monotherapy for acute bipolar depression (both bipolar I and II). Olanzapine's effectiveness has been established only when combined with fluoxetine. None of the conventional antidepressants have been approved for this indication, and their usefulness remains a matter of debate. Although lamotrigine is often rated high for this indication, most placebo-controlled studies have been negative. There have been no studies of adequate size to establish the value of valproate.

Thase ME, Macfadden W, Weisler RH, Chang W, et al: Efficacy of quetiapine monotherapy in bipolar I and II depression: a double-blind, placebo-controlled study (The Bolder II Study). J Clin Psychopharmacol 2006; 26:600–609
Fountoulakis KN, Grunze H, Panagiotidis P, Kaprinis G: Treatment of bipolar depression: an update. J Affect Disord 2008; 109:21–34
Calabrese JR, Huffman RF, White RL, Edwards S, et al: Lamotrigine in the acute treatment of bipolar depression: results of five double-blind, placebo-controlled clinical trials. Bipolar Disord 2008; 10: 323–333

162 A patient reports feeling that he has always had to please others and that if he is not liked by everyone, he will never be successful. Which of the following statements would be characteristic of a cognitive-behavioral approach to the patient's problem?

A. "Let's draw out your circle of friends and examine which ones you feel you must please."
B. "Feeling you must please others is acting more out of an emotional mind than a rational mind."
C. "Tell me about your experience that you can only be successful by pleasing others."
D. "Is it possible that feeling you're not being liked by everyone is a way to ease the pressure of having to be successful?"

The correct response is option C: "Tell me about your experience that you can only be successful by pleasing others."

Option C attempts to elucidate maladaptive cognitions. Option A demonstrates one of the first techniques in interpersonal therapy. Emotional and rational mind are concepts of dialectical behavioral therapy. Option D starts to examine defense mechanisms, which is part of psychodynamic psychotherapy.

Hales RE, Yudofsky SC, Gabbard GO (eds): The American Psychiatric Publishing Textbook of Psychiatry, 5th ed, Arlington,VA, American Psychiatric Publishing, 2008, pp 1176–1177, 1194, 1227

163 A 32-year-old woman presents with a history of frequent, unanticipated panic attacks. Which of the following medications is most likely to be of benefit for treating her disorder?

A. Bupropion.
B. Aripiprazole.
C. Gabapentin.
D. Clonazepam.
E. Buspirone.

The correct response is option D: Clonazepam.

According to the APA Practice Guideline for the Treatment of Patients With Panic Disorder, "SSRIs, SNRIs, TCAs, and benzodiazepines appear roughly comparable in their efficacy...." Bupropion, gabapentin, and buspirone have not been found to be effective, and aripiprazole has not been studied adequately.

American Psychiatric Association Practice Guideline for the Treatment of Patients with Panic Disorder, 2nd ed., 2009, p 11. http://psychiatryonline.org/guidelines.aspx

---

164 Which of the following is the best established psychosocial intervention for the treatment of panic disorder?

A. Dialectical behavioral therapy.
B. Interpersonal psychotherapy.
C. Psychodynamic psychotherapy.
D. Marital and family therapy.
E. Cognitive-behavioral therapy.

The correct response is option E: Cognitive-behavioral therapy.

Cognitive-behavioral therapy is the most widely studied and best validated psychosocial treatment for panic disorder. According to Roy-Byrne et al., "two large meta-analyses reported large effect sizes of 1.55 (response of 63%) and 0.90." Unfortunately, as they point out, "Although the nature of the evidence is robust, such approaches are underused in the USA, compared with drug treatment." There are limited data suggesting that psychodynamic psychotherapy may be useful and less data supporting the use of family and marital therapy. Although exercise and psychoeducation may be of value for patients, there are slight data investigating the efficacy of either of these as a monotherapy.

Mitte K. A meta-analysis of the efficacy of psychoand pharmacotherapy in panic disorder with and without agoraphobia. J Affect Disord 2005; 88:22–45
Roy-Byrne PP, Craske MG, Stein MG. Panic disorder. Lancet 2006; 368:1023–1032
American Psychiatric Association Practice Guideline for the Treatment of Patients With Panic Disorder, 2nd ed (2009). http://psychiatryonline.org/guidelines.aspx
Perrin M, Vandeleur CL, Castelao E, Rothen S, et al.: Determinants of the development of post-traumatic stress disorder, in the general population. Soc Psychiatry Psychiatr Epidemiol. 2013 Sep 11

---

165 A patient with a history of substance dependence and depression treated with tranylcypromine presents to the emergency room with hypertension, tachycardia, chest pain, and severe occipital headache. The patient says he had a relapse of his drug use. Which of the following substances is the most likely contributor to his clinical presentation at this time?

A. Vodka.
B. Methamphetamine.
C. PCP.
D. Marijuana.
E. Inhalants.

The correct response is option B: Methamphetamine.

While aged foods are commonly known to potentially cause hypertensive crisis with MAOIs, there are also several drugs that will also do this. These include ephedrine, pseudoephedrine, amphetamine, cocaine, guanethidine, methyldopa, reserpine, meperidine, and dextromethorphan.

Rapaport MH: Dietary restrictions and drug interactions with monoamine oxidase inhibitors: the state of the art. Journal of Clinical Psychiatry 2007; 68 Suppl 8:42–6

---

166 Trazodone exerts its hypnotic effects by interaction with which of the following neurotransmitter receptors?

A. Dopamine.
B. GABA.
C. Histamine.
D. α_2.
E. Acetylcholine.

The correct response is option C: Histamine.

The sedation caused by trazodone is thought to be due to histamine$_1$ and α_1 receptors antagonism. Muscarinic cholinergic blockade can also lead to drowsiness, but trazodone does not have significant direct cholinergic effects. Dopamine interaction is not associated with sedation.

Stahl SM: Stahl's Essential Psychopharmacology, 3rd ed. New York, Cambridge University Press, 2008, pp 338–341, 845

---

167 Based on the results of Phase 1 of the Clinical Antipsychotic Trials of Intervention Effectiveness (CATIE) study, which of the following antipsychotic medications is most likely to be associated with the development of metabolic complications?

A. Olanzapine.
B. Quetiapine.
C. Risperidone.
D. Ziprasidone.
E. Perphenazine.

The correct answer is option A: Olanzapine.

During the CATIE study, olanzapine was associated with greater weight gain and increases in measures of glucose and lipid metabolism. Patients in the olanzapine group gained more weight than patients in any other group, with an average weight gain of 2 lb (0.9 kg) per month. Furthermore, 30% of patients in the olanzapine group gained 7% or more of their baseline body weight. Olanzapine use also was associated with greater increases in glycosylated hemoglobin, total cholesterol, and triglycerides even after adjustment for the duration of treatment in the study.

Buckley PF, Foster A, Miller B. Schizophrenia host vulnerability and risk of metabolic disturbance during treatment with antipsychotics. FOCUS: Schizophrenia. Spring 2008; 6(2):172–179
Lieberman JA, Stroup TS, McEvoy JP, Swartz MS, et al: Clinical Antipsychotic Trials of Intervention Effectiveness (CATIE) Investigators. Effectiveness of antipsychotic drugs in patients with chronic schizophrenia. N Engl J Med. 2005; 353(12):1209–23
Nasrallah HA. The roles of efficacy, safety, and tolerability in antipsychotic effectiveness: practical implications of the CATIE schizophrenia trial. J Clin Psychiatry. 2007; 68 Suppl 1:5–11

---

168 Which of the following SSRIs is designated as FDA pregnancy category D?

A. Fluoxetine.
B. Paroxetine.
C. Sertraline.
D. Citalopram.
E. Escitalopram.

The correct response is option B: Paroxetine.

All SSRIs are pregnancy category C with the exception of paroxetine, which has been associated with increased risk of fetal cardiovascular malformations, primarily ventricular septal defects and atrial septal defects, when given during the first trimester.

Current Categories for Drug Use in Pregnancy

Category	Description
A	Adequate, well-controlled studies in pregnant women have not shown an increased risk of fetal abnormalities.
B	Animal studies have revealed no evidence of harm to the fetus; however, there are no adequate and well-controlled studies in pregnant women. or Animal studies have shown an adverse effect, but adequate and well-controlled studies in pregnant women have failed to demonstrate a risk to the fetus.
C	Animal studies have shown an adverse effect, and there are no adequate and well-controlled studies in pregnant women. or No animal studies have been conducted, and there are no adequate and well-controlled studies in pregnant women.
D	Studies, adequate, well-controlled, or observational, in pregnant women have demonstrated a risk to the fetus. However, the benefits of therapy may outweigh the potential risk.
X	Studies, adequate, well-controlled, or observational, in animals or pregnant women have demonstrated positive evidence of fetal abnormalities. The use of the product is contraindicated in women who are or may become pregnant.

U.S. Food and Drug Administration (FDA). FDA Advising of Risk of Birth Defects with Paxil. http://www.fda.gov/bbs/topics/NEWS/2005/NEW01270.html

U.S. Food and Drug Administration (FDA), Pregnancy and Lactation Labeling http://www.fda.gov/cder/regulatory/pregnancy_labeling/ default.htm

169 According to the National Comorbidity Survey (NCS), which of the following experiences is most frequently associated with PTSD in women in the United States?

A. Being in a life-threatening accident.
B. Combat exposure.
C. Being involved in a natural disaster.
D. Sexual assault.
E. Witnessing someone being badly injured or killed.

The correct response is option D: Sexual assault.

In the NCS, which was carried out in the early 1990s, the most common stressor precipitants for women were sexual assault with physical attack, being threatened with a weapon, and childhood physical abuse, respectively. Combat exposure was the most common stressor for men. A recent review points out that PTSD lifetime prevalence in the NCS was twice as high in women as men and that combat exposure accounts for a significant proportion of PTSD in U.S. men. It also emphasizes that the main PTSD burden in the United States stems not from war but from criminal victimization, motor vehicle accidents, intimate partner violence, and childhood maltreatment. Women are more likely to have experienced sexual abuse, and men are more likely to have encountered physical violence, whether in the United States or while at war. Surveys have been conducted more recently and support the findings of the NCS that women exposed to sexual abuse and assaultive violence are at the highest risk for developing PTSD.

Hales RE, Yudofsky SC, Gabbard GO (eds): The American Psychiatric Publishing Textbook of Psychiatry, 5th ed. Washington, DC, American Psychiatric Publishing, 2008. pp 565–567

Kessler RC, Sonnega A, Bromet E, Hughes M, Nelson CB: Posttraumatic stress disorder in the National Comorbidity Survey. Arch Gen Psychiatry 1995; 52:1048–1060

Nemeroff CB, Bremner JD, Foa EB, Mayberg HS, North CS, Stein MB. Posttraumatic stress disorder: a state-of-the-science review. J Psychiatr Res. 2006; 40(1):1–21. Reprinted in FOCUS 2009; 7(2):254–273

Breslau N. The epidemiology of trauma, PTSD, and other posttrauma disorders. Trauma Violence Abuse. 2009 Jul 10(3):198–210

170 The core techniques of open-ended questions, affirmation, reflective statements, and summary statements (OARS) are central to which one of the following therapies?

A. Cognitive-behavioral.
B. Interpersonal.
C. Motivational interviewing.
D. Twelve-step facilitation.
E. Prolonged exposure.

The correct response is option C: Motivational interviewing.

Although some of these techniques may be used in a variety of psychotherapeutic modalities, together they represent the four core techniques, or "microskills," of motivational interviewing.

Galanter M, Kleber HD (eds): The American Psychiatric Publishing Textbook of Substance Abuse Treatment, 3rd ed. Washington DC, American Psychiatric Publishing, 2004, pp 371–2

171 Which of the following is the most common sleep problem in persons with major depressive disorder?

A. Vivid mood congruent dreams.
B. Hypersomnia.
C. Restless leg syndrome.
D. Insomnia.
E. Sleep phase disorder.

The correct response is option D: Insomnia.

The most common type of sleep disorder associated with depression is insomnia of some type—usually middle or late insomnia. Eighty percent of patients complain of insomnia, whereas roughly 10% of depressed patients describe hypersomnia. Less frequently, individuals will have initial insomnia, hypersomnia in the form of prolonged sleep episodes, or increased daytime sleepiness. Sleep studies in major depression have shown prolonged sleep latency, shortened total sleep, and increased arousals during the night. Slow-wave sleep is usually reduced. Restless leg syndrome is usually associated with increased age and may be related to metabolic, vascular, and neurological causes.

American Psychiatric Association: Diagnostic and Statistical Manual of Mental Disorders, 5th Edition. Arlington, VA, American Psychiatric Association, 2013, p 368

Sadock BJ, Sadock VA, Ruiz P (eds): Kaplan & Sadock's Comprehensive Textbook of Psychiatry, 9th ed. Philadelphia, Lippincott Williams & Wilkins, 2009, pp 2152–53, 4047

172 Which of the following psychotherapeutic techniques has the greatest body of evidence supporting it as a first-line treatment for PTSD?

A. Hypnosis.
B. Eye movement desensitization and reprocessing (EMDR).
C. Prolonged exposure therapy.
D. Stress inoculation training.
E. Systematic desensitization.

The correct response is option C: Prolonged exposure therapy.

Prolonged exposure therapy involves repeated exposure to the same traumatic memory over a series of sessions and is considered a first-line treatment for PTSD. EMDR remains controversial but has been shown in some studies to have benefits. Hypnosis has been used to induce relaxation to help with autonomic arousal symptoms. Stress inoculation training involves the combination of relaxation, elements of distraction, thought stopping, and self-guided dialogue. Systematic desensitization is effective for a phobic anxiety associated with PTSD. Cognitive processing/restructuring has been shown to have comparative effectiveness to prolonged exposure.

Hales RE, Yudofsky SC, Gabbard GO (eds): The American Psychiatric Textbook of Psychiatry, 5th ed. Washington, DC, American Psychiatric Publishing, 2008. pp 579–580

Nemeroff CB, Bremner JD, Foa EB, Mayberg HS, North CS, Stein MB. Posttraumatic stress disorder: a state-of-the-science review. J Psychiatr Res. 2006; 40(1):1–21. Reprinted in FOCUS 2009; 2:254–273

Foa EB. Psychosocial therapy for posttraumatic stress disorder. J Clin Psychiatry 2006; 67 Suppl 2:40–45

173 Which of the following is most characteristic of symptoms of PTSD?

A. Persist long after the precipitating event is over.
B. Exist only while the trauma is present.
C. Directly proportional to the magnitude of the trauma.
D. Occur only in response to certain types of trauma.
E. Develop immediately upon experiencing the trauma.

The correct response is option A: Persist long after the precipitating event is over.

Although duration of the symptoms varies, recovery within 3 months occurs in approximately half of adults, whereas some individuals remain symptomatic for many years. PTSD can develop in anyone exposed to a traumatic event and is not limited to veterans or certain types of trauma. Symptoms usually begin within 3 months.

American Psychiatric Association: Diagnostic and Statistical Manual of Mental Disorders, 5th Edition. Arlington, VA, American Psychiatric Association, 2013, p 276–277

---

174 A 38-year-old woman with a history of estrogen receptor-positive breast cancer is currently taking tamoxifen to reduce the risk of recurrence. However, she has become increasingly tearful, withdrawn, and anergic over the past month. She also notes difficulty with sleep and concentration as well as distressing hot flashes since initiating tamoxifen. Which one of the following medications is most appropriate to treat her symptoms?

A. Venlafaxine.
B. Paroxetine.
C. Gabapentin.
D. Fluoxetine.
E. Duloxetine.

The correct response is option A: Venlafaxine.

Potent CYP2D6 inhibitors should be avoided in women taking tamoxifen. Of the antidepressants listed, only venlafaxine does not inhibit CYP2D6. Gabapentin is not an appropriate treatment for depression.

Henry NL, Stearns V, Flockhart DA, Hayes DF, Riba M: Drug interactions and pharmacogenomics in the treatment of breast cancer and depression. Am J Psychiatry 2008; 165:1251–1255

---

175 Which of the following distinguishes acute stress disorder from PTSD?

A. Impairment in functioning.
B. Time course.
C. Dissociative symptoms.
D. Reexperiencing.

The correct response is option B: Time course.

Acute stress disorder is time-limited up to 1 month after the precipitating event. Both acute stress disorder and PTSD cause impairment in functioning. For the diagnosis of acute stress disorder, at least nine of the symptoms from five cardinal symptom clusters (intrusion symptoms, negative mood, dissociative symptoms, avoidance symptoms, arousal symptoms) must be present.

American Psychiatric Association: Diagnostic and Statistical Manual of Mental Disorders, 5th Edition. Arlington, VA, American Psychiatric Association, 2013, pp 280–284

---

176 Which of the following symptoms meets DSM-5 criteria for alcohol use disorder?

A. Consuming enough alcohol to become intoxicated.
B. Daily drinking.
C. Repeatedly driving while intoxicated.
D. Recent ingestion of alcohol.
E. Slurred speech.

The correct response is option C: Repeatedly driving while intoxicated.

In DSM-5, the DSM-IV distinction between substance abuse and substance dependence has been eliminated. Alcohol use disorder is a problematic pattern of alcohol use leading to clinically significant impairment or distress, as manifested by at least 2 of the 11 diagnostic criteria. There is also a code based on current severity. A diagnosis of alcohol use disorder requires presence of a maladaptive pattern of alcohol use leading to impairment as manifested by 2 of the 11 criteria within a 12-month period: failure to fulfill major role obligations because of substance use, use in physically hazardous situations (e.g., driving while intoxicated, craving or substance use despite social or interpersonal problems, tolerance, withdrawal, more use than intended, or unsuccessful effort to cut down use).

American Psychiatric Association: Diagnostic and Statistical Manual of Mental Disorders, 5th Edition. Arlington, VA, American Psychiatric Association, 2013, pp 490–499

177 A psychiatrist is asked by the local school to consult on a 13-year-old boy who has exhibited problems with compulsive eating and failure to make academic progress. The boy's parents report that he has always eaten "everything in sight" and has been delayed in his development. Medical history is remarkable for poor muscle tone and failure to thrive as an infant. Physical examination reveals hypotonia, obesity, hypogonadism, a narrow-appearing forehead, down-slanting palpebral fissures, small-appearing hands and feet, and downturning of the corners of the mouth. Intelligence testing is consistent with mental retardation. What is the MOST LIKELY cause of the patient's signs and symptoms?

A. Childhood degenerative disorder.
B. Congenital rubella infection.
C. Homocystinuria.
D. Prader-Willi syndrome.
E. Tuberous sclerosis.

The correct response is option D: Prader-Willi syndrome.

Prader-Willi Syndrome is characterized by hypotonia, obesity, developmental and behavioral problems (including mental retardation), hyperphagia (typically after the first year of life), hypogonadism in males, and dysmorphic features, including a narrow-appearing forehead, down-slanting palpebral fissures, small-appearing hands and feet, and downturning of the corners of the mouth. Children often present in the neonatal period with low muscle tone and failure to thrive. DNA analysis enables molecular confirmation of the diagnosis in most cases.

Essentials of Child and Adolescent Psychiatry, Dulcan MK, Wiener JM American Psychiatric Publishing, 2006, pp 129–130

178 Which of the following psychosocial treatments for social phobia has the most evidence supporting effectiveness?

A. Cognitive-behavioral therapy (CBT).
B. Interpersonal psychotherapy (IPT).
C. Psychodynamic psychotherapy.
D. Family-focused therapy.
E. Group psychoeducation.

The correct response is option A: Cognitive-behavioral therapy.

Several controlled studies have demonstrated the effectiveness of CBT for treatment of social phobia. These have involved both individual and group CBT. A central feature of such treatments involves exposure to feared situations. There have been several small studies suggesting that IPT may be an effective treatment for social phobia. At this time, there is no evidence supporting the efficacy of psychodynamic or family-focused therapy or group psychoeducation.

Foa EB. Social anxiety disorder treatments: psychosocial therapies. J Clin Psychiatry 2006; 67(suppl 12):27–30

Van Ameringen M, Allgulander C, Bandelow B, Greist JH, et al: WCA recommendations for the long-term treatment of social phobia. CNS Spectrums 2003; 8:40–52

Hales RE, Yudofsky SC, Gabbard GO (eds): The American Psychiatric Publishing Textbook of Psychiatry, 5th ed. Arlington, VA, American Psychiatric Publishing, 2008. p 544–5

179 A 62-year-old woman presents for assessment and treatment of a 3-year history of mild but persistent depressive symptoms. One year ago, she was named board chairman of her association and also began a new relationship with a very wealthy individual. The relationship is going well emotionally and sexually, but she sometimes feels inadequate in her new social circles. She misses her former partner particularly when she feels socially awkward. After a discussion of treatment options for improving her overall level of functioning and self-satisfaction, she and her psychiatrist decide upon a structured, time-limited course of interpersonal psychotherapy (IPT). Which ONE of the following would be the most appropriate focus of the IPT?

A. Analysis of transference.
B. Delayed grief.
C. Interpersonal deficits.
D. Role dispute.
E. Role transition.

The correct response is option E: Role transition.

IPT focuses on the interpersonal rather than primarily on one's own psychology. Therefore, focusing on transference is not the vehicle of IPT. The remaining four options can be the focus in IPT; in this case, role transition is the best answer because it aligns well with her main goal of treatment: functioning in her new role as board chairman and in her new romantic relationship. Delayed grief might be a focus if that is what the patient were experiencing. She does not present with interpersonal deficits in the IPT sense.

Weissman, MM, Markowitz, JC, & Klerman, GL: Clinician's Quick Guide to Interpersonal Psychotherapy. New York, Oxford University Press, 2007. http://www.interpersonalpsychotherapy.org/

Markowitz JC: The clinical conduct of interpersonal psychotherapy. Focus 2006; 4(2): 179–84

---

180 Which of the following congenital abnormalities is associated with maternal use of carbamazepine in the first trimester of pregnancy?

A. An increased risk of Ebstein's anomaly, the downward displacement of the tricuspid valve into the right ventricle and variable levels of right ventricular hyperplasia.
B. Craniofacial defects, fingernail hypoplasia, and developmental delay.
C. Fetal development of skin rash in a neonate who has antigen characteristics different from those of the mother.
D. Impaired temperature regulation and apnea.

The correct response is option B: Craniofacial defects, fingernail hypoplasia, and developmental delay.

In the first trimester of pregnancy, carbamazepine is associated with craniofacial defects, fingernail hypoplasia, and developmental delay; lithium is associated with an increased risk of Ebstein's anomaly; valproate is associated with neural tube defects secondary to the failure of the neural tube to close, and lamotrigine is associated with fetal development of skin rash in a neonate who has antigen characteristics different from those of the mother. Benzodiazepines are only rarely associated with organ dysgenisis but have been associated with impaired temperature regulation, apnea, hypotonia, and lower Apgar scores at birth.

Yonkers KA, Wisner KL, Stowe Z, Leibenluft E, et al: Management of bipolar disorder during pregnancy and the postpartum period. Am J Psychiatry 2004; 161:608–20

American Psychiatric Association Practice Guideline for the Treatment of Patients with Bipolar Disorder, 2nd ed (2002). http://psychiatryonline.org/guidelines.aspx

---

181 When initiating treatment with long-acting injectable haloperidol every 4 weeks, what period of time is required to reach steady state?

A. 4 weeks.
B. 8 weeks.
C. 12 weeks.
D. 16 weeks.
E. 20 weeks.

The correct response is option E: 20 weeks.

Five injection intervals are required to reach steady state. Haloperidol is typically dosed every 4 weeks; it therefore takes 20 weeks to reach steady state. Five half-lives are required to reach steady state.

Hales RE, Yudofsky SC, Gabbard GO (eds): The American Psychiatric Publishing Textbook of Psychiatry, 5th ed. Washington DC; American Psychiatric Publishing, 2008. p 1104

---

182 In addition to pharmacotherapy, psychotherapy plays an important role in treating bipolar disorder. Which ONE of the following circumstances best describes when cognitive-behavioral therapy (CBT) is most effective in the adjunctive treatment of bipolar disorder?

A. Acutely ill, depressed.
B. Acutely ill, manic.
C. After four or more episodes.
D. Moderately or acutely ill states.
E. Recovered from acute episode.

The correct response is option E: Recovered from acute episode.

Miklowitz (2008) reports on when and which types of psychotherapy are most useful in the adjunctive treatment of bipolar disorder. He reviewed 18 trials of individual and group psychoeducation, systematic care, family therapy, interpersonal therapy, and CBT. Among his findings are that family therapy, interpersonal therapy, and systematic care were most effective in preventing recurrences when initiated after an acute episode, whereas CBT and group psychoeducation were most effective when initiated during a period of recovery. Psychotherapies that emphasize medication adherence and early recognition of mood symptoms have stronger effects on mania, whereas treatments that emphasize cognitive and interpersonal coping strategies have stronger effects on depression. He also cited a five-site U.K. study that showed CBT was effective in delaying recurrences among patients with fewer than 12 prior episodes.

Miklowitz DJ: Adjunctive psychotherapy for bipolar disorder: state of the evidence. Am J Psychiatry 2008; 165:1408–1419

---

183 Behavioral approaches such as the Semans pause maneuver, the start-stop method of Kaplan, and the pause-squeeze technique of Masters and Johnson have been employed to treat which of the following?

A. Male erectile disorder.
B. Female sexual arousal disorder.
C. Premature ejaculation.
D. Hypoactive sexual desire disorder.
E. Female orgasmic disorder.

The correct response is option C: Premature ejaculation.

These behavioral techniques were developed to treat premature ejaculation, a condition considered to be the most prevalent sexual dysfunction in men. They would not be appropriate treatments for the other options.

Gabbard GO (ed), Gabbard's Treatment of Psychiatric Disorders, 4th ed., Washington, DC, American Psychiatric Press. 2007, pp 641–655

---

184 A 25-year-old man with no past history of abnormal involuntary movements is being treated with haloperidol. He should be evaluated for abnormal involuntary movements every

A. 1 month.
B. 3 months.
C. 6 months.
D. 12 months.
E. 18 months.

The correct response is option C: 6 months.

Individuals taking first-generation (typical) neuroleptics are at increased risk for developing tardive dyskinesia. The APA Practice Guideline for Schizophrenia recommends: "Clinical assessment of abnormal involuntary movements every 6 months in patients taking first-generation antipsychotics and every 12 months in those taking second-generation antipsychotics." In patients at increased risk, assessment should be done every 3 months and every 6 months with treatment using first- and second-generation antipsychotics, respectively. Patients at increased risk for developing abnormal involuntary movements include elderly patients and patients who experience acute dystonic reactions, other clinically significant extrapyramidal side effects, or akathisias."

American Psychiatric Association Practice Guideline for the Treatment of Patients with Schizophrenia, 2nd ed (2004), pp 586–587. http://psychiatryonline.org/guidelines.aspx

---

185 A 19-year-old private in the U.S. Army loses his left leg after his vehicle drives over an improvised explosive device. Two months later he reports ongoing recurrent and intrusive recollections of the event, nightmares and flashbacks to the explosion, avoidance of any activities that remind him of the event, irritability, and disturbed sleep. Which of the following psychotherapeutic interventions is MOST likely to be effective in alleviating his symptoms?

A. Biofeedback.
B. Eye movement desensitization and reprocessing.
C. Exposure-based cognitive-behavior therapy.
D. Guided imagery therapy.
E. Hypnotherapy.

The correct response is option C: Exposure-based cognitive-behavior therapy.

In response to increased attention on U.S. military veterans returning from combat in Iraq and Afghanistan, the Institute of Medicine reviewed and summarized the evidence supporting treatment for PTSD. The 2007 report recognizes that there is evidence for the pharmacological treatment of combat-related PTSD but states that this evidence is not as strong as the evidence for treatment of other trauma-related PTSD. In particular, the report states that large randomized controlled trials, considered a standard of evidence in other areas of medicine, are lacking from the evidence base. The report concludes that existing evidence is sufficient only to establish the efficacy of exposure-based psychotherapies in the treatment of PTSD.

Institute of Medicine (2007). Treatment of posttraumatic stress disorder: An assessment of the evidence. Washington DC: National Academy of Sciences. Available at http://books.nap.edu/catalog.php?record_id=11955#toc

---

186 A 40-year-old patient is taking clozapine for treatment-resistant schizophrenia. Assuming no abnormal laboratory results, after what period of time could complete blood count monitoring be reduced to every 4 weeks?

A. 3 months.
B. 6 months.
C. 12 months.
D. 18 months.
E. 24 months.

The correct response is option C: 12 months.

After initiating clozapine, weekly complete blood count (CBC) monitoring is required. If the white blood cell (WBC) count remains 3500/mm^3 and the absolute neutrophil count (ANC) 2000/mm^3 during the first 6 months of therapy, then the monitoring frequency may be decreased to every 2 weeks. If the WBC count remains 3500/mm^3 and the ANC 2000/mm^3 for another 6 months, then the monitoring frequency may be decreased to every 4 weeks.

According to the APA Practice Guideline for the Treatment of Patients With Schizophrenia, the risk of agranulocytosis (ANC 500/mm^3) has been estimated at 1.3% of patients per year of treatment with clozapine. The risk is highest in the first 6 months of treatment. Weekly WBC and neutrophil monitoring is required. After 6 months, monitoring may occur every 2 weeks, as the risk of agranulocytosis appears to diminish. WBC counts must remain above 3000/mm^3 during clozapine treatment, and absolute neutrophil counts must remain above 1500/mm^3.

Clozaril® package insert, Novartis Pharmaceuticals Corporation, East Hanover, NJ, 2005 http://www.pharma.us.novartis.com/ product/pi/pdf/Clozaril.pdf.
American Psychiatric Association Practice Guideline for the Treatment of Patients with Schizophrenia, 2nd ed (2004). pp 636. http://psychiatryonline.org/guidelines.aspx

---

187 For patients with functional gastrointestinal disorders, which of the following medications would be most likely to alleviate the visceral pain associated with irritable bowel syndrome?

A. Bupropion.
B. Clonazepam.
C. Fluoxetine.
D. Quetiapine.
E. Amitriptyline.

The correct response is option E: Amitriptyline.

Patients with functional gastrointestinal disorders are frequently disabled by visceral pain. Antidepressants have been commonly used for this, and the analgesic properties appear to be independent of the antidepressant effect. Among the antidepressants, the ones that have dual actions on both serotonin and norepinephrine, such as the tricyclic antidepressants, appear to be the most effective in relieving the pain associated with functional gastrointestinal disorders. Amitriptyline is the best studied among them; however, several others such as trimipramine and doxepin have also shown positive results. Desipramine has shown more equivocal results; this may be due to the drug's somewhat more selective affinity for norepinephrine reuptake. Studies with selective serotonin reuptake inhibitors have not been as positive (although some more recent data showed positive results for paroxetine), and bupropion generally has not been used in this context.

Jones MP, Crowell MD, Olden KW, Creed F. Functional gastrointestinal disorders: an update for the psychiatrist. Psychosomatics. 2007; 48(2):93–102

---

188 A 56-year old man with major depression is prescribed paroxetine. One month later, he complains of significant nausea. His dose is lowered from 20 to 10 mg/day; however, he continues to feel nauseated. He is motivated to remain on the medication if possible since he feels it has been enormously helpful for his depression. A genotyping of the cytochrome P450 2D6 gene reveals that he has one inactive copy and one partially inactive copy. Which of the following would be the most appropriate step to take?

A. Discontinue paroxetine immediately and wait 1 month.
B. Attempt even lower doses of paroxetine.
C. Discontinue paroxetine and begin fluoxetine.
D. Discontinue paroxetine and begin citalopram.
E. Continue paroxetine but add ondansetron.

The correct response is option B: Attempt even lower doses of paroxetine.

Although not currently clinical standard practice to conduct genetic analysis, the CYP450 2D6 has particular clinical relevance; it is involved in the primary metabolism of more than 70 medications. The 2D6 gene, which codes for this enzyme, has a high degree of allelic variability, with more than 100 variations of the gene having been recorded. It is also unique in that multiple copies of the gene can occur on the same chromosome. Alleles are classified by their degree of activity, and the number of active alleles directly affects the enzymes' ability to metabolize substances. Individuals with at least two active copies are able to tolerate those medications metabolized by the enzyme at regular doses; those with three or more active copies are considered "ultra-rapid metabolizers" and may need higher doses of medication. Those with two inactive copies are considered to be poor metabolizers and may not be able to tolerate medications metabolized by this enzyme. However, there is an intermediate group of slow metabolizers who have one inactive copy of the allele and one partially inactive copy. These individuals may be able to tolerate 2D6 substrate medications but in lower than average doses; often the doses would be considered subtherapeutic in those with normal metabolism. In the case above, given the robust response to the medication, an attempt to continue the patient on paroxetine is indicated. Although ondansetron is effective for nausea, it would not be indicated here as it is also metabolized by 2D6. Should the patient fail a trial of paroxetine, duloxetine (which can be metabolized by other pathways if 2D6 is not available) and citalopram (which is not metabolized by this enzyme) would be reasonable alternatives.

Mrazek DA. Psychiatric pharmacogenomics. FOCUS 2006;4:339–343

de Leon J. AmpliChip CYP450 Test: personalized medicine has arrived in psychiatry. Expert Rev. Mol. Diagn 2006; 6:277–286

189 Which symptom is characteristically seen in patients with factitious disorder?

A. Thoughts of death.
B. Pathological lying.
C. Fear of pain.
D. Perceptual disturbances.
E. Feelings of inadequacy.

The correct response is option B: Pathological lying.

Patients with factitious disorder usually have a history of multiple hospitalizations, wandering from hospital to hospital (peregrination), and pathological lying (pseudologia fantastica, the telling of dramatic tales that merge truth and falsehood).

Hales RE, Yudofsky SC, Gabbard GO (eds): The American Psychiatric Publishing Textbook of Psychiatry, 5th ed. Washington, DC, American Psychiatric Publishing, 2008, p 429

American Psychiatric Association: Diagnostic and Statistical Manual of Mental Disorders, 5th Edition. Arlington, VA, American Psychiatric Association, 2013, pp 324–325

190 A patient with bipolar disorder is receiving maintenance treatment with extended-release divalproex. How many hours should elapse between his last dose and drawing of the trough level of valproic acid?

A. 4 hours.
B. 8 hours.
C. 12 hours.
D. 18 hours.

The correct response is option D: 18 hours.

A trough level of valproate occurs 21–24 hours after the last dose of the extended-release preparation. Blood drawn 12–15 hours later will have a concentration 18%–25% higher than trough. It appears that samples drawn 18–21 hours later will deviate from trough by only 3%–13%, which is felt to be clinically acceptable. In practice, giving this preparation as a single daily dose in the morning and having blood drawn prior to the next morning dose will result in consistent trough levels.

Reed RC, Dutta S: Does it really matter when a blood sample for valproic acid concentration is taken following once-daily administration of divalproex-ER? Ther Drug Monit 2006; 28:413–418

191 A woman presents for help in coping with stress. During the assessment, it becomes clear that she is excessively preoccupied with her appearance, particularly her face. She spends hours a day examining and caring for her face. She is convinced that her cheekbones are uneven and make her look like a freak. Her appearance is unremarkable. After the assessment is complete, the psychiatrist's best initial approach is to:

A. Reassure the patient about her appearance.
B. Agree that the situation is quite distressing.
C. Point out that her thinking is quite distorted.
D. Agree that her appearance is a problem.
E. Explain the benefits of medication.

The correct response is option B: Agree that the situation is quite distressing.

Patients with body dysmorphic disorder tend to have difficulty acknowledging that they have a psychiatric disorder that needs treatment. The recommended initial steps in treatment are to empathize with the patient and engage them in treatment. At the same time, it is important not to agree with the patient's view of her appearance.

Phillips KA, Hollander E. Treating body dysmorphic disorder with medication: evidence, misconceptions, and a suggested approach. Body Image. 2008; 5:16

Hales RE, Yudofsky SC, Gabbard GO (eds): The American Psychiatric Publishing Textbook of Psychiatry, 5th ed. Washington, DC, American Psychiatric Publishing, 2008, p 634

Phillips KA. Clinical features and treatment of body dysmorphic disorder. FOCUS. 2005; 2:179–183

192 Which of the following is a common symptom of the depressive disorders specifier with seasonal pattern?

A. Light sensitivity.
B. Somatic complaints.
C. Insomnia.
D. Overeating.
E. Impulsiveness.

The correct response is option D: Overeating.

Major depressive episodes that occur in a seasonal pattern are often characterized by hypersomnia, overeating, weight gain, and a craving for carbohydrates.

American Psychiatric Association: Diagnostic and Statistical Manual of Mental Disorders, 5th Edition. Arlington, VA, American Psychiatric Association, 2013, p 187

---

193 Which of the following techniques is commonly used in motivational interviewing?

A. Confrontation.
B. Interpretation of transference.
C. Identification of cognitive distortions.
D. Decision balance.
E. Relaxation training.

The correct response is option D: Decision balance.

During the process of motivational interviewing, decision balance is used to help the patient increase self-awareness, self-efficacy, and the intention to change. Confrontation is to be avoided in motivational interviewing. Interpretation of transference is a technique of psychoanalysis, identification of cognitive distortions is a technique of cognitive therapy, and relaxation training is a technique used in behavior therapy.

Hales RE, Yudofsky SC, Gabbard GO (eds): The American Psychiatric Publishing Textbook of Psychiatry, 5th ed. Arlington, VA, American Psychiatric Publishing, 2003, pp 1267–8, 1160, 1230
Galanter M, Kleber HD (eds): The American Psychiatric Publishing Textbook of Substance Abuse Treatment, 4th ed. Arlington, VA, American Psychiatric Publishing, 2008, pp 353–4

---

194 Which of the following factors best differentiates acute stress disorder from PTSD?

A. Chronicity.
B. Traumatic event severity.
C. Presence of nightmares.
D. Level of functional impairment.
E. Severity of subjective response to the event.

The correct response is option A: Chronicity.

DSM-5 criteria require that the symptoms of PTSD must be present for more than 1 month. Acute stress disorder is distinguished from PTSD because the symptom pattern in acute stress disorder must occur within 4 weeks of the traumatic event and resolve within that 4-week period. If the symptoms persist for more than 1 month and meet criteria for PTSD, the diagnosis is changed from acute stress disorder to PTSD.

American Psychiatric Association: Diagnostic and Statistical Manual of Mental Disorders, 5th Edition. Arlington, VA, American Psychiatric Association, 2013, pp 280–281

---

195 Which of the following best describes the mechanism of action of flumazenil in the treatment of benzodiazepine overdose?

A. Flumazenil blocks benzodiazepines from crossing the blood-brain barrier.
B. Flumazenil competes with benzodiazepines at central synaptic GABA receptor sites.
C. Flumazenil decreases the influx of chloride ions into GABAergic neurons preventing hyperpolarization.
D. Flumazenil increases the influx of sodium ions into GABAergic neurons causing depolarization.
E. Flumazenil increases the rate of oxidative metabolism of benzodiazepines.

The correct response is option B: Flumazenil competes with benzodiazepines at central synaptic GABA receptor sites.

Flumazenil is a potent benzodiazepine-specific antagonist that competes at central synaptic GABA receptor sites in a dose-dependent manner.

Hales RE, Yudofsky SC: Substance use disorders in The American Psychiatric Publishing Textbook of Clinical Psychiatry. Washington DC, American Psychiatric Publishing, 2003, pp 343–4

196 A 22-year-old woman was involved in a severe motor vehicle accident in which several people were significantly injured. She had difficulty recalling portions of the accident, nightmares, and difficulty falling asleep. She refused to drive her car, had difficulty concentrating, and felt emotionally numb. She was unable to attend work. Her symptoms spontaneously resolved after a month, and she was able to return to work. The most likely diagnosis is:

A. Acute stress disorder.
B. Adjustment disorder.
C. Posttraumatic stress disorder.
D. Panic disorder.
E. Brief psychotic disorder.

The correct response is option A: Acute stress disorder.

The symptoms of acute stress disorder include marked symptoms of anxiety or increased arousal, difficulty sleeping, irritability, poor concentration, hypervigilance, exaggerated startle response, and motor restlessness. Acute stress disorder occurs within 4 weeks of the traumatic event and resolves within 4 weeks.

American Psychiatric Association: Diagnostic and Statistical Manual of Mental Disorders, 5th Edition. Arlington, VA, American Psychiatric Association, 2013, p 280

197 Which of the following is the most common form of affective illness in families of patients with bipolar disorder?

A. Bipolar disorder.
B. Unipolar depression.
C. Dysthymia.
D. Premenstrual dysphoric disorder.
E. Cyclothymia.

The correct response is option B: Unipolar depression.

Mood disorders have a strong genetic component, with the greater the presence in families, the greater the risk to the child. Bipolar disorder has a particularly high degree of familial association. Although a family history of bipolar disorder confers a greater risk of mood disorders on the child, it is unipolar, and not bipolar disorder (or any of the others listed), that is the most common mood disorder in families of bipolar patients.

Sadock BJ, Sadock VA (eds): Kaplan & Sadock's Synopsis of Psychiatry: Behavioral Sciences/Clinical Psychiatry, 10th ed. Philadelphia, Lippincott Williams & Wilkins, 2007, p 532

Fanous AH, Kendler KS. Genetic heterogeneity, modifier genes, and quantitative phenotypes in psychiatric illness: Searching for a framework. Molecular Psychiatry 2005;10:6–13. Reprinted with permission in FOCUS 2006; 4:423–430

198 The use of bright light treatment has been shown to be efficacious and safe for the treatment of:

A. Dysthymia.
B. Nonseasonal depression.
C. Bipolar disorder.
D. PTSD.

The correct response is option B: Nonseasonal depression.

A meta-analysis by Golden et al. found that bright light treatment and dawn simulation was efficacious for seasonal affective disorder and for nonseasonal depression, with effect sizes equivalent to those in most antidepressant pharmacotherapy trials. Bright light therapy has caused some patients with bipolar disorder to switch into mania and is therefore contraindicated.

Golden RN, Bradley N, Gaynes R, Ekstrom D, et al: The efficacy of light therapy in the treatment of mood disorder: A review and meta-analysis of the evidence. Am J Psychiatry. Apr 2005; 162(4):656–662

199 Stimulus control treatment for insomnia works by:

A. Reassuring patients that a quiet environment will help them fall asleep.
B. Reestablishing an automatic connection between going to bed and falling asleep.
C. Subtly punishing the patient for failure to fall asleep.
D. Making both bedtimes and rising times more regular.

The correct response is option B: Reestablishing an automatic connection between going to bed and falling asleep.

Psychological and behavioral treatments of insomnia, especially cognitive-behavioral treatment (CBT-I), have been effective for both primary insomnia and insomnia that is comorbid with other conditions. Stimulus control treatment (SCT) aims to overcome the conditioned arousal, which besets many insomniacs upon retiring to bed. SCT helps the patient reestablish an automatic connection between the bed/bedroom/bedtime and falling asleep. Bedroom activities other than sleep—television, computer work, phone calls, eating, or planning—are avoided; sexual activity is the only exception. If the patient is not asleep within 10–20 minutes of bedtime, he or she leaves the bedroom. The reward for those who persist in SCT is gradually shorter sleep latency and increased confidence about falling asleep easily and automatically.

Byrne B. Psychological and behavioral treatments for insomnia. FOCUS Winter 2014, Vol. XII, No. 1 p 31–37

200 Which of the following is one of the standards used to determine mental capacity in decision making?

A. Absence of psychosis.
B. Agreement with the medical recommendations.
C. Severity of psychiatric illness.
D. Rational decision making.
E. Presence of abstract thought.

The correct response is option D: Rational decision making.

Case law and the literature generally describe four standards for determining mental capacity in decision making: communication of choice, understanding of relevant information provided, appreciation of available options and consequences, and rational decision making.

Simon RI. The law and psychiatry. FOCUS: Forensic and Ethical Issues; Fall 2003; 4:363–367

201 Which of the following treatments has the best body of evidence in preventing poststroke depression in older populations?

A. Escitalopram.
B. Mianserin.
C. Sertraline.
D. Problem-solving therapy.
E. Cognitive-behavioral therapy.

The correct response is option A: Escitalopram.

In a 2008 published double-blind placebo-controlled trial of nondepressed patients in their 60s with recent stroke, patients receiving escitalopram or problem-solving therapy for a year were less likely to develop depression than patients receiving placebo; however, using an intention-to-treat conservative method of analyzing the data, problem-solving therapy was not significantly better than placebo, whereas escitalopram continued to be superior to placebo. Studies using mianserin (not available in the United States) and sertraline to prevent poststroke depression have been unsuccessful, as have studies with cognitive-behavioral therapy.

Robinson RG, Jorge RE, Moser DJ, Acion L, et al: Escitalopram and problem-solving therapy for prevention of poststroke depression: a randomized controlled trial. JAMA. 2008; 299(20): 2391–2400
Robinson RG, Jorge RE, Arndt S. Escitalopram, problem-solving therapy, and poststroke depression—reply. JAMA. 2008; 300(15): 1758–1759

202 A single mother reports that her 12-year-old child has become increasingly defiant with parental requests, at times becoming physically aggressive by kicking doors and hitting walls. She notes that the child does not exhibit these problems with the father. Which of the following is the most appropriate treatment?

A. Inoculation techniques, such as boot camp.
B. Contingency management.
C. Medication management.
D. Send the child to live with the father temporarily.
E. Brief hospitalization.

The correct response is option B: Contingency management.

The child is displaying signs of oppositional defiant disorder (ODD). One of the most effective approaches to managing disruptive behavior associated with ODD is training parents to use contingency management techniques. Inoculation techniques, such as boot camp, have no evidence of efficacy and have been shown to be harmful in some cases. Medication management should not be used as the primary treatment for ODD. Sending the child to live with his father would provide no therapeutic benefit for the interactions between the child and his mother. Hospitalization at this time is unwarranted.

Steiner H, Remsing L (2007). Practice Parameter for the Assessment and Treatment of Children and Adolescents with Oppositional Defiant Disorder. J Am Acad Child Adolesc Psychiatry 46; 1:126–41

203 A 22-year-old man with chronic schizophrenia developed gynecomastia after being treated with risperidone for many months. His prolactin level is markedly elevated and you want to switch him to the antipsychotic drug that is less likely to cause this problem. Which one of the following would be the most appropriate choice?

A. Aripiprazole.
B. Olanzapine.
C. Perphenazine.
D. Haloperidol.
E. Paliperidone.

The correct response is option A: Aripiprazole.

Dopamine release from the hypothalamus stimulates dopamine D_2 receptors in the anterior pituitary gland and has an inhibiting effect on prolactin secretion. Antipsychotic drug-induced hyperprolactinemia is due to blockade of D_2 receptors. Unlike the other options that block D_2 receptors, aripiprazole is a partial D_2 receptor agonist, and it does not elevate serum prolactin levels.

Haddad PM, Wieck A: Antipsychotic-induced hyperprolactinaemia: mechanisms, clinical features and management. Drugs 2004; 64:2291–2314
Wood M, Reavill C: Aripiprazole acts as a selective dopamine D2 receptor partial agonist. Expert Opin Investig Drugs 2007; 16: 771–775

204 A 70-year-old man presents to a clinic with progressive memory loss. Which of the following findings is most representative of cortical dementia in this patient?

A. Apathy.
B. Aphasia.
C. Decreased attention.
D. Bradyphrenia.
E. Mood lability.

The correct response is option B: Aphasia.

Cortical dementias arise from disorders that affect the cerebral cortex (Alzheimer's, Creutzfeldt-Jakob). Cortical dementia is characterized by impairment in recall and recognition; language deficits including aphasia, apraxia, and agnosia; and visuospatial deficits. In general, cortical dementias are not associated with prominent motor signs. Subcortical dementias are associated with greater impairment in recall memory, a decrease in verbal fluency without anomia, bradyphrenia (slowed thinking), depressed mood, affective lability, apathy, and decreased attention/concentration.

Sadock BJ, Sadock VA (eds): Kaplan and Sadock's Synopsis of Psychiatry: Behavioral Sciences/Clinical Psychiatry (Synopsis of Psychiatry), 10vth ed. Philadelphia, Lippincott Williams and Wilkins, 2007. pp 1353

205 A psychiatrist is asked to determine if a very ill, delirious, and possibly senile patient has the capacity to make a new will. Which of the following features must be present to determine that the patient has the capacity?

A. Orientation to time and place.
B. Unimpaired attention span.
C. Awareness that she is making a will.
D. Choice of beneficiary that is not frivolous.
E. Ability to recognize family.

The correct response is option C: Awareness that she is making a will.

The capacity to make a will has the fewest cognitive requirements of any legal document. All that is needed is awareness that a will is being made, knowledge of who the rightful heirs should be, and some idea of the value of the estate. Knowing who the rightful heirs should be does not mean that they must be named as the beneficiaries. The patient could in fact choose a beneficiary that others might consider frivolous. Neither unimpaired orientation nor attention span is necessary if the patient can cooperate to the extent needed for the cognitive requirements. Even if the patient is delusional or hallucinating, the will can be written, as long as the symptoms do not interfere with decision making as regards the will.

Rosner R, (Ed) Principles and Practice of Forensic Psychiatry, 2 nd ed, London, Arnold, 2003 p 309

206 Which of the following types of therapy used to treat schizophrenia is based on the premise that attempting to suppress or control mental events is NOT helpful?

A. Traditional cognitive-behavioral therapy (CBT).
B. Compliance therapy.
C. Acceptance and commitment therapy (ACT).
D. Supportive psychotherapy.
E. Illness education.

The correct response is option C: Acceptance and commitment therapy (ACT).

ACT is a variation of CBT originally developed for the treatment of nonpsychotic conditions. In contrast with traditional CBT, which aims to change the individual's cognitions and to facilitate the development of a more rational perspective, the goal in ACT is to modify the individual's relationship to his or her thinking more broadly. ACT is based on the premise that attempting to suppress or control mental events is not helpful and rather encourages persons to accept and to experience thoughts and feelings nonjudgmentally or mindfully.

Dickerson FB, Lehman AF: Evidence-based psychotherapy for schizophrenia. J of Nervous & Mental Disease. 2006; 194:3–9

207 A 45-year-old patient requests a medication to treat symptoms consistent with generalized anxiety disorder (GAD). The patient has a history of heavy drinking. Which of the following medications would be most appropriate to prescribe?

A. Clonazepam.
B. Bupropion.
C. Quetiapine.
D. Diazepam.
E. Venlafaxine.

The correct response is option E: Venlafaxine.

The most appropriate option is venlafaxine, which is an efficacious treatment for GAD. Although benzodiazepines, such as clonazepam, alprazolam, and diazepam, are effective in treating GAD, the risk of benzodiazepine abuse or dependence among alcohol abusers limits their utility. Bupropion is not generally considered to be a first-line treatment for GAD. Quetiapine is not an approved treatment for GAD.

Schatzberg AF, Nemeroff CB (eds): Essentials of Clinical Psychopharmacology, 2nd ed, Washington, DC, American Psychiatric Publishing, 2006, pp 141–4, 189, 542–5
Tyrer T, Baldwin D. Generalized anxiety disorder. Lancet 2006; 368:2156–2166
Hoge EA, Oppenheimer JE, Simon NM: Generalized anxiety disorder. FOCUS: Anxiety Disorders, Summer 2004; 3:353–354

208 A bus driver calls in sick whenever there is inclement weather such as rain or light snow. He has never had an accident while driving, nor does he know anyone personally who had an accident due to inclement weather. He also avoids driving his own car in poor weather and attempts to convince his family members to do the same. He admits he is very cautious about many things, which interferes with his sleep, causes fatigue, and makes him irritable. Which of the following is the most likely diagnosis?

A. Panic disorder.
B. Social phobia: situational.
C. Posttraumatic stress disorder.
D. OCD.
E. Generalized anxiety disorder.

The correct response is option E: Generalized anxiety disorder.

The bus driver's excessive concern about driving in inclement weather, as well as his worry over others driving under those conditions, plus his report that he is very cautious suggests that generalized anxiety disorder is the most likely choice. In addition, the report that he is cautious suggests there are other areas of his life in which he worries excessively. Insomnia, fatigue, and irritability are also part of the diagnostic picture. Panic disorder is unlikely because his worries are so generalized (a cautious man) with no history of panic attacks or evidence of typical agoraphobia. Similarly, social phobia is unlikely because his driving avoidance relates to weather and not meeting bus passengers. There is no evidence of a trauma that could explain his avoidance (PTSD). Finally, he reports no rituals and his worries, unlike many obsessions, are reasonable but excessive.

American Psychiatric Association: Diagnostic and Statistical Manual of Mental Disorders, 5th Edition. Arlington, VA, American Psychiatric Association, 2013

209 A 20-year-old woman was brought to the emergency department by police after disrupting one of her university classes. She was agitated and demanded that her intellectual abilities be acknowledged. She had pressured speech and her affect alternated between periods of euphoria and irritability. Her roommate told the emergency staff that the patient had been very energetic, had been unable to sleep for a week, and had previously been admitted to hospital for a similar episode. Which of the following diagnoses is most likely?

A. Cocaine intoxication.
B. Cyclothymia.
C. Bipolar I disorder.
D. Bipolar II disorder.
E. Schizophrenia.

The correct response is option C: Bipolar I disorder.

For bipolar I disorder to be diagnosed, criteria must be met for a manic episode, lasting at least 1 week. This is a distinct period of abnormally elevated expansive or irritable mood and abnormally increased energy lasting at least 1 week and present most of the day—or any duration if hospitalization is necessary—with additional criteria met from criterion B: inflated self-esteem or grandiosity, decreased need for sleep, pressure of speech, flight of ideas, distractibility, agitation, and disinhibition. According to DSM-5, bipolar II disorder is defined by diagnostic criteria being met for both a current or past hypomanic episode and a current or past major depressive episode.

American Psychiatric Association: Diagnostic and Statistical Manual of Mental Disorders, 5th Edition. Arlington, VA, American Psychiatric Association, 2013, p 123–132

210 Children and adolescents are considered a vulnerable population in the conduct of research because they:

A. Cannot consent.
B. Suffer more adverse effects.
C. Are in riskier studies.
D. Cannot assent.
E. Do not benefit.

The correct response is option A: Cannot consent.

Children and adolescents are considered a vulnerable population in terms of research because of their inability to consent and the risk that they will be exploited. Children and adolescents are expected to give assent depending on their age and capabilities. Studies involving children and adolescents are not necessarily more risky, and subjects do not necessarily suffer more adverse effects. Subjects may directly benefit depending on the study.

Levine RJ. Respect for children as research subjects, in Lewis' Comprehensive Textbook of Child and Adolescent Psychiatry. Martin A, Volkmar FR, eds. Philadelphia, Lippincott Williams & Wilkins, 2007. p 143

211 A 53-year-old man presents asking for help with problem drinking. He reports frequent swelling of his ankles and says that when he goes to the corner store, he has to walk slowly or he'll get too short of breath. He says he's supposed to be taking "some heart pills" but hasn't had any for a number of months and can't remember their names. He has attempted to quit drinking on two prior occasions and was treated with diazepam for "the shakes." He has been drinking 1–2 pints of rum daily for the past 10 months. His last drink was several hours ago. What would be the most appropriate initial referral?

A. Medical hospitalization.
B. Partial hospitalization program.
C. Intensive outpatient program.
D. Office-based program.
E. Therapeutic community.

The correct response is option A: Medical hospitalization.

The patient's physical symptoms and history are strongly suggestive of significant untreated cardiac disease. His history also suggests that with continued abstinence he will go through alcohol withdrawal. His initial treatment should be in a setting where he can be closely medically monitored and his heart disease treated as needed.

Mee-Lee D, Shulman G, Fishman M, et al. (eds): ASAM Patient Placement Criteria for the Treatment of Substance-Related Disorders, 2nd ed, revised. Chevy Chase, MD, American Society of Addiction Medicine, 2001

212 A 46-year-old man is begun on citalopram 20 mg daily for a major depressive episode. After 4 weeks, he returns to his psychiatrist citing little if any change in his symptoms. Which of the following would be the most appropriate next step in the patient's treatment?

A. Increase the patient's dosage to 40 mg/day of citalopram.
B. Discontinue citalopram and begin venlafaxine.
C. Continue citalopram but add lithium.
D. Begin vagal nerve stimulation.
E. Continue citalopram and begin aripiprazole.

The correct response is option A: Increase the patient's dosage to 40 mg/day of citalopram.

The management of "difficult to treat" depression remains a challenge, with various strategies suggested, including switching to different antidepressants, augmenting with various medications, and nonpharmacological treatments such as electroconvulsive therapy and vagal nerve stimulation. Before such approaches are considered, however, one wants to make sure that the patient has had an adequate trial of his or her initial antidepressant, defined as a sufficient dose for a sufficient duration. In the STAR*D trial, the mean dose of citalopram needed for remission was 40 mg/day. Similarly, of the patients in STAR*D who remitted while taking citalopram, only 30% responded within 4 weeks, and another 30% who remitted did not do so until 10 weeks or more. In general, if no improvement in depressive symptoms is seen on an SSRI after 4 weeks, a trial of a higher dose may be warranted. However, higher doses tend not to be more effective than standard doses.

Zisook S: Ask the Expert: Psychopharmacology: major depressive disorder. FOCUS 2006;4:484–486

Yudofsky SC, Hales RE (eds): The American Psychiatric Publishing Textbook of Neuropsychiatry and Behavioral Sciences, 5th ed. Arlington, VA, American Psychiatric Publishing, 2008, pp 1058–1061

---

213 Which of the following features would be most predictive of a favorable response to lithium maintenance in bipolar disorder?

A. Euthymic intervals.
B. Rapid cycling.
C. Mixed episodes.
D. Substance abuse.
E. Psychosis.

The correct response is option A: Euthymic intervals.

Features predictive of a good response to lithium include euphoric mania, full interepisode remission (euthymia), the absence of comorbidity, few lifetime episodes, the absence of rapid cycling, and a mania-depression-euthymia sequence of clinical course.

Jefferson JW, Greist JH: Lithium, in Kaplan & Sadock's Comprehensive Textbook of Psychiatry, 9th ed. Edited by Sadock BJ, Sadock VA, Ruiz P. Philadelphia, Lippincott Williams & Wilkins, 2009, pp 3132–45

Grof P: Responders to long-term lithium treatment, in Lithium in Neuropsychiatry: The Comprehensive Guide. Edited by Bauer M, Grof P, Müller-Oerlinghausen B Abingdon, UK, Informa Healthcare, 2006, pp 157–178

---

214 Which of the following medications has shown the most evidence for reducing suicide risk in the long-term treatment of bipolar disorder?

A. Carbamazepine.
B. Divalproex.
C. Gabapentin.
D. Lithium.
E. Olanzapine.

The correct response is option D: Lithium.

Lithium has more research evidence than any other anitmanic agent regarding its effect on reducing suicide and suicidal acts during long-term treatment of bipolar disorder. Lithium has been shown to be more effective than any other antimanic agent in reducing suicide risk. Patients treated with other antimanic agents likely have lower suicide risk than bipolar persons not medicated at all.

Tondo L, Isacsson G, Baldessarini RJ: Suicidal behavior in bipolar disorder: risk and prevention. CNS Drugs 2003; 17:491–511

Goodwin FK, Fireman B, Simon GE, Hunkeler EM, et al: Suicide risk in bipolar disorder during treatment with lithium and divalproex. JAMA 2003; 290:1467–1473

Cipriani A, Pretty H, Hawton K, Geddes JR. Lithium in the prevention of suicidal behavior and all-cause mortality in patients with mood disorders: A systematic review of randomized trials. Am J Psychiatry, Oct 2005; 162:1805–1819

215 A 56-year-old man with a history of cancer presents with confusion, pure amnestic syndrome, and affective symptoms. Diagnostic studies are consistent with paraneoplastic limbic encephalitis. Which of the following cancers is the most common cause of this paraneoplastic syndrome?

A. Pancreatic cancer.
B. Prostate cancer.
C. Renal cancer.
D. Small cell lung cancer.
E. Testicular cancer.

The correct response is option D: Small cell lung cancer.

Paraneoplastic "limbic encephalitis" results from an immunological cross-reaction between tumor antigens and antigens within the CNS. It can cause a range of psychiatric presentations including cognitive deficits, confusional states, a pure amnestic syndrome, and affective symptoms. Small cell carcinoma of the lung is the most common cause of paraneoplastic syndrome.

Levenson JL (ed): Essentials of Psychosomatic Medicine. American Psychiatric Publishing, Washington, DC, 2007. p 323

216 A 24-year-old man on lithium maintenance therapy develops severe, persistent polyuria and polydipsia. Which of the following medications is most likely to be effective in treating these side effects without requiring administration of supplemental electrolytes?

A. Amiloride.
B. Furosemide.
C. Hydrochlorothiazide.
D. Metolazone.
E. Torsemide.

The correct response is option A: Amiloride.

The most common renal effect of lithium is impaired concentrating capacity caused by reduced renal response to antidiuretic hormone (ADH), manifested as polyuria, polydipsia, or both. Although the polyuria associated with early lithium treatment may resolve, persistent polyuria may occur. Concurrent administration of a thiazide diuretic such as hydrochlorothiazide may be helpful. However, potassium levels must be monitored, and potassium replacement may be necessary. Amiloride, a potassium-sparing diuretic, is reported to be effective in treating lithium-induced polyuria and polydipsia. Its advantages are that it does not alter lithium levels and does not require administration of supplemental potassium.

American Psychiatric Association Practice Guideline for the Treatment of Patients with Bipolar Disorder, 2nd Edition (2002). Reprinted in FOCUS: Bipolar Disorder, 2003; 1:81–82. http://psychiatryonline.org/guidelines.aspx

217 A 17-year-old patient diagnosed with anorexia nervosa at age 14 is brought to a psychiatrist by her parents. They are concerned because she is 65% of her expected body weight. The most appropriate intervention is to:

A. Suggest a group therapy program.
B. Initiate treatment with an antidepressant.
C. Restore the patient's nutritional state.
D. Refer the patient and family for counseling.
E. Provide cognitive therapy.

The correct response is option C: Restore the patient's nutritional state.

The immediate aim of treatment should be to restore the patient's nutritional state to normal. Emaciation can cause irritability, depression, preoccupation with food, and sleep disturbance. It is exceedingly difficult to achieve behavioral change with psychotherapy in a patient who is experiencing the psychological effects of emaciation.

Hales RE, Yudofsky SC, Gabbard GO (eds): The American Psychiatric Publishing Textbook of Psychiatry, 5th ed. Washington, DC, American Psychiatric Publishing, 2008. p 980

218 According to the results of the Clinical Antipsychotic Trials of Intervention Effectiveness (CATIE) study, which antipsychotic medication had the lowest all-cause discontinuation rate?

A. Olanzapine.
B. Quetiapine.
C. Risperidone.
D. Ziprasidone.
E. Perphanazine.

The correct response is option A: Olanzapine.

The most prominent finding of the CATIE study was the 74% all-cause discontinuation rate before 18 months. The causes for discontinuation included lack of tolerability, lack of efficacy, clinician decision (due to safety concerns), and patient decision (electing to terminate). Among the atypical antipsychotics, the time to discontinuation was significantly longer for patients treated with olanzapine compared with those on risperidone and quetiapine but not compared to those on perphanazine or ziprasidone. In addition, completion rates for the 18-month study were olanzapine 36%, perphanazine 25%, quetiapine 18%, risperidone 26%, and ziprasidone 21%.

Lieberman JA, Stroup TS, McEvoy JP, Swartz MS, et al: Effectiveness of antipsychotic drugs in patients with chronic schizophrenia. N Engl J Med. 2005; 353:1209–23

219 Which of the following medication combinations for individuals with OCD comorbid with tic disorder is supported best by evidence?

A. Fluoxetine plus clonazepam.
B. Sertraline plus buspirone.
C. Mirtazapine plus naltrexone.
D. Fluvoxamine plus haloperidol.

The correct response is option D: Fluvoxamine plus haloperidol.

Evidence indicates that individuals with OCD and comorbid tic disorder respond better to fluvoxamine plus haloperidol. Whereas SSRIs are typical first-line treatments for OCD, clonazepam has not consistently demonstrated effectiveness for OCD nor for OCD with a tic disorder. The combination of clomipramine and risperidone can be helpful in treating difficult cases of OCD, but it is not as effective as an SSRI plus haloperidol for OCD comorbid with a tic disorder. The combination of mirtazapine plus naltrexone is not studied for OCD.

Fineberg NA, Gale TM, Sivakumaran T. A review of antipsychotics in the treatment of obsessive compulsive disorder. J Psychopharmacology 2006; 20:97–103. Reprinted in FOCUS: OCD summer 2007 3
Hales RE, Yudofsky SC, Gabbard GO (eds): The American Psychiatric Publishing Textbook of Psychiatry, 5th ed. Arlington, VA, American Psychiatric Publishing, 2008, pp 558–63
Schatzberg AF, Nemeroff CB (eds): Essentials of Clinical Psychopharmacology, 2nd ed, Washington, DC, American Psychiatric Publishing, 2006, p 536
Geller DA, Biederman J, Stewart SE, et al. Which SSRI? A meta-analysis of pharmacotherapy trials in pediatric obsessivecompulsive disorder. Am J Psychiatry 2003; 160:1919–1928

220 Studies of the neurobiological correlates of borderline personality disorder have revealed hyperactivity in which one of the following?

A. Amygdala.
B. Prefrontal cortex.
C. Tegmental area.
D. Cingulate.
E. Accumbens.

The correct response is option A: Amygdala.

The amygdala, prefrontal and preorbital cortex, and the anterior cingulate have all been implicated in the neurobiology of borderline personality disorder. Specifically, the prefrontal cortex and anterior cingulate are hypoactive, whereas the amygdala is hyperactive, in borderline personality disorder. The ventral tegmental area and the nucleus accumbens have not been clearly linked to borderline personality disorder.

Kernberg OF, Michels R: Borderline personality disorder. Am J Psychiatry. 2009; 166:505–8

---

221 A 38-year-old patient with major depressive disorder has had a partial response to 80 mg of citalopram. He states this is the best drug that he has been on, but he continues to experience symptoms despite being on the medication for 7 weeks. He continues to occasionally have suicidal thoughts, which frightens him because he made a suicide attempt 4 years ago. The best intervention at this time is to augment with:

A. Fluoxetin.
B. Lamotrigine.
C. Lithium.
D. Thyroid.
E. Buspirone.

The correct response is option C: Lithium.

The choice of lithium is best for two reasons: it has the best data as being an effective augmentation drug, and it lowers the risk of suicide. Lamotrigine and thyroid are used for augmentation, but the data supporting this use are not as strong as that for lithium, and there are no data on their impact on suicide. Buspirone is a possibility, but lithium is a better choice for the reasons listed above. There is no reason to augment with a second SSRI (fluoxetine) because the serotonin transporters are already inhibited by citalopram.

American Psychiatric Association Practice Guideline for the Treatment of Patients With Major Depressive Disorder, 3rd ed (2010). http://psychiatryonline.org/guidelines.aspx
American Psychiatric Association Practice Guideline for the Treatment of Patients with Suicidal Behaviors, 2nd ed (2000), p 1375. http://psychiatryonline.org/guidelines.aspx

---

222 Which of the following medications for bipolar disorder has been associated with polycystic ovarian syndrome (PCOS)?

A. Topiramate.
B. Divalproex.
C. Carbamazepine.
D. Lamotrigine.
E. Lithium.

The correct response is option B: Divalproex.

In the Systematic Treatment Enhancement Program for Bipolar Disorder (STEP-BD), 230 women ages 18–45 were evaluated for PCOS. Oligoamenorrhea with hyperandrogenism developed in 10.5% of women on valproate, compared with 1.4% of women on lithium or a nonvalproate anticonvulsant. Oligoamenorrhea always had its onset during the first year of valproate therapy. Although not all studies have found such an association, divalproex (valproate) is the only drug of those listed above that has been linked to PCOS.

Joffe H, Cohen LS, Suppes T, McLaughlin WL, et al: Valproate is associated with new-onset oligoamenorrhea with hyperandrogenism in women with bipolar disorder. Biol Psychiatry 2006; 59:1078–1086
Rasgon N: The relationship between polycystic ovary syndrome and antiepileptic drugs: a review of the evidence. J Clin Psychopharmacol 2004; 24:322–334

---

223 The parents of a 4-year-old boy report that a few hours after he goes to sleep, their son will suddenly get up in the bed and look extremely frightened. His heart races; he is diaphoretic and cries out. He is difficult to awaken and has no recall of the event the next morning. Which of the following is the most appropriate next step in the management of this patient?

A. Administer a short-acting hypnotic for 2 weeks.
B. Have the child go to bed at a later time.
C. Obtain an electroencephalogram to rule out temporal lobe epilepsy.
D. Reassure the parents that their son will outgrow the disorder.
E. Suggest to the parents that they allow their son to sleep with them for a temporary period.

The correct response is option D: Reassure the parents that their son will outgrow the disorder.

The patient presents with classic symptoms of night terror. These occur during stage 3 and 4 of non-REM sleep, so they are not associated with nightmares. Because the child is in deep sleep, he will be difficult to arouse and have no recall of a bad dream. The episodes tend to occur during the first third of the night when individuals are most likely to be in stage 3 or 4 of non-REM sleep. Occurrence usually is in childhood. If onset is later, such as adolescence, it may be prudent to obtain an electroencephalogram to rule out temporal lobe epilepsy. This is usually a self-limiting disorder that children outgrow. So, the next best step is to reassure the parents. Rarely is there a need to administer a hypnotic.

Saddock BJ, Saddock VA. Pocket Handbook of Clinical Psychiatry. 4th ed. Philadelphia, PA. Lippincott Williams and Wilkins, 2005. pp 243–244

---

224 A 68-year-old woman being treated for bipolar disorder became semicomatose and incontinent of urine. Her serum sodium concentration was 110 mmol/L. Which of the following medications is the most likely cause?

A. Lithium.
B. Divalproex.
C. Oxcarbazepine.
D. Lamotrigine.
E. Olanzapine.

The correct response is option C: Oxcarbazepine.

Dong and colleagues found that the frequency of hyponatremia (Na+ <134) was 29.9% among 97 oxcarbazepine-treated patients having severe (Na+ <128) hyponatremia. Hyponatremia was much more likely in patients over 40 years of age and in patients treated simultaneously with levetiracetam. Patients whose sodium levels were low at their initial visit after starting oxcarbazepine were much more likely than patients with normal sodium at the initial visit to have persistent hyponatremia.

Dong X, Leppik IE, White J, Rarick J: Hyponatremia from oxcarbazepine and carbamazepine. Neurology 2005; 65:1976–1978

Sachdeo RC, Wasserstein A, Mesenbrink PJ, D'Souza J: Effects of oxcarbazepine on sodium concentration and water handling. Ann Neurol 2002; 51:613–620

---

225 In bipolar disorder, which of the following characteristics BEST differentiates adult-onset bipolar disorder from childhood-onset?

A. Presence of psychotic features.
B. Prolonged early course.
C. Mixed episodes.
D. Recurrent depression.
E. Treatment resistance.

The correct response is option D: Recurrent depression.

Patients with childhood-onset bipolar disorder are more likely to have psychotic features; have a more severe course of illness; be male; have a comorbid substance use disorder; experience fewer remissions; have manic and mixed episodes; have a more prolonged early course; and be treatment-resistant. Patients with adult-onset bipolar disorder are more likely to experience recurrent episodes of depression.

Dulcan MK, Weiner JM. Essentials of Child and Adolescent Psychiatry. Arlington (VA): American Psychiatric Publishing, 2006. pp 273–274

---

226 A psychiatrist's neighbor tells her that he is having trouble sleeping due to work-related stresses. He asks for recommendations and some medication until he can get an appointment with his internist. What ethical problem results if the psychiatrist gives the neighbor the medication?

A. Prescribing medication creates a doctor-patient relationship.
B. The assistance may be ineffective, straining the relationship.
C. Providing free care can foster resentment.
D. Assisting this neighbor creates an expectation that the psychiatrist will treat other neighbors.

The correct response is option A: Prescribing medication creates a doctor-patient relationship.

Giving advice and medication may create a doctor-patient relationship with an associated expectation of duty of care.

Simon RI. Quick reference for forensic and ethical issues in psychiatry, FOCUS: Forensic and Ethical Issues; Fall 2003; 4:345

---

227 A local radio talk show host comes to see you for psychotherapy because you were described as "the best doctor at the clinic" by one of his friends. He spends most of the hour talking about problems he is having with a workmate who he feels is treating him rudely. At the end of the session, he asks to be seen at a special time to accommodate his work schedule. When you tell him you will be unavailable at that time, he becomes dismissive and angry. These traits are suggestive of which ONE of the following personality disorders?

A. Schizoid.
B. Antisocial.
C. Obsessive-compulsive.
D. Narcissistic.
E. Borderline.

The correct response is option D: Narcissistic.

Criteria for narcissistic personality disorder can include having a grandiose sense of self-importance, believing that one is special and can only be understood by other special people, and a sense of entitlement including unreasonable expectations of favorable treatment.

American Psychiatric Association: Diagnostic and Statistical Manual of Mental Disorders, 5th Edition. Arlington, VA, American Psychiatric Association, 2013. pp 669–671

---

228 In DSM-5, in what way are the criteria for anorexia nervosa revised from DSM-IV?

A. The amenorrhea requirement is lifted.
B. A subtype related to atypical anorexia is added.
C. The "significantly low body weight" requirement is removed.
D. The diagnostic criteria for anorexia nervosa were not revised.

The correct response is option A: The amenorrhea requirement is lifted.

In DSM-5 criteria for anorexia nervosa, the DSM-IV Criterion D requiring amenorrhea, or the absence of at least three menstrual cycles, has been deleted. This criterion cannot be applied to males, premenarchal females, females taking oral contraceptives, and postmenopausal females. In some cases, individuals exhibit all other symptoms and signs of anorexia nervosa but still report some menstrual activity.

American Psychiatric Association: Diagnostic and Statistical Manual of Mental Disorders, 5th Edition. Arlington, VA, American Psychiatric Association, 2013, Highlights of Changes From DSM-IV-TR to DSM-5. Eating Disorders, p 813

---

229 Which of the following traumatic events is MOST likely to induce PTSD in exposed individuals?

A. Unexpected death.
B. Natural disasters.
C. Motor vehicle accidents.
D. Witness to violence.
E. Sexual assault.

The correct response is option E: Sexual assault.

Individuals exposed to interpersonal violence tend to have higher rates of PTSD. Although PTSD can occur after any type of trauma, some types of trauma are more likely to be problematic.

American Psychiatric Association Practice Guideline for the Treatment of Patients with Acute Stress Disorder and Posttraumatic Stress Disorder. 2004. http://psychiatryonline.org/guidelines.aspx

230 A 9-year-old boy is brought by his mother at the insistence of the school for the assessment of behavior problems. The diagnosis of attention-deficit/hyperactivity (ADHD) disorder is made, along with the recommendation to start stimulant medication. The mother is concerned that stimulant medication might put her son at risk for developing substance use problems. Regarding the risk of developing substance use problems, what is known about stimulant treatment for ADHD?

A. Increased risk of drug dependence only.
B. Increased risk of both alcohol and drug dependence.
C. Decreased risk of drug dependence only.
D. Decreased risk of both alcohol and drug dependence.
E. Unchanged risk for both alcohol and drug dependence.

The correct response is option D: Decreased risk of both alcohol and drug dependence.

Treatment of childhood ADHD with psychostimulant medication reduces the risk of both alcohol and drug use disorders during adolescence and adulthood. Individuals with untreated ADHD are at greater risk for developing substance use disorders.

Wilens TE, Faraone SV, Biederman J, et al.: Does stimulant therapy of attention-deficit/hyperactivity disorder beget later substance abuse? A meta-analytic review of the literature. Pediatrics 2003; 111:179–85

Biederman J, Wilens T, Mick E, et al.: Is ADHD a risk factor for psychoactive substance use disorders? Findings from a four-year prospective follow-up study. J Am Acad Child Adolesc Psychiatry 1997; 36:21–29. Reprinted in FOCUS: Substance Related Disorders; Spring 2003.; 2:96–204

Groenman AP, Oosterlaan J, Rommelse NN, et al: Stimulant treatment for attention-deficit hyperactivity disorder and risk of developing substance use disorder. Br J Psychiatry. 2013 Aug;203(2):112–119

231 Which of the following disorders must be considered specifically in the differential diagnosis of individuals with late-onset (after the age of 45 years) OCD?

A. Huntington's disease.
B. Autism spectrum disorder.
C. Delusional disorder.
D. Body dysmorphic disorder.
E. Schizophrenia.

The correct response is option A: Huntington's disease.

Individuals diagnosed with OCD after the age of 45 years (late onset) should specifically be evaluated for neurodegenerative illnesses (e.g., Huntington's disease), traumatic injury, or neoplastic and vascular causes. Early symptoms of Huntington's disease may include instability of mood, irritability, or compulsive behaviors. Symptoms of autism spectrum disorders are present from early childhood. The other answers should be considered at any age at onset.

Martis B, Keuthen NJ, Wilson KA, Jenike M. Obsessive-compulsive disorder, in Clinical Manual of Anxiety Disorders. Edited by Stein DJ. American Psychiatric Publishing, Washington DC, 2004, p 94

232 A psychiatrist has been seeing a terminally ill woman in psychotherapy. The patient has become too ill to come to the office, so the psychiatrist elects to make a house call. In committing this boundary crossing, he should:

A. Act in a more social manner.
B. Discuss this variation from usual practice with a lawyer before going.
C. Discuss the implications of this change of venue with the patient.
D. Never go to the patient's home.

The correct response is option C: Discuss the implications of this change of venue with the patient.

The psychiatrist should act professionally, discuss the situation with his patient, and document the discussion.

Gutheil TG. Boundary issues in: American Psychiatric Publishing Textbook of Personality Disorders, edited by Oldham J, Skodol AE, Bender DS. American Psychiatric Publishing, 2005, p 428

---

233 Which of the following is the most common psychiatric symptom found in patients with fibromyalgia?

A. Anorexia.
B. Psychosis.
C. Hypersomnia.
D. Mania.
E. Depression.

The correct response is option E: Depression.

Patients with fibromyalgia commonly have depression, anxiety, and insomnia. Individuals with this disorder also tend to have a family or prior history of depression and antidepressant use.

Arnold LM. Management of fibromyalgia and comorbid psychiatric disorders. J Clin Psychiatry. 2008; 69(supplement 2):14

---

234 Which type of treatment program has the best short-term outcomes for cocaine dependence?

A. Voucher-based contingency management.
B. Psychodynamic group psychotherapy.
C. Interpersonal psychotherapy.
D. Twelve-step groups (without other counseling).
E. Cue exposure therapy.

The correct response is option A: Voucher-based contingency management.

Voucher-based contingency management has yielded good outcomes in a number of studies with diverse populations. The psychodynamically based psychotherapies, group and interpersonal psychotherapy, have shown good outcomes predominantly in case series, so they do not have a sufficient evidence base to recommend them in this situation. Attendance at 12-step groups alone has not been shown to be an acceptable alternative to more formal treatment. Twelve-step facilitation therapy and individual drug counseling both use 12-step principles and encourage group participation; these modalities have been shown to have good outcomes. Cue exposure therapy, although not extensively studied, has been shown to be not effective.

American Psychiatric Association Practice Guideline for the Treatment of Patients with Substance Use Disorders, 2nd Edition (2006), pp 449–451. http://psychiatryonline.org/guidelines.aspx

Pechnick RN, Glasner-Edwards S, Hrymoc M, Wilkins, JN. Preclinical development and clinical implementation of treatments for substance abuse disorders. FOCUS: Substance Abuse: Spring 2007; 2:158–159

---

235 A patient in therapy has recently been told that his psychiatrist may change jobs and will be transferring his care to another psychiatrist. He has always needed a great deal of reassurance but now calls almost daily asking for opinions on decisions he is trying to make in his life. He often worries his ill wife will die before he does. Each time he is advised to attend day treatment to get further support; he often agrees to do so but does not follow through. On the basis of this vignette, which of the following personality disorders is most likely?

A. Dependent.
B. Antisocial.
C. Paranoid.
D. Borderline.
E. Narcissistic.

The correct response is option A: Dependent.

Criteria for dependent personality disorder include unrealistic fears of abandonment, urgently seeking another relationship as a source of support when a close relationship ends, difficulty in expressing disagreements with others, and difficulty initiating projects on one's own.

American Psychiatric Association: Diagnostic and Statistical Manual of Mental Disorders, 5th Edition. Arlington, VA, American Psychiatric Association, 2013, pp 675–678

---

236 During an initial evaluation, a patient complains of multiple episodes of having palpitations, sweating, and intense anxiety. Information that would be most supportive of panic disorder is that the episodes occur when the patient:

A. Is reminded of a past assault.
B. Must use a public bathroom.
C. Attends a large party.
D. Is in essentially any setting.
E. Must use an elevator.

The correct response is option D: Is in essentially any setting.

Panic episodes can occur in multiple types of settings, and panic disorder should not be diagnosed if these episodes occur within the context of another anxiety disorder. Panic episodes also can occur due to medical causes or substances. Option A is suggestive of posttraumatic stress disorder. Option B may indicate OCD. Option C may be social phobia. Option D is most indicative of panic disorder. Option E may be a simple phobia or agoraphobia.

Kinrys G, Pollack MH. Panic disorder and agoraphobia, in Clinical Manual of Anxiety Disorders. Edited by Stein DJ. American Psychiatric Publishing, Washington DC, 2004, 13–16

---

237 Which of the following statements most accurately describes the benefits of SSRIs in the treatment of PTSD? SSRIs have been shown to

A. Ameliorate core PTSD and other associated symptoms.
B. Treat primarily the comorbid psychiatric disorders.
C. Improve primarily hyperarousal symptoms.
D. Improve the effectiveness of α_2-adrenergic agonists.
E. Act only to augment psychotherapy in PTSD.

The correct response is option A: Ameliorate core PTSD and other associated symptoms.

SSRIs have been demonstrated in randomized, double-blind controlled studies to be effective in the treatment of PTSD because of their effectiveness in treating the core symptoms of PTSD, the disorders typically comorbid with PTSD, the associated problematic behavioral symptoms, and their side-effect profile. SSRIs are considered the first-line medication treatment for PTSD.

American Psychiatric Association Practice Guideline for the Treatment of Patients with Acute Stress Disorder and Posttraumatic Stress Disorder. Am J Psychiatry. 2004; 161(11):17. http://psychiatryonline.org/guidelines.aspx

---

238 Which of the following factors will increase the potential for toxicity with lithium?

A. Cigarette smoking.
B. Concomitant administration of mirtazapine (Remeron).
C. Drinking a lot of water.
D. Exercising outdoors on a hot day.

The correct response is option D: Exercising outdoors on a hot day.

Exercise leads to dehydration and reduced volume of distribution (and therefore lithium toxicity). A first response to lithium toxicity is to encourage drinking water. Lithium is excreted through the kidney and not the liver. Antidepressants are generally safely administered with lithium. Cigarette smoking has known effects on cytochrome P450 enzymes in liver, but lithium is venally secreted without hepatic involvement.

Sadock BJ, Sadock VA, Ruiz P (eds): Kaplan & Sadock's Comprehensive Textbook of Psychiatry, 9th ed. Philadelphia, Lippincott Williams & Wilkins, 2009, pp 1353–59

---

239 An individual with a history of opiate dependence admits to daily use of opiates, but a confirmatory urine toxicology screen is negative. Which of the following opiates is the patient most likely using?

A. Hydrocodone.
B. Morphine.
C. Codeine.
D. Heroin.
E. Opium.

The correct response is option A: Hydrocodone.

In testing for opioids, urine toxicology screens primarily test for drugs derived from opium, such as morphine, codeine, and heroin. Synthetic opioids such as hydrocodone, methadone, and oxycodone may not be detected by standard tests.

Center for Substance Abuse Treatment. Detoxification and Substance Abuse Treatment. Treatment Improvement Protocol (TIP) Series 45. DHHS Publication No. (SMA) 06-4131. Rockville, MD: Substance Abuse and Mental Health Services Administration, 2006, pp 50–1. Also available at http://www.ncbi.nlm.nih.gov/books/NBK64115/pdf/TOC.pdf

---

240 A 72-year-old man with severe chronic obstructive airway disease complains of anxiety, muscle tension, and a general feeling of uneasiness. The most appropriate psychotropic medication for this patient's condition would be:

A. Clonazepam.
B. Diazepam.
C. Alprazolam.
D. Lorazepam.
E. Buspirone.

The correct response is option E: Buspirone.

In treating anxiety disorders in patients with significant respiratory problems, it is often important to consider respiratory function. Anxiolytics may depress respiratory drive and further aggravate the patient's condition. Because buspirone produces no respiratory depression, it is an option to be considered in treating anxiety in these patients.

Schatzberg AF, Nemeroff CB (eds): Textbook of Psychopharmacology, 4th ed. Arlington, VA, American Psychiatric Publishing, 2009, pp 491–94

---

241 Which of the following statements best describes the mechanism of action of acamprosate thought to occur in the treatment of alcohol use disorder?

A. Acamprosate blocks the reuptake of chloride ions in central GABAergic neurons.
B. Acamprosate competes with alcohol for central GABAergic neurons in a dose-dependent fashion.
C. Acamprosate affects μ opiate receptors blocking the centrally mediated reinforcing effects of alcohol.
D. Acamprosate inhibits aldehyde dehydrogenase, resulting in the accumulation of toxic levels of acetaldehyde.
E. Acamposate reduces neuronal hyperactivity during early alcohol recovery.

The correct response is option E: Acamprosate reduces neuronal hyperactivity during early alcohol recovery.

Acamprosate is a small, flexible molecule that resembles GABA and decreases glutamatergic neurotransmission, perhaps by acting as an *N*-methyl-D-aspartate antagonist. It has been proposed that this medication helps sustain abstinence in detoxified alcohol-dependent individuals by reducing neuronal hyperactivity during early recovery.

American Psychiatric Association Practice Guideline for the Treatment of Patients with Substance Use Disorders, Second Edition, (2006). pp 383–384. http://psychiatryonline.org/guidelines.aspx

Mason B. Acamprosate for alcohol dependence: an update for the clinician. FOCUS: Psychopharmacology Fall 2006; 4:505–506

Dermatis H, Galanter M. Clinical advances in pharmacological and integrated treatment approaches for alcohol and drug use disorders. FOCUS: Substance Abuse Spring 2007:2:142

---

242 Which of the following substances is associated with an increase in the long-term risk of developing psychotic disorder?

A. Alcohol.
B. Cannabis.
C. Nicotine.
D. Opiates.
E. Inhalants.

The correct response is option B: Cannabis.

A large meta-analysis demonstrated that cannabis use increases the risk of psychotic outcomes independent of transient intoxication. Although other substances may cause psychotic symptoms during periods of intoxication, no evidence exists to support an independent risk for psychosis as a result of using these other substances.

Moore THM, Zammit S, Lingford-Hughes A, Barnes TRE, et al: Cannabis use and risk of psychotic or affective mental health outcomes: a systematic review. Lancet 2007; 370:319–28

Veen ND, Selten J, Van der Tweel I, Feller WG, et al: Cannabis Use and Age at Onset of Schizophrenia. Am J Psychiatry. 2004;161:501–506

Davis GP, Compton MT, Wang S, Levin FR, Blanco C. Association between cannabis use, psychosis, and schizotypal personality disorder: findings from the National Epidemiologic Survey on Alcohol and Related Conditions. Schizophr Res. 2013 Dec;151(1–3):197–202

---

243 A psychiatrist may terminate care of a patient in which of the following circumstances?

A. Patient has not paid a bill.
B. Patient has failed to be cooperative in treatment.
C. Patient has consultation with another psychiatrist.
D. Patient misses two appointments and does not return the psychiatrist's calls.
E. Patient is hospitalized on an inpatient unit and care is permanently transferred.

The correct response is option E: The patient is hospitalized on an inpatient unit and care is permanently transferred.

If a patient is hospitalized and his/her care is permanently transferred to another physician, then termination is legal and ethical. However, unless the patient is being permanently transferred to the care of the hospitalizing psychiatrist, failure to attend to a patient during hospitalization may be considered abandonment. Mere nonpayment of a bill, failure to be cooperative, consultation with another mental health professional, or failure to keep an appointment are not appropriate causes for termination if the patient continues to need treatment.

Simon RI, Shuman DW. Clinical Manual of Psychiatry and Law. Arlington, VA, American Psychiatric Publishing, 2007, pp 28–34

---

244 Which of the following medications, commonly used in alcohol treatment to decrease craving, has been shown to be more effective if given after a period of sobriety?

A. Acamprosate.
B. Disulfiram.
C. Gabapentin.
D. Naltrexone.
E. Topiramate.

The correct response is option A: Acamprosate.

The goal of using acamprosate is to decrease the relapse rate after an initial abstinence period has been achieved. In European clinical trials, acamprosate has been shown to be most effective in those who have achieved a period of abstinence from alcohol (usually 7–10 days). U.S. studies have not replicated this finding. However, it is suspected that this is because of a difference in the psychotherapies provided. The European studies tended to use more formalized counseling as opposed to the medication management visit approach used in the U.S. studies.

American Psychiatric Association Practice Guideline for the Treatment of Patients with Substance Use Disorders, 2nd ed. 2006, pp 383–384. http://psychiatryonline.org/guidelines.aspx

Connery HS, Kleber HD. Guideline Watch: Practice Guideline for the Treatment of Patients with Substance Use Disorders, 2nd ed. April 2007. http://psychiatryonline.org/guidelines.aspx

Mason B. Acamprosate for alcohol dependence: an update for the clinician. FOCUS: Psychopharmacology Fall 2006; 4:507–508

---

245 Which of the following is characteristic of social anxiety disorder (social phobia)?

A. Spontaneous uncued panic attacks.
B. Avoiding public speaking because of trembling.
C. Fear of humiliation when speaking in a group setting.
D. Fainting while having blood drawn.
E. Avoiding parties because of fear of contamination.

The correct response is option C: Fear of humiliation when speaking in a group setting.

According to DSM-5, "the essential feature of social phobia is a marked and persistent fear of social or performance situations in which the individual is exposed to possible scrutiny by others." Although panic attacks can be associated with social phobia, they tend to be cued by the social situation and are not spontaneous or uncued as seen in panic disorder. Social avoidance because of concern about a potentially embarrassing manifestation of a medical disorder (e.g., tremor of Parkinson's disease) is more appropriately diagnosed as anxiety disorder, not otherwise specified. Fainting during a blood draw would be diagnosed a as specific phobia, blood-injection-injury type. Avoidance due to fear of contamination would be characteristic of obsessive-compulsive disorder.

American Psychiatric Association: Diagnostic and Statistical Manual of Mental Disorders, 5th Edition. Arlington, VA, American Psychiatric Association, 2013, pp 202–207

---

246 A patient with OCD and fears of contamination insists that his family remove their shoes when they enter his living space. Which of the following concepts best describes this behavior?

A. Repetition compulsion.
B. Displacement.
C. Ritual by proxy.
D. Projection.
E. Reaction formation.

The correct response is option C: Ritual by proxy.

As rituals become an essential act to control anxiety, patients may attempt to get family members to partake in the behavior. Called "ritual by proxy," the patient's demands may extend to insisting the family have "outside" and "inside" clothes. Sometimes the patient insists the family reassure him that he has completed a task that will avoid a "dangerous" outcome; for example, "Did I turn off the gas?" The family must tell him that he did, numerous times. The treatment for such behavior is "ritual prevention" in which the family reminds the patient that the psychiatrist has told the family not to comply. The other choices are defense mechanisms that are not specific to OCD.

Stein DJ, Hollander E, Rothbaum BO (eds): Textbook of Anxiety Disorders, 2nd ed. Arlington, VA, American Psychiatric Publishing, 2010, p 343

---

247 A 48-year-old woman is brought to the emergency department after being found unconscious. Examination reveals respiratory depression, extreme miosis, stupor, coma, and pulmonary edema. The patient's presentation is MOST consistent with an overdose of:

A. Alcohol.
B. Cannabis.
C. Inhalants.
D. Opioids.
E. Sedative-hypnotics.

The correct response is option D: Opioids.

The syndrome of acute opioid overdose is recognized by extreme miosis or in severe cases by mydriasis (due to anoxia), drowsiness, slurred speech, and impairment in attention and memory and sometimes pulmonary edema. Overdose is a medical emergency and can result in coma, shock, and death. Naloxone is an opioid receptor antagonist that can be used to reverse the effects of opiates used in overdose.

Hales RE, Yudofsky SC: Substance use disorders, in The American Psychiatric Publishing Textbook of Psychiatry, 5th ed. Arlington, VA, American Psychiatric Publishing, 2008, pp 384–87

---

248 Patients with obsessive-compulsive disorder are most likely to respond to which of the following therapy modalities?

A. Psychoanalysis.
B. Dynamic psychotherapy.
C. Dialectical behavior therapy.
D. Motivational enhancement therapy.
E. Exposure and response prevention.

The correct response is option E: Exposure and response prevention.

Behavioral treatment, in particular exposure therapy, to decrease anxiety associated with obsessions and response prevention to decrease the frequency of rituals or obsessions has been demonstrated to be very effective in the treatment of OCD. There are no controlled studies that demonstrate effectiveness of dynamic psychotherapy or psychoanalysis in dealing with the core symptoms of OCD. Dialectical behavior therapy is a specialized form of therapy developed for the treatment of borderline personality disorder, and motivational enhancement therapy is a type of therapy developed for the treatment of substance use disorders.

American Psychiatric Association Practice Guideline for the Treatment of Patients with Obsessive-Compulsive Disorder 2007. http://psychiatryonline.org/guidelines.aspx
Hales RE, Yudofsky SC, Gabbard GO (eds): The American Psychiatric Publishing Textbook of Psychiatry, 5th ed. Arlington, VA, American Psychiatric Publishing, 2008, pp 374, 564–65, 842, 1235

---

249 Which of following is the most common fear during the dying process?

A. Loneliness.
B. Abandonment.
C. Pain.
D. Uncertainty.

The correct response is option C: Pain.

All of the above choices are important to the dying patient, but fear of physical suffering appears to be the most common. It is the issue most often mentioned in the definition of a "good death." There is increased attention paid to pain relief currently; hospital staff members are required to ask patients to rate their pain on a scale of 1 (least) to 10 (unbearable). Staff should make efforts to keep the pain level at 5 or below.

Roberts LW, Dyer AR: A Concise Guide to Ethics in Mental Health Care, Washington, DC, American Psychiatric Publishing, 2004, pp 187–188

Wise MG, Rundell JR (eds): Textbook of Consultation-Liaison Psychiatry., 2nd ed. Washington, DC, American Psychiatric Publishing, 2002, pp 772–773

Levenson JL (ed): Textbook of Psychosomatic Medicine. Arlington, VA, American Psychiatric Publishing, 2005, pp 981–82

---

250 A 38-year-old woman is admitted to the hospital with a severe manic episode. On examination, she is noted to have motor excitement, mutism, and stereotypic movements. Which of the following medications would be the most appropriate in treating this patient?

A. Carbamazepine.
B. Haloperidol.
C. Lamotrigine.
D. Lorazepam.
E. Olanzapine.

The correct response is option D: Lorazepam.

Motor excitement, mutism, and stereotypic movements are consistent with catatonia. Catatonic features may develop in up to one-third of patients during a manic episode. In treating catatonia, neuroleptics have generally exhibited poor efficacy and may be associated with an increased likelihood of neuroleptic malignant syndrome. In contrast, prospective studies have demonstrated the efficacy of lorazepam in the treatment of catatonic syndromes, including those associated with mania.

American Psychiatric Association Practice Guideline for the Treatment of Patients with Bipolar Disorder, 2nd ed. (2002). http://psychiatryonline.org/guidelines.aspx

Taylor MA, Fink M. Catatonia in psychiatric classification: a home of its own. Am J Psychiatry. 2003 Jul;160(7):1233–41

Bush G, Fink M, Petrides G, Dowling F, Francis A: Catatonia. II. Treatment with lorazepam and electroconvulsive therapy. Acta Psychiatr Scand. 1996 Feb;93(2):137–43

---

251 A 35-year-old man with a history of opiate dependence is brought to the emergency department after being found unconscious. Examination reveals respiratory depression, extreme miosis, stupor, coma, and pulmonary edema. The emergency department physician administers naloxone 1 mg intravenously every 3 minutes until a maximum dosage of 10 mg has been given. However, the patient remains unresponsive. What would be the most appropriate next step?

A. Double the next intravenous dose of naloxone.
B. Increase the frequency with which the naloxone is administered.
C. Reconsider the diagnosis of an opioid overdose.
D. Start a continuous infusion of naloxone.
E. Switch from intravenous naloxone to nasogastric administration of naltrexone.

The correct response is option C: Reconsider the diagnosis of an opioid overdose.

The recommendations for the administration of naloxone are repeated doses every 3 minutes until respiratory or CNS depression is completely reversed or until a maximum dose of 10 mg IV has been given. Because of the poor bioavailability from significant hepatic first-pass effects, naloxone for acute intoxication is typically administered intravenously rather than nasogastrically. After the patient has received 10 mg of naloxone and remains unresponsive, it is very unlikely that the symptoms are due to an opioid overdose, and other diagnoses should be considered.

American Psychiatric Association Practice Guideline for the Treatment of Patients with Substance Use Disorders, 2nd Edition (2006), p 35. http://psychiatryonline.org/guidelines.aspx

Hales RE, Yudofsky SC: Substance use disorders, in The American Psychiatric Publishing Textbook of Psychiatry, 5th ed. Arlington, VA, American Psychiatric Publishing, 2008, pp 384–87

252 The concept that directs child psychiatrists and health care providers to involve children in decisions about their care commensurate with their developmental capacity is referred to as:

A. Cognitive incapacity.
B. Pediatric assent.
C. Pediatric consent.
D. Remaining autonomy.

The correct response is option B: Pediatric assent.

Informed consent applies to patients who have reached adulthood, except when the patient has been determined to lack capacity. As argued by the American Academy of Pediatrics Committee on Bioethics, decision making involving the health care of older children and adolescents should include, to the greatest extent possible, the assent of the patient as well as the participation of the parents and the physician. Pediatricians should not necessarily treat children as rational autonomous decision makers (pediatric consent) but should give serious consideration to each patient's developing capacities (vs. incapacities) for participating in decision making, including rationality and autonomy. "Remaining autonomy" refers to patients who are becoming increasingly impaired in cognition.

American Academy of Pediatrics, Committee on Bioethics. Informed consent, parental permission, and assent in pediatric practice. Pediatrics 1995; 95:314–317

Coverdale J, McCullough LB, Molinari V, Workman R. Ethically justified clinical strategies for promoting geriatric assent. Int J Geriatr Psychiatry 2006; 21:151–7

253 Which of the following syndromes is the most common form of inherited intellectual disability?

A. Fragile X syndrome.
B. Williams syndrome.
C. Rett syndrome.
D. Prader-Willi syndrome.
E. Angelman syndrome.

The correct response is option A: Fragile X syndrome.

Fragile X syndrome is the most common cause of inherited intellectual disability. It is reported to occur in 1 in 4,000 males and 1 per 8,000 females. Fragile X is caused by dysfunction of FMR1 gene at Xq27.3. It is characterized by large testicles, connective tissue disease, large head with prominent forehead and jaw, long face with large ears, and intellectual disability usually in the moderate to severe range.

The other entities listed are also genetic syndromes associated with intellectual disability; their rates of occurrence are approximately:

Williams syndrome: 1 in 7,500;
Rett syndrome: 1 in 10,000;
Angelman syndrome: 1 in 10,000 to 20,000;
Prader-Willi syndrome: 1 in 30,000.

Smoller JW, Sheidley BR, Tsuang MT. Psychiatric Genetics: Applications in Clinical Practice. American Psychiatric Publishing, 1st edition, 2008, pp 200–212

Dulcan MK (ed), Dulcan's Textbook of Child and Adolescent Psychiatry. American Psychiatric Publishing, Washington, DC 2010, Chapter 12. Intellectual Disability (Mental Retardation), pp 157–159

254 Hypertensive paroxysms associated with diaphoresis, tachycardia, flushing, nausea, and significant apprehension suggests the presence of which of the following general medical conditions that mimics anxiety?

A. Mitral valve problem.
B. Cocaine withdrawal.
C. Coronary insufficiency.
D. Hyperthyroidism.
E. Pheochromocytoma.

The correct response is option E: Pheochromocytoma.

The question describes the clinical features of pheochromocytoma, also known as chromaffin tumors. These are derived most often from the adrenal medulla, as well as the sympathetic ganglia. The clinical features of these tumors, most commonly hypertensive paroxysms, are predominantly due to the release of catecholamines.

Hales RE, Yudofsky SC, and Gabbard GO (eds): The American Psychiatric Publishing Textbook of Psychiatry, 5th ed. Arlington, VA, American Psychiatric Publishing, 2008. p 522

Kay J, Tasman A. Essentials of Psychiatry. Hoboken, NJ, John Wiley and Sons, 2006. pp 399–401

---

255 Behavioral therapy for a patient with OCD is most difficult when which of the following symptoms are present?

A. Observable rituals.
B. Delusions.
C. Contamination fears.
D. Checking behaviors.

The correct response is option B: Delusions.

Preservation of insight is an OCD hallmark. Although compelled to respond to inappropriate or bizarre rituals, good-prognosis OCD patients retain the awareness that their responses are unreasonable. Observable rituals, checking behaviors, and contamination fears lend themselves readily to behavioral manipulation, and severe symptoms may require extended therapy.

Greist JH, Baer L. Psychotherapy for obsessive-compulsive disorder. In: American Psychiatric Publishing Textbook of Anxiety Disorders. American Psychiatric Publishing, Washington DC 2002. Stein DJ, Hollander E (eds) p 228–229

---

256 A psychiatrist is seeing a 35-year-old patient with schizophrenia who is accompanied by his mother. During a discussion about possible medication options, the psychiatrist turns to the patient and asks "What would you prefer to do?" This question is an example of which ethical principle?

A. Altruism.
B. Respect for autonomy.
C. Beneficence.
D. Nonmaleficence.

The correct response is option B: Respect for autonomy.

Respect for autonomy is honoring the patient's right to make decisions for himself or herself. Altruism in health care delivery is the commitment of service to benefit others even at personal sacrifice. Beneficence is the obligation to try to help patients by relieving their suffering and enhancing their quality of life. Nonmaleficence is the duty to avoid harm.

Roberts LW. Ethical principles and skills in the care of mental illness. FOCUS: Forensic and Ethical Issues in Psychiatry. Fall 2003; 4:339–340

---

257 Which of the following defines the virtue "veracity"?

A. Saying only what is true, never misleading the patient, and pacing disclosure to the patient effectively.
B. Practicing medicine consistent with the highest intellectual and moral standards, both professional and individual.
C. Recognizing, preventing, and relieving pain, suffering, and distress and acting to prevent and relieve pain, suffering, and distress.
D. Not being excessively swayed by potential feared consequence.
E. Taking reasonable risks to one's self-interest (in time, convenience, health, and even life) to protect the interests of patients.

The correct response is option A: Saying only what is true, never misleading the patient, and pacing disclosure to the patient effectively.

Veracity refers to the physician's duty to tell the truth and not mislead through acts of commission or omission. The other options refer to integrity, compassion, courage, and self-sacrifice, respectively.

Roberts LW, Dyer AR, Concise Guide to Ethics in Mental Health Care. American Psychiatric Publishing, Washington D.C., 2004 p 8

Roberts LW. Ethical principles and skills in the care of mental illness. FOCUS: Forensic and Ethical Issues, Fall 2003; 4:340

---

258 A 25-year-old man has a history of facial and truncal tics since childhood. He presents to an outpatient clinic for evaluation of anxiety and is diagnosed as having OCD. Which of the following patterns of OCD symptoms is he most likely to exhibit?

A. Obsessions and checking.
B. Cleanliness and washing.
C. Symmetry and ordering.
D. Hoarding.

The correct response is option C: Symmetry and ordering.

Factor analysis has determined that symptoms of OCD fall into several potentially meaningful subtypes. Chronic tic disorder has repeatedly been found to be associated with the subtype characterized by symmetry and ordering.

Eisen JL, Yip AG, Mancebo MC, Pinto A, Rasmussen SA. Phenomenology of Obsessive-Compulsive Disorder, in American Psychiatric Publishing Textbook of Anxiety Disorders, 2nd ed. Edited by Stein DJ, Hollander E, Rothbaum BO. Arlington, VA, American Psychiatric Publishing, 2010, pp 265–71

Leckman JF, Grice DE, Boardman J, et al: Symptoms of obsessive-compulsive disorder. Am J Psychiatry 1997; 154:911–917

---

259 The starting dose of lamotrigine should be reduced by half if a patient is taking which of the following medications?

A. Carbamazepine.
B. Oral contraceptive.
C. Phenobarbital.
D. Divalproex.
E. Phenytoin.

The correct response is option D: Divalproex.

Divalproex will reduce the clearance of lamotrigine by about 50% resulting in a doubling of lamotrigine blood level. The risk of serious rash will be increased unless appropriate dose adjustments are made. Carbamazepine, oral contraceptives, phenytoin, and phenobarbital are inducers of lamotrigine metabolism and will cause substantial reductions in lamotrigine blood levels.

Kanner AM, Frey M: Adding valproate to lamotrigine: a study of their pharmacokinetic interaction. Neurology 2000; 55:588–591

Weintraub D, Buchsbaum R, Resor SR, Hirsch LJ: Effect of antiepileptic drug comedication on lamotrigine clearance. Arch Neurol 2005; 62:1432–1436

Sidhu J, Job S, Singh S, Philipson R: The pharmacokinetic and pharmacodynamic consequences of the co-administration of lamotrigine and a combined oral contraceptive in healthy female subjects. Br J Clin Pharmacol 2006; 61:191–199

---

260 A 75-year-old man with a history of mild Alzheimer's disease becomes increasingly aggressive at home. In addition, he is noted to have worsening memory and word-finding difficulty, inadequate self-care, and less interest in activities. Which of the patient's symptoms is most likely to be helped by risperidone?

A. Memory.
B. Word finding.
C. Independent functioning.
D. Aggression.
E. Interest in activities.

The correct response is option D: Aggression.

Aggression is a difficult acute symptom in dementia. Drugs should be used only when nonpharmacologic approaches have failed to adequately control behavioral disruption. There is concern regarding the potential for serious adverse outcomes.

The recently published CATIE-AD study reported that in usual care settings among patients continuing Phase I treatment for 12 weeks in comparison to placebo, "antipsychotics may be more effective for particular symptoms, such as anger, aggression and paranoid ideation," but "they do not appear to improve cognition, functioning, care needs or quality of life." According to a June 2009 statement from the APA Council on Aging about the use of antipsychotics in Alzheimer patients, "their use should be preceded by a discussion of risks and benefits with the patient and/or other decision makers. Clinicians should monitor patients closely, prescribe the lowest effective dosages, and discontinue the drugs as soon as possible."

Sultzer DL, Davis SM, Tariot PN, Dagerman KS, et al: CATIE-AD Study Group. Clinical symptom responses to atypical antipsychotic medications in Alzheimer's disease: phase 1 outcomes from the CATIE-AD effectiveness trial. Am J Psychiatry. 2008; 165(7):844–854

Salzman C, Jeste DV, Meyer RE, Cohen-Mansfield J, et al: Elderly patients with dementia-related symptoms of severe agitation and aggression: consensus statement on treatment options, clinical trials methodology, and policy. J Clin Psychiatry. 2008 Jun; 69(6):889–98

Jeste DV, Blazer D, Casey D, Meeks T, et al: ACNP White Paper: update on use of antipsychotic drugs in elderly persons with dementia. Neuropsychopharmacology. 2008 Apr; 33(5):957–70

Ballard C, Corbett A, Chitramohan R, Aarsland D. Management of agitation and aggression associated with Alzheimer's disease: controversies and possible solutions. Curr Opin Psychiatry. 2009 Aug 18

261 Two teenagers randomly fire their guns at a 54-year-old man in their neighborhood. A week later, the patient complains that he can't "get it out of my mind" and is having frequent nightmares about this incident. He is always "on the watch" when he drives down the road and avoids going out alone. The most likely diagnosis for this patient is:

A. Generalized anxiety disorder.
B. Obsessive-compulsive disorder.
C. Acute stress disorder.
D. Social phobia.
E. Posttraumatic stress disorder.

The correct response is option C: Acute stress disorder.

The essential feature of acute stress disorder is exposure to the event and the presence of nine symptoms from five symptom categories: intrusion symptoms, dissociative, negative mood, avoidance, and arousal symptoms that occur within 1 month after exposure to an extreme traumatic stressor. The disturbance lasts for a maximum of 4 weeks after the traumatic event; if symptoms persist beyond 4 weeks, the diagnosis of posttraumatic stress disorder may be applied.

American Psychiatric Association: Diagnostic and Statistical Manual of Mental Disorders, 5th Edition. Arlington, VA, American Psychiatric Association, 2013, pp 280–281

262 A 42-year-old patient complains of a fear of crowded places. This fear is present in any situation in which the patient perceives that escape may be difficult, including riding alone in elevators and cars. As a result of this fear, the patient rarely leaves home. Which of the following is the most likely diagnosis?

A. Social phobia.
B. Agoraphobia.
C. Specific phobia.
D. Avoidant personality disorder.
E. Panic disorder.

The correct response is option B: Agoraphobia.

According to the DSM-5, agoraphobia involves marked fear or anxiety about two or more situations in which escape might be difficult or embarrassing and leads to avoidance of the situation or endurance of the situation with distress. Specific phobia should be considered only if the avoidance is limited to one specific situation, and social phobia should be considered if the avoidance is limited to social situations only. However, this patient avoids all situations in which escape is perceived to be difficult, including situations in which the patient is alone. Agoraphobia may be diagnosed irrespective of the presence of panic symptoms.

American Psychiatric Association: Diagnostic and Statistical Manual of Mental Disorders, 5th Edition. Arlington, VA, American Psychiatric Association, 2013, pp 217–221

---

263 Which of the following is an objective sleep disturbance that occurs in depression?

A. Shortened sleep latency.
B. Decreased nighttime arousal.
C. Increased total sleep time.
D. Shortened REM latency.
E. Increased slow-wave sleep.

The correct response is option D: Shortened REM latency.

The REM latency in depression is shortened. The sleep latency is prolonged, and there is increased nighttime arousal, decreased total sleep time, and decreased slow-wave sleep. There can be increased stage 1 sleep and a prolonged first REM period.

Schiffer RB, Rao SM, Fogel BS (eds): Neuropsychiatry, 2nd ed. Philadelphia, Lippincott, Williams & Wilkins, 2003. p 385

---

264 The main factor of somatic symptom disorder that differentiates it from factitious disorder or malingering is that in somatic symptom disorder:

A. Patients seek to play the sick role.
B. There are external incentives for the behavior.
C. Complaint of symptoms is exaggerated.
D. Patients often have had multiple hospitalizations.
E. Symptoms are not under voluntary control.

The correct response is option E: Symptoms are not under voluntary control.

In somatization, symptoms are not under conscious control of the patient. Patients seek the sick role in factitious disorder, whereas external incentives are the motive in malingering. In both factitious disorder and malingering, symptoms are intentionally feigned or produced. Symptom complaint exaggeration is not a main factor of somatic symptom disorder, and multiple hospitalizations can be present in all three.

American Psychiatric Association: Diagnostic and Statistical Manual of Mental Disorders, 5th Edition. Arlington, VA, American Psychiatric Association, 2013, pp 311–326

---

265 A 38-year-old married woman presents to a psychiatrist complaining of difficulty in her sex life. She reports that for much of her married life, she has had little interest in sexual intercourse with her husband. She has not had any affairs, and she denies any discord in her relationship with her husband aside from the lack of a satisfactory sex life. She does not masturbate and rarely has any sexual fantasies. On the few occasions that she does have intercourse with her husband, she is able to enjoy sex and achieve an orgasm. Which of the following diagnoses is most appropriate?

A. Genito-pelvic pain/penetration disorder.
B. Sexual aversion disorder.
C. Female sexual interest/arousal disorder.
D. Sexual dysfunction due to a general medical condition.
E. Female orgasmic disorder.

The correct response is option C: Female sexual interest/arousal disorder.

Genito-pelvic pain/penetration disorder is new in DSM-5 and represents a merging of the DSM-IV categories of vaginismus and dyspareunia, which were highly comorbid and difficult to distinguish. The diagnosis of sexual aversion disorder has been removed because of rare use and lack of supporting research. Sexual dysfunction due to a general medical condition and the subtype due to psychological versus combined factors have also been deleted because of findings that the most frequent clinical presentation is one in which both psychological and biological factors contribute. Female sexual interest/arousal disorder is characterized by lack of or deficient sexual fantasies and sexual desire, as is present in this patient. Individuals with this disorder often have no dysfunction once they are engaged in intercourse.

American Psychiatric Association: Diagnostic and Statistical Manual of Mental Disorders, 5th Edition. Arlington, VA, American Psychiatric Association, 2013, pp 433, 814

---

266 The age at which a clinician should consider the possibility of early-onset Alzheimer's disease is

A. 35 years.
B. 45 years or below.
C. 55 years or below.
D. 65 years or below.
E. 75 years or below.

The correct response is option D: 65 years or below.

The DSM-IV diagnoses of dementia and amnestic disorder are subsumed in DSM-5 under the entity major neurocognitive disorder. However, the term dementia is not precluded from use in the etiological subtypes, in which that term is standard. Early-onset forms of Alzheimer's disease are seen in the fifth and sixth decades and are often related to known causative mutations.

Meeks TW, Lanouette N, Vahia I, Dawes S, et al: Psychiatric assessment and diagnosis in older adults. FOCUS. 2009 winter; 7(1):3–13

American Psychiatric Association: Diagnostic and Statistical Manual of Mental Disorders, 5th Edition. Arlington, VA, American Psychiatric Association, 2013, p 613, 816

---

267 A 22-year-old woman is driving her boyfriend home. The car hits a tree and he is killed. Six months after the accident, she is still unable to drive, she reports disturbing dreams related to the event and avoids going out, jumps when she hears loud noises, and cannot feel any sadness or happiness. What is the most likely diagnosis for this patient?

A. Adjustment disorder.
B. Agoraphobia.
C. Major depressive disorder.
D. Posttraumatic stress disorder.
E. Acute stress disorder.

The correct response is option D: Posttraumatic stress disorder.

The patient's symptoms are intrusion, avoidance, negative cognitions, and increased arousal. DSM-5 criteria for posttraumatic stress disorder differ significantly from those in DSM-IV. Whereas there were three major symptom clusters in DSM-IV—reexperiencing, avoidance/numbing, and arousal, in DSM-5 there are four symptom criteria: intrusion, avoidance, negative alterations in cognition and mood, and arousal and reactivity. Criterion D, *persistent negative alterations in cognitions and mood,* retains most of the DSM-IV numbing symptoms and also includes new or reconceptualized symptoms, such as persistent negative emotional states.

American Psychiatric Association: Diagnostic and Statistical Manual of Mental Disorders, 5th Edition. Arlington, VA, American Psychiatric Association, 2013, p 271–272

---

268 Which of the following actions is most likely to ease the fears of a dying patient and his family?

A. Postponing the discussion of pain and pain management.
B. Giving the family and patient information on a need to know basis.
C. Telling the patient that only the family's input regarding care will be sought.
D. Educating the patient that he may have discomfort that cannot be alleviated.
E. Obtaining the patient's wishes regarding treatment decisions.

The correct response is option E: Obtaining the patient's wishes regarding treatment decisions.

Conveying a number of important messages to the dying patient and his family allows them to feel more confident and comfortable in dealing with end-of-life issues. These messages as described by Mitka include the following: You will have the best medical treatment, aiming to prevent exacerbation, to improve function and survival, and to ensure comfort. You will never have to endure overwhelming pain, shortness of breath, or other symptoms. Your care will be continuous, comprehensive, and coordinated. You and your family will be prepared for everything that is likely to happen in the course of your illness.

Your wishes will be sought, respected, and followed whenever possible. We will help you consider your personal and financial resources, and we will respect your choices about their use. We will do all that we can to see that you and your family will have the opportunity to make the best of every day.

Sadock BJ, Sadock VA, Ruiz P (eds): Kaplan & Sadock's Comprehensive Textbook of Psychiatry, 9th ed. Philadelphia, Lippincott Williams & Wilkins, 2009, p 2355

Mitka M: Suggestions for help when the end is near. JAMA 2000; 284:2441

---

269 A 26-year-old bystander of a horrific motor vehicle accident is taken to the emergency department after reporting that suddenly she had gone blind. She does not appear to focus on anyone who is talking. However, her eyes are noted to track her reflection when a mirror is waved in front of her. After hospital admission, a complete medical and neurological workup is found to be normal. What should be the first intervention for her condition?

A. Pointing out that she can see as a result of the mirror test.
B. Instituting a reward system for sight improvement.
C. Discussing the stress of the event under amobarbital.
D. Suggesting symptom improvement through hypnosis.
E. Reassuring her that her sight will soon return.

The correct response is option E: Reassuring her that her sight will soon return.

The patient is likely suffering from conversion disorder. Direct confrontation of symptom inconsistency is never recommended. Although hypnosis, behavior therapy and amobarbital interviews can all be beneficial, they should only be tried if reassurance and relaxation are not effective.

Hales RE, Yudofsky SC, Gabbard GO (eds). The American Psychiatric Publishing Textbook of Psychiatry, 5th ed. Arlington, VA, American Psychiatric Publishing, 2008, pp 628–629

---

270 A 48-year-old obese man presents for an evaluation at the prompting of his wife. The wife, who has accompanied the patient to the appointment, complains that the patient snores loudly and keeps her awake at night. She states he sometimes seems to be gasping for air. On questioning, the patient admits to falling asleep easily during the day and even falling asleep while driving on occasion. He also complains of morning headaches and was recently diagnosed with hypertension. Which of the following is the best initial treatment for this patient's condition?

A. Uvulopalatopharyngoplasty.
B. Temazepam.
C. Biofeedback.
D. Modafinil.
E. Nasal continuous positive airway pressure (CPAP).

The correct response is option E: Nasal continuous positive airway pressure (CPAP).

This patient most likely has moderate-severe obstructive sleep apnea. The best initial treatment is nasal CPAP. Uvulopalatopharyngoplasty is a treatment option, though it would not typically be considered first line. Temazepam and biofeedback are not indicated for obstructive sleep apnea, and temazepam may worsen daytime sleepiness, with its associated negative consequences. Although modafinil is used to treat daytime sleepiness, it does not address the underlying condition.

Hales RE, Yudofsky SC, Gabbard GO (eds): The American Psychiatric Publishing Textbook of Psychiatry. 5th ed. American Psychiatric Publishing, Washington, DC. 2008, pp 999–1000

271 A 55-year-old patient with alcohol dependence treated with naltrexone 50 mg daily has been abstinent from alcohol for the past 2 months. The patient has been advised to undergo surgical knee replacement. What is the minimum duration of time prior to the surgery for which naltrexone must be discontinued in order for opiate analgesia to be effective?

A. 24 hours.
B. 72 hours.
C. 5 days.
D. 1 week.
E. 2 weeks.

The correct response is option B: 72 hours.

Naltrexone, which blocks μ opioid receptors, must be discontinued 48–72 hours prior to receiving opiate analgesia.

Anton RF: Naltrexone for the management of alcohol dependence. NEJM 2008; 359:715–21

272 A 35-year-old patient worries obsessively that he will kill his mother. To alleviate the anxiety, he calls her repeatedly throughout the day to hear her voice and reassure himself that he has not harmed her. He has tried adequate trials of high doses of fluoxetine, paroxetine, lorazepam, and clonazepam without improvement. Which of the following medications would be most appropriate to prescribe next?

A. Citalopram.
B. Alprazolam.
C. Bupropion.
D. Lithium.
E. Clomipramine.

The correct response is option E: Clomipramine.

Clomipramine is the next best medication to prescribe. Clomipramine has substantial evidence to support its use in OCD, but because of its side-effect profile, it is not typically prescribed until two SSRIs have failed (as in this patient). Citalopram would not be a good choice given that the patient has already failed therapeutic trials of two SSRIs. Benzodiazepines have not consistently shown efficacy. Bupropion and lithium are not typically prescribed for primary anxiety disorders.

Greist J, Jefferson J. Obsessive-compulsive disorder. FOCUS: OCD: Summer 2007, 3:283–298
Schatzberg AF, Nemeroff CB (eds): Essentials of Clinical Psychopharmacology, 2nd ed, Washington, DC, American Psychiatric Publishing, 2006, pp 144, 185, 337–40
Schruers K, Koning K, Leurmans J, et al. Obsessive-compulsive disorder: a critical review of therapeutic perspectives. Acta Psychiatr Scand 2005; 111:261–271
American Psychiatric Association Practice Guideline for the Treatment of Patients with Obsessive-Compulsive Disorder 2007. http://psychiatryonline.org/guidelines.aspx

273 A 60-year-old man with early Parkinson's disease presents to your office at the urging of his wife. She reports that the patient has begun "acting out" his dreams while asleep, and on at least one occasion this "acting out" led to his assaulting her. Polysomnogram is likely to demonstrate motor artifact and/or lack of complete hypotonia during which phase of sleep?

A. Stage I.
B. Stage II.
C. Stage III.
D. Stage IV.
E. REM sleep.

The correct response is option E: REM sleep.

This patient likely has REM sleep behavior disorder, which is characterized by lack of complete hypotonia during REM sleep. This results in patients displaying motor activity during sleep, often acting out their dreams. Older men with CNS disease, such as Parkinson's, are more likely to manifest this disorder.

Hales RE, Yudofsky SC, Gabbard GO (eds): The American Psychiatric Publishing Textbook of Psychiatry. 5th ed. American Psychiatric Publishing, Washington, DC. 2008. p 2040

---

274 Adding which one of the following medicines can increase the risk of toxicity in a patient stabilized on lamotrigine for bipolar maintenance therapy?

A. Lithium.
B. Valproate.
C. Quetiapine.
D. Topiramate.
E. Olanzapine.

The correct response is option B: Valproate.

When administered with lamotrigine, valproate can result in a twofold increase in lamotrigine levels. This is thought to be due to valproic acids inhibiting of CYPP450 microsomal function. It is the reason why the usual lamotrigine titration level should be decreased by 50% if a patient is on valproic acid.

Schatzberg AF, Cole JO, DeBattista C (eds): Manual of Clinical Psychopharmacology, 7th ed. Arlington, VA, American Psychiatric Publishing, 2010, p 340

---

275 A 52-year-old man presents with a rapidly progressive dementia, visual symptoms, and cerebellar signs. Within a few weeks, he is mute and has myoclonus. He dies 4 months later. Light microscopy of the brain reveals spongiform changes. This presentation is most consistent with which of the following diagnoses?

A. Creutzfeldt-Jakob disease.
B. HIV infection.
C. Huntington's disease.
D. Progressive supranuclear palsy.
E. Wilson's disease.

The correct response is option A: Creutzfeldt-Jakob disease.

The transmissible spongiform encephalopathies are a group of rare dementias caused by an accumulation of abnormal prion protein within the brain. Creutzfeldt-Jakob disease is the most common human transmissible spongiform encephalopathy. It typically presents with a rapidly progressive dementia, and within weeks to months, marked cognitive impairment develops. The median duration of symptom onset to death is only 4 months. Spongiform changes are seen in the brain due to neuronal loss, gliosis, and deposition of "amyloid."

Levenson JL (ed): Essentials of Psychosomatic Medicine, American Psychiatric Publishing, Washington, DC, 2007, p 322

---

276 A family is seen in family therapy. During the process, the therapist attempts to increase differentiation, decrease triangulations, resolve cutoffs, and improve the ability of the family to manage anxiety. This process is MOST consistent with which family therapeutic approach?

A. Behavioral/cognitive-behavioral therapy.
B. Systemic family therapy.
C. Psychodynamic-psychoanalytic psychotherapy.
D. Strategic family therapy.
E. Transgenerational family therapy.

The correct response is option B: Systemic family therapy.

In systemic family therapy, the core concepts are differentiation of the self, triangulation, emotional cutoffs, family emotional system, and sibling position. The goals are to increase differentiation, detriangulation, resolve cutoffs, and improvement in the ability to manage anxiety. In behavioral/cognitive-behavioral family therapy, the core concepts are based on social learning theory with the goal of enhancing communication and problem-solving skills. Psychodynamic-psychoanalytic approaches focus on object relations, projective identification, splitting, and scapegoating. Strategic family therapy aims at resolving the presenting problem. The focus of transgenerational family therapy is the repair of ruptured relationships.

Sadock BJ, Sadock VA, Ruiz P (eds): Kaplan and Sadock's Comprehensive Textbook of Psychiatry, 9th ed. Philadelphia, Lippinicott Williams & Wilkins, 2009, pp 2845–2857

Textbook of Psychotherapeutic Treatments. Gabbard GO (ed). Arlington VA, American Psychiatric Publishing, 2009, p 512

---

277 Which of the following diagnoses has been eliminated in DSM-5?

A. Gender identity disorder.
B. Borderline personality disorder.
C. Gender dysphoria.
D. Pedophilic disorder.
E. Transvestic disorder.

The correct response is option A: Gender identity disorder.

In DSM-5, the diagnosis of gender identity disorder (GID) has been eliminated. DSM-5 focuses on gender dysphoria (which replaces both the former GID and gender incongruence). Gender dysphoria reflects a change in conceptualization of the disorder's defining features by emphasizing the phenomenon of "gender incongruence" rather than cross-gender identification per se. DSM-5 acknowledges the wide variation of gender-incongruent conditions.

American Psychiatric Association: Diagnostic and Statistical Manual of Mental Disorders, 5th Edition. Arlington, VA, American Psychiatric Association, 2013; Highlights of Changes from DSM-IV to DSM-5, p 814

---

278 A 72-year-old patient is admitted to the hospital with a fever of 101.8° F and a urinary tract infection. The patient believes that it is 1974 and that the hospital room is a kitchen. The nursing staff is concerned because the patient is agitated, trying to get out of bed, and trying to pull out the IV. Which of the following medications is the best choice for the patient's agitation?

A. Lorazepam.
B. Haloperidol.
C. Diazepam.
D. Thioridazine.
E. Valproate.

The correct response is option B: Haloperidol.

The initial drug of choice for treatment of delirium is haloperidol because of the low potential for anticholinergic or hypotensive effects, ability to be administered intravenously, and minimal cardiotoxicity. Benzodiazepines are only indicated in delirium because of substance withdrawal (primarily alcohol or sedative-hypnotic withdrawal). Valproate is not indicated for the treatment of delirium.

Wise MG, Rundell JR (eds): Clinical Manual of Psychosomatic Medicine: A Guide to Consultation-Liaison Psychiatry. Arlington VA, American Psychiatric Publishing, 2005, pp 40–44

Sadock BJ, Sadock VA: Kaplan & Sadock's Comprehensive Textbook of Psychiatry, 9th ed. Philadelphia, Lippincott Williams & Wilkins, 2009, p 1165

Maldonado JR: Ask the Expert: Psychosomatic Medicine/Delirium. Focus 2009; 7(3):336–42

---

279 Which of the following stages has been identified by Kübler-Ross as a part of the process for dying patients?

A. Anger.
B. Suicidal ideation.
C. Intellectualization.
D. Visual hallucinations.
E. Disorientation.

The correct response is option A: Anger.

Kübler-Ross postulated five stages that many dying patients pass through from the time they first become aware of their fatal prognosis to their actual death: denial, anger, bargaining, depression, and acceptance.

Sadock BJ, Sadock VA, Ruiz P (eds): Kaplan & Sadock's Comprehensive Textbook of Psychiatry, 9th ed. Philadelphia, Lippincott Williams & Wilkins, 2009, pp 2382–83

---

280 In individuals who partially respond to an SSRI, which of the following is an effective adjunct to SSRIs for the core symptoms of PTSD?

A. Tricyclic antidepressants (TCAs).
B. Atypical antipsychotics.
C. Anticonvulsants.
D. Benzodiazepines.
E. Prolonged exposure therapy.

The correct response is option E: Prolonged exposure therapy.

Studies have shown that partial responders to sertraline showed significant improvement when SSRI treatment was augmented with prolonged exposure. TCAs have been tested sparingly, especially in recent years, as interest has shifted to newer antidepressants, especially because new antidepressants have more benign side-effect profiles than older agents. Atypical antipsychotics have been shown to be helpful only for psychotic symptoms. Because of concerns about toxicity, controlled trials of TCAs have not been done. Benzodiazepines cannot be recommended unless their use can be justified for comorbid disorders. Anticonvulsants have had mixed results as adjuvants in clinical trials.

Friedman MJ. PTSD: Pharmacotherapeutic approaches. Focus. 2013; 11(3):315–320

---

281 The treatment for body dysmorphic disorder that has been shown to be most effective includes which of the following psychotherapeutic techniques?

A. Mindfulness training.
B. Exposure and response prevention.
C. Group psychotherapy.
D. Social skills training.
E. Biofeedback.

The correct response is option B: Exposure and response prevention.

The exposure and response prevention component of CBT has been found to be helpful in the treatment of body dysmorphic disorder. Part of the treatment includes exposing the patient to anxiety-provoking situations while not allowing the rituals to be performed. Group psychotherapy has not been demonstrated to be effective. Social skills training would be beneficial for social anxiety, which is often comorbid with body dysmorphic disorder. However, it would not address the core symptoms of body dysmorphic disorder.

Phillips KA: Clinical features and treatment of body dysmorphic disorder. FOCUS. 2005; 3:179–183
Obsessive-Compulsive Disorder: Core Interventions in the Treatment of Obsessive-Compulsive Disorder and Body Dysmorphic Disorder. National Collaborating Centre for Mental Health (UK). Leicester (UK): British Psychological Society; 2006. National Institute for Health and Clinical Excellence: Guidance.

282 A 69-year-old woman is hospitalized for pyelonephritis, which is successfully treated with antibiotics. Discharge to her home, where she lives alone, is planned. However, her daughter calls and informs the treatment team that she found several bottles of recently prescribed unused medications in the patient's home. The team wonders whether the patient can safely manage her medications at home and asks psychiatry to evaluate her capacity. Which of the following potential reasons for medication noncompliance implies that the patient lacks capacity?

A. The patient was too delirious from her infection to remember to take her medications.
B. The patient's eyesight is too impaired to read the instructions on her pill bottles.
C. The patient is unable to understand the reasons the medications were prescribed.
D. The patient has a long history of noncompliance owing to a general mistrust of doctors.
E. The patient felt too hopeless and depressed to comply with her medication regimen.

The correct response is option C: The patient is unable to understand the reasons the medications were prescribed.

There are many potential reasons for medication noncompliance, and not all of them are reasons to consider a patient incapacitated. Physical reasons, such as arthritis or poor eyesight, can interfere, and these should be addressed with practical measures. Depression and delirium, although temporarily incapacitating a patient, are considered remediable conditions and should be treated before a capacity assessment is finalized. For some patients, noncompliance is consistent with their long-term personality and values. However, a patient's inability to understand the reasons a medication is prescribed during a psychiatric examination (which took place after her acute medical condition was resolved) suggests a more pervasive cognitive deficit affecting her ability to appreciate her condition. This inability to appreciate her illness and her need for medication is one of several generally accepted criteria for the capacity to make decisions.

Lai JM, Karlawish J. Assessing the capacity to make everyday decisions: a guide for clinicians and an agenda for future research. Am J Geriatr Psychiatry. 2007; 15(2):101–111

283 A 35-year-old man presents with memory deficits and emotional lability. Head computed tomography reveals atrophy of the caudate. His father died from the same disorder when he was 38 years old. This presentation is most consistent with which of the following disorders?

A. Alzheimer's disease.
B. Huntington's disease.
C. Progressive multifocal leukodystrophy.
D. Subacute sclerosing panencephalitis.
E. Whipple's disease.

The correct response is option B: Huntington's disease.

Although some Alzheimer's disease has a genetic component, Huntington's disease is inherited; it is transmitted autosomal dominant with complete penetrance. The relationship between the onset of symptoms in the son and the same illness causing the death of his father at a very early age suggests that it is inherited. Huntington's disease causes a combination of progressive motor, cognitive, psychiatric, and behavioral dysfunction. The key pathological processes of Huntington's disease occur in the striatum, caudate, and putamen.

Levenson JL (ed): Essentials of Psychosomatic Medicine. American Psychiatric Publishing, Washington, DC, 2007. p 320

American Psychiatric Association: Diagnostic and Statistical Manual of Mental Disorders, 5th Edition. Arlington, VA, American Psychiatric Association, 2013, pp 613–640

284 A 21-year-old patient has been diagnosed as having panic disorder. She reports that she frequently had difficulties with side effects in starting medications in the past. For this patient, which of the following would be the best beginning daily dose of sertraline?

A. 25 mg.
B. 50 mg.
C. 75 mg.
D. 100 mg.

The correct response is option A: 25 mg.

Patients with panic disorder can be unusually sensitive to the side effects of SSRIs, especially the activation. Adherence becomes a problem because restlessness, jitteriness, insomnia, and agitation cannot be tolerated by the patient. It would be prudent to start this patient on a very low dose so side effects can be minimized as she adapts to the medication. Some psychiatrists initially give small amounts of a benzodiazepine like clonazepam to achieve symptom reduction while waiting the weeks for the SSRI to become effective. The benzodiazepine may treat panic while also reducing SSRI-induced activation symptoms.

Stein DJ, Hollander E, Rothbaum BO (eds): Textbook of Anxiety Disorders, 2nd ed. Arlington, VA, American Psychiatric Publishing, 2010, pp 399–401

---

285 Paranoid personality disorder is marked by pervasive distrust and suspiciousness of others. For this diagnosis, distrust and suspiciousness can be manifested by which ONE of the following?

A. Choosing solitary activities most of the time.
B. Experiencing social anxiety that persists even with familiarity.
C. Experiencing unusual perceptions such as bodily illusions.
D. Reading hidden, threatening meaning into benign events.
E. Showing emotional detachment.

The correct response is option D: Reading hidden, threatening meaning into benign events.

Although a patient with paranoid personality disorder may display any one or more of the other features, they are not criteria for this diagnosis. Choosing solitary activities and showing emotional detachment are diagnostic criteria for schizoid personality disorder; experiencing social anxiety even in familiar contexts and unusual bodily illusions are diagnostic criteria for schizotypal personality disorder.

American Psychiatric Association: Diagnostic and Statistical Manual of Mental Disorders, 5th Edition. Arlington, VA, American Psychiatric Association, 2013, pp 649, 652, 655

---

286 A 50-year-old man with a 20-year history of smoking 1–2 packs per day attempts to quit by using the nicotine patch. He relapses to smoking after 4 days of cessation. He comes for an appointment, saying he knew it was going to be harder than he thought and he's not sure he can go through the process again. The best response would be:

A. "Most people need more than two tries before they successfully quit."
B. "You will need to try harder next time."
C. "With persistence, about 75% of smokers successfully quit."
D. "Let's try the same thing again."
E. "Most smokers require more intensive treatment to quit."

The correct response is option A: "Most people need more than two tries before they successfully quit."

The psychiatrist should help maintain the patient's hope in the face of his demoralization. Most smokers who successfully quit have had 5–7 prior unsuccessful attempts. The 75% estimate is, however, too optimistic—about half of all smokers successfully quit. The next quit attempt should take advantage of lessons learned from this failed attempt and not simply retry the same interventions. Most smokers quit on their own or with minimal treatment.

American Psychiatric Association Practice Guideline for the Treatment of Patients with Substance Use Disorders, 2nd ed., (2006). http://psychiatryonline.org/guidelines.aspx

287 In elderly patients, which of the following conditions is most important to address to prevent depressive symptoms after hip fracture surgery?

A. Postoperative pain.
B. Requiring assistance with mobility.
C. Using benzodiazepines daily.
D. Using >4 medications.

The correct response is option A: Postoperative pain.

Depression after hip fracture surgery in the elderly is both common and a significant cause of morbidity. A number of investigators have looked for factors that might predict depression in an attempt to prevent it. Significant factors predicting postoperative depression in elderly individuals include postoperative anxiety and pain. The other variables listed have not been shown to have a significant effect (mobility problems reach some statistical significance when they are severe; however, this significance is diminished when controlling for pain). These findings are important because pain and anxiety represent treatable problems that should be treated aggressively in elderly postsurgical patients.

Voshaar RC, Banerjee S, Horan M, Baldwin R, et al: Predictors of incident depression after hip fracture surgery. Am J Geriatr Psychiatry. 2007; 15(9):807–814

288 A 36-year-old woman with breast cancer completed radiotherapy. However, 3 months later she continues to complain of disabling fatigue. In evaluating this patient, which of the following symptoms would suggest that the fatigue was directly due to her medical condition rather than depression?

A. Late insomnia.
B. Impaired concentration.
C. Feelings of limb heaviness.
D. Decreased interest in activities.
E. Weight loss.

The correct response is option C: Feelings of limb heaviness.

Fatigue is a common problem with cancer patients, and it can be difficult to distinguish fatigue directly caused by comorbid illnesses such as depression. However, such a differentiation can be important for planning effective treatment. Many symptoms of cancer fatigue, such as insomnia, impaired concentration, lack of interest, and poor appetite and associated weight loss are common to both disorders. However, certain physical symptoms, such as the subjective reports of weakness or limb heaviness, may be associated with cancer fatigue rather than depression.

Levy MR. Cancer fatigue: a neurobiological review for psychiatrists. Psychosomatics. 2008; 49(4):283–291

289 A 24-year-old woman is comatose with generalized myoclonic twitching and is found to have a serum lithium concentration of 4.2 mEq/L. The treatment of choice is:

A. Saline diuresis.
B. Hemodialysis.
C. Exchange transfusion.
D. Plasmapheresis.

The correct response is option B: Hemodialysis.

In the presence of severe lithium poisoning, which generally presents with neurotoxicity, hemodialysis is the treatment of choice because it most rapidly clears lithium from the body. Lithium is a simple structure (an element) that is water-soluble and is neither protein-bound nor metabolized; hence, it is readily dialyzable. Following dialysis, lithium redistribution from tissues may result in a rebound increase in blood level, which, in turn, may necessitate further dialysis.

Jefferson JW, Greist JH: Lithium, in Kaplan & Sadock's Comprehensive Textbook of Psychiatry, 9th ed. Edited by Sadock BJ, Sadock VA, Ruiz P. Philadelphia, Lippincott Williams & Wilkins, 2009, pp 3132–45

290 A 72-year-old man is referred by his primary care doctor to a geriatric psychiatrist for treatment of depression. Two weeks earlier, the man had seen his primary care doctor, who started citalopram 20 mg daily. The patient continues to report severe depressive symptoms. On interview, it becomes apparent that this is the man's first episode of depression, and he has no history of any prior psychiatric disorder. The psychiatrist should advise that the patient:

A. Discontinue citalopram and begin nortriptyline.
B. Discontinue citalopram and begin venlafaxine.
C. Continue citalopram but add lithium.
D. Continue the current treatment as prescribed.
E. Increase the citalopram to 40 mg daily.

The correct response is option D: Continue the current treatment as prescribed.

Late-onset depression is often thought to have a different course than early-onset depression, and it is speculated that the approach should be different as well; however, there are few data to support this. The Sequenced Treatment Alternatives to Relieve Depression (STAR*D) study, when looking at late-onset depression, did not find any difference in treatment response when compared with younger patients. Until new data suggest otherwise, the approach to late life depression should be similar to that for depression in younger individuals, which in this case would be to continue the citalopram as prescribed, because there remains a good possibility that the patient will respond in subsequent weeks without additional intervention. The addition of adjunctive medications as well as a premature dose increase would only increase the risk of side effects without increasing the chance of response.

Kozel FA, Trivedi MH, Wisniewski SR, Miyahara S, et al: Treatment outcomes for older depressed patients with earlier versus late onset of first depressive episode: a Sequenced Treatment Alternatives to Relieve Depression (STAR*D) report. Am J Geriatr Psychiatry. 2008; 16(1):58–64

291 In addition to being effective in treating major depression, interpersonal psychotherapy (IPT) has been shown to be highly effective in the treatment of which of the following disorders?

A. Substance use disorder.
B. Bulimia nervosa.
C. Obsessive-compulsive disorder.
D. Schizophrenia.
E. Persistent depressive disorder.

The correct response is option B: Bulimia nervosa.

The bulk of evidence for IPT is for the treatment of major depression; however, it has also been shown to be helpful in the treatment of bulimia, and IPT is included as an option in the American Psychiatric Association's Practice Guidelines for both disorders. Studies of IPT for substance use disorder have not demonstrated efficacy. IPT experts have suggested that the treatment is less likely to be helpful for internally focused illnesses, such as schizophrenia and obsessive-compulsive disorder; however, this opinion has not been systematically tested.

Markowitz JC: The clinical conduct of interpersonal psychotherapy. FOCUS 2006; 4:179–184
Yager J, Devlin MJ, Halmi KA, et al.: Guideline Watch (August 2012): Practice Guideline for the Treatment of Patients With Eating Disorders, 3rd Edition. American Psychiatric Association. http://psychiatryonline.org/content.aspx?bookid=28&sectionid=39113853

292 A decrease of which neuropeptide has been linked most closely to narcolepsy?

A. Neurotensin.
B. Oxytocin.
C. Somatostatin.
D. Hypocretin.
E. Melanocyte-stimulating hormone.

The correct response is option D: Hypocretin.

Patients with narcolepsy and cataplexy have low CSF concentrations of hypocretin, a peptide produced in the lateral hypothalamus. A narcolepsy-like condition has been produced in hypocretin receptor knockout mice.

Dauvilliers Y, Arnulf I, Mignot E. Narcolepsy with cataplexy. Lancet. 2007; 369:499–511

Moore DP. Textbook of Clinical Neuropsychiatry, 2nd ed. London, Hodder Arnold, 2008. pp 575–577

---

293 Which of the following antidepressants could be prescribed for a depressed patient who has major concerns about the possible effects of medication on sexual functioning?

A. Sertraline.
B. Venlafaxine.
C. Paroxetine.
D. Bupropion.
E. Trazodone.

The correct response is option D: Bupropion.

Bupropion has a favorable side-effect profile, in part because of its low affinity for muscarinic, adrenergic, and histaminic receptors. Sexual dysfunction and weight gain are rare side effects and are less frequent than with the other antidepressants listed. Bupropion has also been used in combined treatments with other antidepressants, particularly with SSRIs for treating patients with SSRI-induced sexual dysfunction.

Schatzberg AF, Nemeroff CB (eds): Essentials of Clinical Psychopharmacology, 2nd ed. Arlington, VA, American Psychiatric Publishing, 2006. pp 85–90

Hales RE, Yudofsky SC, Gabbard GO (eds): The American Psychiatric Publishing Textbook of Psychiatry, 5th ed. Washington, DC, American Psychiatric Publishing, 2008. pp 1060–1061

---

294 Which of the following disorders was previously included in DSM-IV as an anxiety disorder and is included in DSM-5 in its own chapter/category with specific criteria for children?

A. Selective mutism.
B. Separation anxiety.
C. PTSD.
D. Agoraphobia.

The correct response is option C: PTSD.

In DSM-5, the chapter on anxiety disorders no longer contains PTSD (trauma- and stressor-related disorders) or OCD. Anxiety disorders include disorders that share features of excessive fear and anxiety-related behavioral disturbances. In DSM-5, PTSD is developmentally sensitive in that diagnostic thresholds have been lowered for children and adolescents, and separate criteria have been added for children age 6 years or younger.

American Psychiatric Association: Diagnostic and Statistical Manual of Mental Disorders, 5th Edition. Arlington, VA, American Psychiatric Association, 2013, pp 271–274

Martin A, Volkmar FR (eds) Lewis's Comprehensive Textbook Child and Adolescent Psychiatry, 4th ed. Philadelphia, Lippincott Williams & Wilkins, 2007. p 706

Sheeringa MS, Zeanah CH, Myers L, Putnam FW. New findings on alternative criteria for PTSD in preschool children. J Am Acad Child Adolesc Psychiatry. 2003; 42(5):564–565

---

295 When compared with individuals with Parkinson's disease dementia (PD-D), individuals with Alzheimer's disease dementia (AD-D) typically show more severe impairment in:

A. Apraxia.
B. Visual hallucinosis.
C. Depressive symptoms.
D. Visuospatial dysfunction.

The correct response is option A: Apraxia.

In DSM-5, the DSM-IV diagnoses of dementia and amnestic disorder are subsumed under the newly named entity major neurocognitive disorder. However, the term dementia is not precluded from use in the etiological subtypes, in which that term is standard. Diagnostic criteria for neurocognitive disorder are followed by diagnostic criteria for the different etiological subtypes. Whereas AD-D and PD-D can occur simultaneously, AD-D alone has a neuropsychological profile distinct from PD-D. In early and moderate stages, AD-D findings are predominantly cortical, whereas PD-D findings are prefrontal and subcortical. All deficits except for apraxia are more likely to appear earlier and more severely in PD-D than AD-D, whereas apraxia, along with agitation, disinhibition, irritability, and euphoria, is more common in AD-D.

Emre M. What causes mental dysfunction in Parkinson's disease? Mov Disord. 2003; 18 Suppl 6: S63–S71
American Psychiatric Association: Diagnostic and Statistical Manual of Mental Disorders, 5th Edition. Arlington, VA, American Psychiatric Association, 2013, p 816

---

296 Generally, restraint and seclusion are considered appropriate treatment interventions when the patient is at imminent risk to harm himself or others AND:

A. The patient is refusing medication.
B. No less restrictive alternative is available.
C. The hospital prefers physical to chemical restraint.
D. The time period is expected to be brief.
E. A physician is present to write the order.

The correct response is option B: No less restrictive alternative is available.

Generally, the courts have held that restraints and seclusion can be used only when the patient is at risk to harm himself or others and no less restrictive alternative exists. Most states have laws regulating the use of restraints, specifying the circumstances in which restraints can be used.

Simon RI. The law and psychiatry. FOCUS: Forensic and Ethical Issues in Psychiatry; Fall 2003; 4:365

---

297 A bus carrying students from a local high school is swept down the side of the mountain following a mudslide. Despite rescue attempts, all the youth on the bus either die or are seriously injured. On the basis of prevalence data, which of the following groups of individuals is most likely to develop PTSD symptoms after the disaster?

A. Family members.
B. First responders.
C. Guidance counselors.
D. Classmates.
E. Teachers.

The correct response is option B: First responders.

In a systematic review of posttraumatic stress disorder following disasters, the highest prevalence of PTSD was found among survivors and first responders. The prevalence of PTSD among first responders assessed following involvement in rescue, recovery, and cleaning efforts was especially high.

Neria Y, Nandi A, Galea S. Post-traumatic stress disorder following disasters: a systematic review. Psychol Med. 2008; 38(4):467–480

---

298 In association with research leading up to DSM-5, the core features of personality disorders were reexamined. Investigators assessed which characteristics were stable, trait-like, and "attitudinal" and which tend to vary with life stresses over time. For which one of the following personality disorder diagnoses were rigidity and problems delegating found to be the least changeable criteria?

A. Schizotypal personality disorder.
B. Narcissistic personality disorder.
C. Borderline personality disorder (BPD).
D. Avoidant personality disorder.
E. Obsessive-compulsive personality disorder (OCPD).

The correct response is option E: Obsessive-compulsive personality disorder (OCPD).

Leading up to DSM-5, investigators reexamined core features of PD diagnoses. Investigators tracked the course of individual diagnostic criteria of four DSM-IV diagnoses, borderline, schizotypal, avoidant, and obsessive-compulsive personality disorders, in 474 patients who completed 24 months of a longitudinal study. The least changeable criteria for BPD were affective instability, impulsivity, and anger; for schizotypal PD, paranoid ideation and unusual thinking; for avoidant PD, feelings of inadequacy and social ineptness; and for OCPD, rigidity and problems delegating. Each diagnosis was found to be composed of both stable personality trait-like and "attitudinal" criteria and criteria that vary with life stresses over time.

McGlashan TH, Grilo CM, Sanislow CA, Ralevski E, et al: Two-year prevalence and stability of individual DSM-IV criteria for schizotypal, borderline, avoidant, and obsessive-compulsive personality disorders: toward a hybrid model of axis II disorders. Am J Psychiatry, 2005; 162:883–889

---

299 Which of the following antiepileptic drugs has been shown to be effective in treating binge-eating disorder associated with obesity in short-term, placebo-controlled studies?

A. Topiramate.
B. Lamotrigine.
C. Oxcarbazepine.
D. Valproate.
E. Tiagabine.

The correct response is option A: Topiramate.

The anticonvulsant medication topiramate is effective for binge reduction and weight loss, although adverse effects may limit its clinical utility for some individuals. In short-term trials, topiramate has been shown to significantly reduce binge frequency. In one study, 58% of patients on topiramate reached remission versus 29% on placebo.

McElroy SL, Hudson JI, Capece JA, Beyers K, et al: Topiramate Binge Eating Disorder Research Group. Topiramate for the treatment of binge eating disorder associated with obesity: a placebo-controlled study. Biol Psychiatry. 2007; 61(9): 1039–1048

Yager J, Devlin MJ, Halmi KA, et al.: Guideline Watch (August 2012): Practice Guideline for the Treatment of Patients With Eating Disorders, 3rd ed. American Psychiatric Association. http://psychiatryonline.org/content.aspx?bookid=28&sectionid=39113853

---

300 A 32-year-old man is admitted to the hospital with a severe episode of bipolar disorder, mixed. Which of the following would be the best first-line pharmacologic treatment for him?

A. Lithium alone.
B. Lithium plus a benzodiazepine.
C. Lithium plus an antidepressant.
D. Lithium plus an antipsychotic.
E. Lithium plus valproate.

The correct response is option D: Lithium plus an antipsychotic.

The first-line pharmacological treatment for more severe manic or mixed episodes is the initiation of lithium plus an antipsychotic or valproate plus an antipsychotic. For less ill patients, monotherapy with lithium, valproate, or an antipsychotic such as olanzapine may be sufficient. Short-term adjunctive treatment with a benzodiazepine may also be helpful.

American Psychiatric Association Practice Guideline for the Treatment of Patients with Bipolar Disorder, 2nd ed (2002), in FOCUS: Bipolar Disorder, Winter 2003, 1:64.

301 Which of the following medications has the strongest body of evidence for the treatment of bulimia nervosa?

A. Bupropion.
B. Fluoxetine.
C. Duloxetine.
D. Paroxetine.
E. Venlafaxine.

The correct response is option B: Fluoxetine.

In November 1996, the FDA approved fluoxetine for the treatment of moderate to severe bulimia nervosa based on the results of two 8-week and one 16-week placebo-controlled trials.

Yager J, Devlin MJ, Halmi KA, et al.: Guideline Watch (August 2012): Practice Guideline for the Treatment of Patients With Eating Disorders, 3rd Edition. American Psychiatric Association. http://psychiatryonline.org/content.aspx?bookid=28&sectionid=39113853

302 Which of the following patterns is most likely to be seen on an EEG of a delirious patient?

A. Generalized slowing.
B. Increased alpha.
C. Decreased theta.
D. Triphasic sharp waves.
E. Focal high-frequency spikes.

The correct response is option A: Generalized slowing.

Delirious patients have progressive disorganization of rhythms and generalized slowing. There is slowing of the peak and average frequencies in addition to increased theta and delta but decreased alpha rhythms.

Hales RE, Yudofsky SC, Gabbard GO (eds): The American Psychiatric Publishing Textbook of Psychiatry, 5th ed. Washington, DC, American Psychiatric Publishing, 2008. p 864
Fearing MA, Inouye SK. Delirium. American Psychiatric Publishing Textbook of Geriatric Psychiatry. 2009. Blazer DG, Steffens DC (eds). Reprinted in FOCUS. 2009; 1:53–63

303 Which of the following types of psychotherapy focuses on a patient's current social functioning within one of four problem areas (reaction, interpersonal disputes, role transition, or interpersonal deficits)?

A. Supportive psychotherapy.
B. Interpersonal psychotherapy.
C. Cognitive therapy.
D. Psychodynamic psychotherapy.
E. Psychoanalytic psychotherapy.

The correct response is option B: Interpersonal psychotherapy.

Interpersonal psychotherapy was developed out of the work of Henry Stack Sullivan by Klerman and colleagues to focus on interpersonal functioning in four common problem areas. The focus tends to be on current relationships and can include the teaching of new behavioral skills.

Hales RE, Yudofsky SC (eds): The American Psychiatric Publishing Textbook of Psychiatry. 4th ed. American Psychiatric Publishing, Washington, DC. 2008, pp 1186–1188
Markowitz JC: The clinical conduct of interpersonal psychotherapy. Focus 2006; 4(2): 179–84

304 A patient with a long history of successful treatment with 20 mg of fluoxetine has been found to be HIV+ and has begun antiretroviral therapy. The patient sees you because of a return of symptoms of depression. Which of the following is the most likely pharmacologic cause?

A. As the patient gained weight from an increased appetite, more of the fluoxetine became bound to fat cells.
B. The protease inhibitor caused lipodystrophy, which decreased fluoxetine levels.
C. The protease inhibitor began to compete with fluoxetine for protein-binding sites.
D. The protease inhibitor induced the activity of an enzyme that enhanced the metabolism of fluoxetine and norfluoxetine.
E. The protease inhibitor has a direct interaction on the fluoxetine, causing it to lose efficacy.

The correct response is option D: The protease inhibitor induced the activity of an enzyme that enhanced the metabolism of fluoxetine and norfluoxetine.

Some protease inhibitors induce the activity of cytochrome P450 2D6, which increases the metabolism of many medications like fluoxetine and TCAs. Induction of this enzyme would decrease the plasma concentration of fluoxetine and norfluoxetine. Lipodystrophy is a complication of antiretroviral therapy but would not occur immediately after initiating treatment. Displacement of fluoxetine from protein would increase, not decrease, fluoxetine levels. Current highly active antiretroviral therapy (HAART) treatment is not believed to cause direct drug interactions that would decrease fluoxetine's effectiveness.

Hales RE, Yudofsky SC, Gabbard GO (eds): The American Psychiatric Publishing Textbook of Psychiatry, 5th ed. Arlington, VA, American Psychiatric Publishing, 2008, pp 1055–1057

---

305 A 24-year-old man is arrested after repeated episodes of rubbing his genitals against women's buttocks while riding on the subway. The most likely paraphilic diagnosis is which of the following?

A. Fetishistic disorder.
B. Frotteuristic disorder.
C. Exhibitionism.
D. Voyeurism.
E. Sexual masochism.

The correct response is option B: Frotteuristic disorder.

According to DSM-5, "The paraphilic focus of Frotteuristic disorder involves touching or rubbing against a nonconsenting person." The behavior typically takes place in crowded locations from which escape is more likely. Fetishistic disorder involves recurrent, sexually arousing fantasies, sexual urges, or behaviors involving the use of nonliving objects or specific focus on nongenital body parts.

American Psychiatric Association: Diagnostic and Statistical Manual of Mental Disorders, 5th Edition. Arlington, VA, American Psychiatric Association, 2013, pp 691, 700

---

306 Which ONE of the following is the most consistently agreed upon characteristic of supportive psychotherapy?

A. It is a form of psychodynamic psychotherapy.
B. It is based on the use of transference or other interpretation.
C. It is best for patients with Axis II disorders.
D. Its practice requires only common sense, interpersonal skills, and a capacity for empathy.
E. It serves primarily to strengthen the patient's self-esteem.

The correct response is option E: It serves primarily to strengthen the patient's self-esteem.

A number of texts on supportive psychotherapy are available, but no universally agreed upon definitions of supportive psychotherapy and its methods exist. Agreed upon elements of supportive psychotherapy include 1) that it strengthens the patient's self-esteem and 2) that it enhances the therapeutic alliance.

Douglas CJ: Teaching supportive psychotherapy to psychiatric residents. Am J Psychiatry 2008; 165:445–452
Hellerstein DJ, Markowitz JC: Developing supportive psychotherapy as evidence-based treatment. Am J Psychiatry 2008; 165: 1355-–1356

---

307 Which of the following treatments has the greatest body of evidence demonstrating efficacy for treatment of specific phobia?

A. Eye movement desensitization and reprocessing (EMDR).
B. In vivo exposure therapy.
C. Hypnotherapy.
D. Pharmacotherapy.
E. Imaginal exposure therapy.

The correct response is option B: In vivo exposure therapy.

The best data support exposure therapy as the most reliable treatment. "Imaginal exposure" therapy uses an imagined picture of the feared object. It has not proved to be as effective as in vivo treatment. EMDR uses an imagined phobic object as well, but with horizontal eye movements stimulated by hand movements of the therapist. It has not been successful. Studies of pharmacotherapy and hypnotherapy are inconclusive.

Stein DJ, Hollander E, Rothbaum BO (eds): Textbook of Anxiety Disorders, 2nd ed. Arlington, VA, American Psychiatric Publishing, 2010, pp 533–35

---

308 A 23-year-old man is the sole survivor of a fire aboard a crowded plane. In the immediate aftermath of exposure to the trauma, which of the following interventions is most likely to be successful in preventing psychological sequelae?

A. Encourage him to imagine positive emotions.
B. Have the man ventilate about how he is feeling.
C. Normalize the stress reaction.
D. Prescribe a short-acting benzodiazepine.
E. Use critical incident debriefing.

The correct response is option C: Normalize the stress reaction.

For both those who develop more severe stress reactions and the general population of exposed individuals, normalization of stress reactions is a key intervention principle to enhance calming. A major reason why ventilation and psychological debriefing have been criticized is that they serve to enhance arousal in the immediate aftermath of trauma exposure. Benzodiazepines are effective for acute symptom relief and immediate calming but have been shown to increase the likelihood of PTSD among symptomatic trauma survivors when used as monotherapy. Exposure therapy is only effective when the event can be paired with freedom from anxiety.

Hobfoll SE, Watson P, Bell CC, Bryant RA, et al: Five essential elements of immediate and mid-term mass trauma intervention: empirical evidence. Psychiatry. 2007; 70(4):283–315. Reprinted in FOCUS. 2009; 2:221–242

American Psychiatric Association Practice Guideline for the Treatment of Patients with Acute Stress Disorder and Posttraumatic Stress Disorder. 2004. http://psychiatryonline.org/guidelines.aspx

---

309 Following survival of a tornado that killed 38 people in a local community, a woman is provided with education and training in coping skills that includes deep-muscle relaxation, breathing control, assertiveness, role-playing, covert modeling, thought stopping, positive thinking, and self-talks. The intervention described is:

A. Aversion therapy.
B. Insight-oriented psychotherapy.
C. Interpersonal therapy.
D. Stress inoculation training (SIT).

The correct response is option D: Stress inoculation training (SIT).

SIT is a type of cognitive-behavioral therapy that can be thought of as a toolbox, or set of skills, for managing anxiety and stress. A number of studies have found SIT to be effective with rape victims, accident survivors, and soldiers experiencing combat stress reactions.

Hobfoll SE, Watson P, Bell CC, Bryant RA, et al: Five essential elements of immediate and mid-term mass trauma intervention: empirical evidence. Psychiatry. 2007; 70(4):283–315. Reprinted in FOCUS. 2009; 2:221–242

---

310 Which of the following symptoms is most consistent with a medication side effect of an antipsychotic medication rather than progression of Huntington's disease?

A. Flowing movements.
B. Postural instability.
C. Effects on swallowing.
D. Akathisia.
E. Facial apraxia.

The correct response is option D: Akathisia.

Characteristics specific to side effects of antipsychotic medications, but not Huntington's disease, are akathisia and marching in place. Characteristics specific to Huntington's disease include forehead chorea, flowing movements, facial apraxia, oculomotor defects, gait disorder, postural instability, and effects on swallowing.

Gabbard GO (ed): Treatments of Psychiatric Disorders 4th ed. American Psychiatric Publishing, Washington, DC. 2007. p 486

Scott B. Movement Disorders. American Psychiatric Publishing Textbook of Geriatric Psychiatry. 2009. Blazer DG, Steffens DC (eds).

---

311 The hormone that masculinizes the human brain during uterine life is:

A. Testosterone.
B. Dihydrotestosterone.
C. Estrone.
D. Estradiol.
E. Progesterone.

The correct response is option D: Estradiol.

Whereas the fetal testis is required to produce the testosterone that serves as precursor, the actual hormone of masculinization is estradiol, produced from testosterone by the enzyme aromatase. The developing female brain is ordinarily exposed neither to testosterone nor to estrogen derivatives. A second breakdown product of testosterone—dihydrotestosterone—is responsible for the development of male genitalia—testes, scrotum, and penis—from female anlagen initially found in all embryos. In the absence of dihydrotestosterone, the female habitus is the default option.

Schwarz JM, McCarthy MM: Steroid-induced sexual differentiation of the developing brain: multiple pathways, one goal. J Neurochem. 2008; 105:1561–1572

Bostwick JM, Martin KA: A man's brain in an ambiguous body: a case of mistaken gender identity. Am J Psychiatry. 2007; 164: 1499–1505

---

312 Which of the following cognitive abilities is preserved in normal aging?

A. Working memory.
B. Perceptual-motor skills.
C. Vocabulary.
D. Fluency.
E. Logical problem solving.

The correct response is option C: Vocabulary.

Whereas perceptual-motor skills, working memory, fluency, and logical problem solving all decline with increasing age, vocabulary may stay stable or even increase with age.

Spar JE, La Rue A. Normal aging. In Spar JE, La Rue A (eds). Clinical Manual of Geriatric Psychiatry, 1st ed. Arlington, VA: American Psychiatric Publishing, 2006. pp 213–214

Meeks TW, Lanouette N, Vahia I, Dawes S, et al: Psychiatric assessment and diagnosis in older adults. FOCUS. 2009; 7:3–16

---

313 Explicit feelings of shame, shame proneness, and self-stigma associated with higher ratings of anger and hostility have been empirically demonstrated to be increased in patients with which of the following disorders?

A. Social phobia.
B. Borderline personality disorder.
C. Histrionic personality disorder.
D. Persistent depressive disorder.
E. Paranoid personality disorder.

The correct response is option B: Borderline personality disorder.

Shame proneness is common in patients with borderline personality disorder and is related to anger-hostility, lower quality of life, and low self-esteem. Clinicians have long recognized that shame is an important characteristic of patients with borderline personality disorder (BPD) often associated with suicidality, self-harm, rage, and impulsivity, and some have even suggested that BPD is largely a chronic shame response. A recent study compared women with BPD, social phobia, and normal healthy control subjects, using self-report measures to assess "explicit shame" (i.e., consciously accessible self-cognitions) and "implicit shame" or shame proneness (i.e., measures of implicit or automatic self concepts and attitudes based on speed and closeness of word and phrase associations evoked in response to vignettes of potentially embarrassing and anxiety-provoking situations). In general, measures of explicit and implicit shame were not highly correlated. In comparison to the other groups, women with BPD scored higher in measures of shame and shame proneness and in contrast to the other groups were more prone to associate with shame than anxiety in response to the vignettes. After controlling for depression, shame proneness was associated with lower quality of life and lower self-esteem and positively correlated with measures of anger-hostility. Empirical studies of these constructs in patients with other personality disorders have not yet been conducted or published.

Rüsch N, Lieb K, Göttler I, Hermann C, et al: Shame and implicit self-concept in women with borderline personality disorder. Am J Psychiatry, September 2007 164:500–508

Rüsch N, Hölzer A, Hermann C, Schramm E, et al: Self-stigma in women with borderline personality disorder and women with social phobia. J Nerv Ment Dis. 2006 Oct; 194(10):766–73

---

314 Following a massive hurricane, the occupants of a city are placed in a temporary refugee camp until other housing can be obtained. Which of the following ways of organizing the refugee camp is likely to be most successful in preventing PTSD?

A. Bring in citizen leaders from nearby cities to run the camp.
B. Develop the camp into a village with a village council.
C. Have the military oversee operation of the camp.
D. Organize the camp along racial, religious, and ethnic divisions.
E. Provide individuals with their own tents.

The correct response is option B: Develop the camp into a village with a village council.

Large-scale interventions in the majority of countries consistently find that efforts to promote social support networks in temporary refugee camps are effective in preventing PTSD symptoms. This is related to self-efficacy and collective efficacy. This is best embodied in the idea of developing the camp into a village with village councils, welcoming committees, places of worship, places to for services, etc. Further, citizens of the village, rather than outsiders, fill the social roles and do so within their natural cultural traditions and practices. If people spend most of their time alone in their own tents, they are not as likely to be as connected to others.

Hobfoll SE, Watson P, Bell CC, Bryant RA, et al: Five essential elements of immediate and mid-term mass trauma intervention: empirical evidence. Psychiatry. 2007; 70(4):283–315. Reprinted in FOCUS. 2009; 2:221–242

---

315 Which of the following signs and symptoms is most reliable in distinguishing between delirium and dementia?

A. Orientation.
B. Short-term memory.
C. Long-term memory.
D. Sleep pattern.
E. Level of consciousness.

The correct response is option E: Level of consciousness.

Memory impairment, sleep disruption, and other cognitive disturbances may be present in both dementia and delirium. The characteristic feature of delirium is a disturbance of arousal or level of consciousness; this is typically not present in dementia. Other features that characterize delirium are disorientation, development of perceptual disturbance, attention deficits, disordered sleep-wake, fluctuation in presentation (waxing and waning), and changes in psychomotor activity, depending on the type of delirium.

Maldonado JR. Ask the Expert: Delirium. FOCUS. 2009; 3:336–342

Sadock BJ, Sadock VA, Ruiz P (eds): Kaplan & Sadock's Comprehensive Textbook of Psychiatry, 9th ed. Philadelphia, Lippincott Williams & Wilkins, 2009, pp 4069–70

---

316 A 64-year-old patient is hospitalized for an injury that occurred while he was inebriated. Three days after admission, the patient is disoriented, hallucinating, and has a grand mal seizure. His blood pressure is 160/100, with a pulse of 105. Which of the following medications is most appropriate for managing this patient's condition?

A. Haloperidol.
B. Sertraline.
C. Quetiapine.
D. Lorazepam.
E. Propranolol.

The correct response is option D: Lorazepam.

This patient has developed delirium secondary to alcohol withdrawal (i.e., delirium tremens). The most appropriate initial treatment for alcohol withdrawal delirium is a benzodiazepine. Antipsychotic medications may be appropriate in combination with benzodiazepines, but caution must be used because antipsychotic agents can lower the seizure threshold. The patient's age and history of alcohol use suggest that a drug with a shorter half-life and renal clearance would be of greatest benefit. Antidepressants are not indicated in alcohol withdrawal.

American Society of Addiction Medicine (ASAM). Principles of Addiction Medicine, 3rd ed. ASAM, 2003; pp 626, 630

Hales RE, Yudofsky SC, Gabbard GO (eds): The American Psychiatric Publishing Textbook of Psychiatry, 5th ed. Washington, DC, American Psychiatric Publishing, 2008, p 571

---

317 Which of the following chromosomal abnormalities is associated with an increased risk of early-onset Alzheimer's dementia?

A. Angelman syndrome (deletion of the 15q11-q13 region of chromosome 15).
B. Down syndrome (trisomy 21).
C. Turner syndrome (monosomy X).
D. Klinefelter syndrome (46, xy/47, xxy mosaicism).

The correct response is option B: Down syndrome (trisomy 21).

Down syndrome (trisomy 21) has been associated with an increased risk for dementia. Such a risk has not been identified with chromosome 15 deletions (Angelman syndrome), monosomy X (Turner syndrome), 46, xy/47, xxy mosaicism (Klinefelter syndrome).

Coppus AM, Evenhuis HM, Verberne GJ, Visser FE, et al: The impact of apolipoprotein E on dementia in persons with Down's syndrome. Neurobiol Aging. 2008; 29(6): 828–835

National Institutes of Health, US Department of Health & Human Services: Your Guide to Understanding Genetic Conditions Handbook. http://ghr.nlm.nih.gov/handbook/genetics

---

318 Which of the following is the most common psychiatric diagnosis among patients with cancer who have no prior psychiatric history?

A. Posttraumatic stress disorder.
B. Major depressive disorder.
C. Acute stress disorder.
D. Adjustment disorder.
E. Generalized anxiety disorder.

The correct response is option D: Adjustment disorder.

Although the other disorders listed may occur in patients with cancer, the largest group of psychiatric disorders present in cancer patients are the adjustment disorders (with depressed mood, anxious mood, and/or mixed features).

Sadock BJ, Sadock VA, Ruiz P (eds): Kaplan & Sadock's Comprehensive Textbook of Psychiatry, 9th ed. Philadelphia, Lippincott Williams & Wilkins, 2009, p 2322

---

319 A 40-year-old woman with bipolar I disorder complains of a lengthy, paralyzing period of depression following an episode of mania that led to hospitalization. Her symptoms have not responded to treatment with lamotrigine alone. Which of the following medications has the best evidence for efficacy as monotherapy to treat this patient's depression?

A. Aripiprazole.
B. Haloperidol.
C. Quetiapine.
D. Valproic acid.

The correct response is option C: Quetiapine.

Quetiapine monotherapy has been shown in a large randomized, double-blind placebo-controlled trial to be effective in treatment of bipolar I or II depression. Although valproic acid would be an appropriate choice for maintenance therapy in a patient with bipolar I disorder, it would be expected to have limited utility in acutely treating bipolar depression. Aripiprazole monotherapy has evidence for efficacy in the acute treatment of manic or mixed episodes but has not been sufficiently studied to recommend its use in the acute treatment of bipolar depression. Haloperidol also does not have evidence for efficacy, and extrapyramidal side effects could be associated with an apparent worsening of depressive symptoms.

Hirschfeld RMA: "Guideline Watch: Practice Guideline for the Treatment of Patients with Bipolar Disorder, 2nd Edition" APA Practice Guidelines pp 3–4, November 2005. Reprinted in FOCUS, Winter 2007,1:36. http://psychiatryonline.org/guidelines.aspx

American Psychiatric Association Practice Guideline for the Treatment of Patients with Bipolar Disorder, 2nd ed (2002). http://psychiatryonline.org/guidelines.aspx

American Psychiatric Association Practice Guideline for the Treatment of Patients with Schizophrenia, 2nd ed (2004). http://psychiatryonline.org/guidelines.aspx

---

320 A 28-year-old man presents with the chief complaint of excessive daytime sleepiness. He reports the sudden onset of brief periods of daytime sleep that are very restful. On a few occasions, he has experienced brief muscle paralysis after laughter. Recently, he has had two episodes of temporary paralysis when he awakens during the morning accompanied by vivid visual hallucinations. A polysomnogram is most likely to show which of the following?

A. Episodes of decreased blood oxygen saturation in spite of ventilatory effort.
B. Sleep-onset REM periods (SOREMPS) within 15 minutes of falling asleep.
C. Increased sleep spindles and K-complexes in stage 2 non-REM sleep.
D. Multiple awakenings during stage 3 and 4 of non-REM sleep.
E. Prolonged episodes of REM sleep in the first half of the night.

The correct response is option B: Sleep-onset REM periods (SOREMPS) within 15 minutes of falling asleep.

The patient presents with classic symptoms of narcolepsy including excessive daytime somnolence, cataplexy, sleep paralysis, hypnagogic and hypnopompic hallucinations, and SOREMPS. On the polysomnogram, the most common finding is SOREMPS within 15 minutes of falling asleep (normal is 90 minutes).

Saddock BJ, Saddock VA. Pocket Handbook of Clinical Psychiatry. 4th ed. Philadelphia, PA. Lippincott Williams and Wilkins, 2005. pp 238–239

---

321 Which of the following is most likely to be predictive of a good prognosis in schizophrenia?

A. Early age at onset of symptoms.
B. Presence of predominantly negative symptoms.
C. Acute onset with underlying precipitating factors.
D. Presence of neurological signs and symptoms.
E. Low IQ.

The correct response option C: Acute onset with underlying precipitating factors.

Factors that may indicate a good prognosis for schizophrenia include good premorbid functioning, older age at the time of first symptoms, acute onset with precipitating factors, female gender, being married, good support system, higher IQ, family history of affective disorder, absence of obvious negative symptoms, and no significant history of drug or alcohol use.

Lauriello J, Bustillo JR, Shingler KC: The first interview of a patient with psychosis: symptoms, safety, and stabilization. FOCUS: Schizophrenia. Winter 2004; 2(1):7–12

Hales RE, Yudofsky SC, Gabbard GO (eds): The American Psychiatric Textbook of Psychiatry, 5th ed. Arlington, VA, American Psychiatric Publishing, 2008, pp 424–426

322 Which of the following medications is considered to be a first-line pharmacological treatment for delirium?

A. Lorazepam.
B. Haloperidol.
C. Quetiapine.
D. Trazodone.
E. Hydroxyzine.

The correct response is option B: Haloperidol.

Nonpharmacological treatments should be implemented as the first line of treatment of delirium. Pharmacological management should only be used in patients with severe agitation that interferes with medical treatment or in patients who pose a danger to themselves, other patients, or staff. When such pharmacological treatment becomes necessary, neuroleptics are the first-line treatment. Among them, haloperidol is the most widely used and studied. Atypical antipsychotics such as quetiapine may be helpful but have only been tested in small, uncontrolled studies and may be associated with higher mortality. Benzodiazepines typically lead to oversedation and confusion. Antidepressants generally have not been shown to be useful, and the heterocyclic antidepressants may worsen delirium. Similarly, antihistamines such as diphenhydramine and hydroxyzine can cause or worsen delirium.

Hales RE, Yudofsky SC, Gabbard, GO (eds): The American Psychiatric Publishing Textbook of Psychiatry, 5th ed. Washington, DC, American Psychiatric Publishing, 2008. pp 1462

Fearing MA, Inouye SK: Delirium, in The American Psychiatric Publishing Textbook of Geriatric Psychiatry. Edited by Blazer DG, Steffens DC. Washington, DC, American Psychiatric Publishing, 2009, pp 229–241. Reprinted in FOCUS. 2009; 7:53–63

323 A 67-year-old woman presents with visual hallucinations, memory loss, apathy, and extrapyramidal symptoms. The patient's extrapyramidal symptoms increase markedly when given olanzapine 2.5 mg. This presentation is most consistent with:

A. Vascular dementia.
B. Dementia of the Alzheimer's type.
C. Lewy body dementia.
D. Dementia due to HIV.
E. Dementia due to Huntington's disease.

The correct response is option C: Lewy body dementia.

Lewy body dementia presents with well-formed visual hallucinations, delusions, depression, apathy, anxiety, and extrapyramidal symptoms. Patients with Lewy body dementia are extremely sensitive to the extrapyramidal effects of antipsychotic medication.

Hales RE, Yudofsky SC, Gabbard GO (eds): The American Psychiatric Publishing Textbook of Psychiatry, 5th ed, Washington, DC, American Psychiatric Publishing, 2008. pp 330–331

324 A 70-year-old woman presents with a history of a fixed belief that her arms and legs are infested with bugs that are crawling and biting her. She has no known associated medical condition and is physically healthy. Which of the following is best supported as a treatment of her condition?

A. Methylphenidate.
B. Imipramine.
C. Pimozide.
D. Selegiline.
E. Fluoxetine.

The correct response is option C: Pimozide.

The patient appears to be suffering from delusional parasitosis, which is a fixed belief of being infested with living organisms despite a lack of medical evidence of such infestation. It is often associated with various medical conditions such as tuberculosis, syphilis, polycyathemia vera, congestive heart failure, diabetes mellitus, vitamin B_{12} deficiency, renal and hepatic disorders, dementia, and Huntington's disease. It can also be caused by use of amphetamines, cocaine, etc. Delusional parasitosis can present as a monosymptomatic hypochondriacal psychosis and labeled as delusional disorder, somatic type. Patients with this condition respond to the potent antipsychotic pimozide, which also serves as an opiate antagonist and possibly decreases pruritis and pain by that mechanism. Other antipsychotics, such as haloperidol and risperidone, have also been used in such trials. Methylphenidate may worsen the symptoms, while there are no positive studies reported with imipramine, selegiline, and psychotherapy.

Gupta AK. Psychocutaneous disorders, in Kaplan & Sadock's Comprehensive Textbook of Psychiatry, 9th ed. Edited by Sadock BJ, Sadock VA, Ruiz P. Philadelphia, Lippincott Williams & Wilkins, 2009, pp 2435–36

---

325 For the treatment of genito-pelvic pain/penetration disorder (vaginismus), which of the following interventions in combination with education and counseling would be most effective?

A. A short-acting benzodiazepine prior to intercourse.
B. Guided imagery during intercourse.
C. Limiting intercourse to the female superior position.
D. Use of a vibrator applied to the clitoris to induce orgasm.
E. Vaginal dilation exercises using plastic dilators.

The correct response is option E: Vaginal dilation exercises using plastic dilators.

Genito-pelvic pain/penetration disorder is new in DSM-5 and represents a merging of the DSM-IV categories of vaginismus and dyspareunia, which were highly comorbid and difficult to distinguish. Vaginismus is an involuntary muscle constriction of the outer third of the vagina that interferes with penile insertion and intercourse. This dysfunction most frequently affects women following sexual trauma. For treatment, women are advised to dilate their vaginal opening with their fingers or dilators.

Saddock BJ, Saddock VA. Pocket Handbook of Clinical Psychiatry. 4th ed. Philadelphia, PA. Lippincott Williams and Wilkins, 2005. pp 214, 218

American Psychiatric Association: Highlights of Changes from DSM-IV to DSM-5, in Diagnostic and Statistical Manual of Mental Disorders, 5th Edition. Arlington, VA, American Psychiatric Association, 2013, pp 810–816

---

326 Which antidepressant group is most likely to induce significant anticholinergic side effects that should be considered when treating late-life depression?

A. Serotonin norepinephrine reuptake inhibitors.
B. Monoamine oxidase inhibitors.
C. Selective serotonin reuptake inhibitors.
D. Reversible monoamine oxidase inhibitors.
E. Tricyclic antidepressants.

The correct response is option E: Tricyclic antidepressants.

The geriatric population is particularly susceptible to anticholinergic-induced urinary retention and confusional states. Tricyclics have significant anticholinergic effects that can also result in dry mouth, constipation, and blurred vision.

Schatzberg AF, Nemeroff CB (eds): Essentials of Clinical Psychopharmacology, 2nd ed., Washington, DC, American Psychiatric Publishing, 2006. pp 64

Schatzberg AF, Cole JO, DeBattista C (eds): Manual of Clinical Psychopharmacology, 6th ed. Washington, DC. American Psychiatric Publishing, 2007. pp 112–115

327 A 69-year-old man with chronic obstructive pulmonary disease, cirrhosis of the liver, benign prostatic hypertrophy, and alcohol dependence is prescribed acamprosate as part of his comprehensive treatment plan for his alcoholism. Which of the following laboratory tests would be most appropriate to obtain in order to determine the best starting dose of acamprosate?

A. Alanine aminotransferase.
B. Electrolytes.
C. Creatinine clearance.
D. Serum osmolality.
E. Serum total protein.

The correct response is option C: Creatinine clearance.

The dose of acamprosate will need to be adjusted for patients with renal impairment as determined by creatinine clearance. Acamprosate absorption across the gastrointestinal tract is moderate, slow, and sustained. Acamprosate is not protein-bound. An extensive portion of the drug is eliminated via the gastrointestinal tract with the feces. The portion of the drug that is absorbed does not undergo metabolism. Acamprosate is excreted in the urine as acamprosate. There is a linear relationship between renal clearance and plasma half-life of the drug.

Sadock BJ, Sadock VA (eds): Kaplan and Sadock's Comprehensive Textbook of Psychiatry, 9th ed. Philadelphia, Lippincott Williams & Wilkins, 2009, pp 3102–3104

328 Social rhythm therapy for bipolar disorder is based on which of the following types of psychotherapy?

A. Cognitive-behavioral therapy.
B. Family therapy.
C. Group therapy.
D. Interpersonal therapy.
E. Psychodynamic psychotherapy.

The correct response is option D: Interpersonal therapy.

Social rhythm therapy is an adaptation of Klerman and Weissman's interpersonal psychotherapy as an individual psychotherapy for the treatment for bipolar disorder. It proposes that sleep-wake cycle abnormalities found in bipolar disorder may be responsible for some of the symptomatic manifestations of the illness. Both positive and negative life events may cause disruptions in patients' social rhythms that, in turn, alter sleep-wake cycles and lead to the development of bipolar symptoms. Features of the therapy include having the patient regularize their daily routines, diminish interpersonal problems, and adhere to medication regimens.

Frank E, Kupfer DJ, Thase ME, Mallinger AG, et al: Two-year outcomes for interpersonal and social rhythm therapy in individuals with bipolar I disorder. Archives of General Psychiatry. 2005; 62:996–1004
Frank E, Swartz HA, Kupfer DJ: Interpersonal and social rhythm therapy: managing the chaos of bipolar disorder. Biological Psychiatry 2000; 48:593–604
American Psychiatric Association Practice Guideline for the Treatment of Patients with Bipolar Disorder, 2nd Edition (2002). http://psychiatryonline.org/guidelines.aspx

329 A 15-year-old girl is diagnosed with anorexia nervosa. She has had symptoms for 18 months. Her medical status is stable, and she maintains an acceptable weight. The treatment that would be most beneficial for ongoing care is:

A. Behavioral management.
B. Psychodynamic psychotherapy.
C. Cognitive-behavioral therapy.
D. Family therapy.
E. Dialectical behavior therapy.

The correct response is option D: Family therapy.

Understanding the current evidence supporting psychotherapeutic interventions for anorexia nervosa is important for clinical practice. In controlled trials, anorexics who were younger than 16 years old, with symptoms less than 3 years, benefited more from family therapy than individual therapy.

Yager J, Devlin MJ, Halmi KA, et al.: Guideline Watch (August 2012): Practice Guideline for the Treatment of Patients With Eating Disorders, 3rd Edition. American Psychiatric Association. http://psychiatryonline.org/content.aspx?bookid=28&sectionid=39113853

---

330 Which one of the following medications is associated with causing Ebstein's anomaly in the newborn if taken regularly by pregnant women?

A. Lithium.
B. Valproic acid.
C. Carbamazepine.
D. Lamotrigine.
E. Aripiprazole.

The correct response is option A: Lithium.

Lithium use in the first trimester of pregnancy is associated with Ebstein's anomaly, a serious defect in the formation of the tricuspid valve of the heart. Valproic acid and carbamazepine in the first trimester are associated with an increased risk of neural tube defects. Lamotrigine use in pregnancy is of concern because of the theoretical risk the fetus could get Stephens-Johnson syndrome, but the mother would not get it and so not be aware of the need to stop the lamotrigine. There are not a lot data on the use of atypical antipsychotics as mood stabilizers during pregnancy.

Hales RE, Yudofsky SC, Gabbard GO (eds): The American Psychiatric Publishing Textbook of Psychiatry, 5th ed. Arlington, VA, American Psychiatric Publishing, 2008, p 1500

---

331 A 42-year-old woman receiving chemotherapy for non-Hodgkin's lymphoma develops anorexia-cachexia syndrome. She is started on a medication to address her symptoms. A few weeks later she returns with reports of an increase in her sense of well-being and decreased pain and nausea. However, she has gained no weight and has new-onset muscle weakness. Which of the following agents is most likely responsible?

A. Corticosteroids.
B. Cyproheptadine.
C. Medroxyprogesterone acetate.
D. Metoclopramide.
E. Ondansetron.

The correct response is option A: Corticosteroids.

Anorexia-cachexia syndrome occurs frequently in patients with cancer. There are a number of agents available for treatment. Corticosteroids increase the sense of well-being and often decrease pain and nausea. However, they are associated with osteoporosis, muscle weakness, immunosuppression, and delirium and have no demonstrated effects on body weight. Cyproheptadine increases appetite but does not prevent weight loss. Medroxyprogesterone acetate increases appetite and body weight but does not impact the overall sense of well-being or reduction of pain. Metoclopramide only addresses emesis. Ondansetron does not prevent weight loss.

Levenson JL (ed): Essentials of Psychosomatic Medicine. American Psychiatric Publishing, Washington, DC, 2007. pp 114–115

---

332 A 42-year man is being treated with cognitive-behavior therapy (CBT) for depression. He describes several mistakes he made at work and voices the belief that "No matter what I try, I always fail." This is an example of:

A. Automatic thought.
B. Maladaptive schema.
C. Full consciousness.
D. Modified cognition.
E. Unconscious conflict.

The correct response is option B: Maladaptive schema.

Schemas are defined as "fundamental rules or templates for information processing that are shaped by developmental influences and other life experiences." They are the deepest level of cognition as defined by CBT and are an important target for the therapy. The other two levels are full consciousness, the state of full awareness in which decisions are made, and automatic thoughts, rapid, automatic thoughts that occur in one's stream of consciousness that are not generally evaluated carefully by the thinker. Identifying cognitive errors and modifying cognition are among the goals of CBT.

Jesse H. Wright. Cognitive behavior therapy: basic principles and recent advances. FOCUS 2006; 4:173–178

Textbook of Psychotherapeutic Treatments. Gabbard GO (ed). Arlington VA, American Psychiatric Publishing, 2009, pp 170–72

---

333 Which of the following mood stabilizers is FDA-approved for acute mania in children older than 12 years?

A. Lithium.
B. Sodium valproate.
C. Carbamazepine.
D. Lamotrigine.
E. Topiramate.

The correct response is option A: Lithium.

Lithium is approved for acute mania and maintenance therapy for children older than 12 years. Although all mood stabilizers and antipsychotic agents are commonly used for early-onset bipolar disorder in clinical settings, none of these agents has been well studied in the pediatric population. The few double-blind placebo-controlled studies of lithium in this population are generally positive, but they are limited by very small sample sizes and diagnostic variability. The FDA approval of lithium for use in children older than 12 years was largely based on the response in adult studies.

McClellan J, Kowatch R, Findling RL; Work Group on Quality Issues. Practice parameter for the assessment and treatment of children and adolescents with bipolar disorder. J Am Acad Child Adolesc Psychiatry. 2007; 46(1):107–25

---

334 A 66-year-old man being treated for bipolar disorder is noted to have asymptomatic hypercalcemia and elevated levels of parathyroid hormone. Which of the following medications is the most likely cause?

A. Divalproex.
B. Lamotrigine.
C. Lithium.
D. Topiramate.
E. Olanzapine.

The correct response is option C: Lithium.

Lithium is the only psychiatric medication for which there is well-documented evidence for causing hypercalcemia and hyperparathyroidism. Although quite uncommon, this side effect has, on occasion, led to surgical intervention to remove hyperplastic or adenomatous parathyroid glands.

Jefferson JW, Greist JH: Lithium, in Kaplan & Sadock's Comprehen sive Textbook of Psychiatry, 9th ed. Edited by Sadock BJ, Sadock VA, Ruiz P. Philadelphia, Lippincott Williams & Wilkins, 2009, pp 3132–45

Abdullah H, Bliss R, Guinea AI, Delbridge L: Pathology and outcome of surgical treatment for lithium-associated hyperparathyroidism. Br J Surgery 1999; 86:91–93

McHenry CR, Lee K: Lithium therapy and disorders of the parathyroid glands. Endocrine Practice 1996; 2:103–109

---

335 A 28-year-old hospitalized patient is started on an antipsychotic medication for schizophrenia. Within 3 weeks, the patient complains of chest pain, shortness of breath, and swelling of the lower extremities. Which medication is the patient most likely taking?

A. Fluphenazine.
B. Quetiapine.
C. Risperidone.
D. Aripiprazole.
E. Clozapine.

The correct response is option E: Clozapine.

The patient's symptoms are suggestive of cardiac dysfunction. Of the choices listed, only clozapine has been associated with myocarditis and cardiomyopathy, typically in the early stages of treatment. A study of 213 cases of myocarditis indicated that 85% of these occurred at the recommended dosage of clozapine in the first 2 months of therapy. The presence of eosinophilia in many of the reported cases indicates that an immunoglobulin E medicated hypersensitivity reaction may have been involved.

Clozaril® package insert, Novartis Pharmaceuticals Corporation, East Hanover, NJ, 2005. http://www.pharma.us.novartis.com/ product/pi/pdf/ Clozaril.pdf.

Hales RE, Yudofsky SC and Gabbard GO (eds): The American Psychiatric Publishing Textbook of Psychiatry, 5th ed. Arlington, VA, American Psychiatric Publishing, 2008. pp 1097–1098

Schatzberg AF, Nemeroff CB (eds): Textbook of Psychopharmacology, 3rd ed. Arlington, VA, American Psychiatric Publishing, 2006. p 449

336 A requirement in the United States for initiating hospice care is that the patient must have:

A. A cognitive-impairing terminal illness.
B. A health care power of attorney.
C. A prognosis ≤6 months to live.
D. No family members able to provide care.
E. Medicare and/or Medicaid benefits.

The correct response is option C: A prognosis of ≤6 months to live.

Although a Medicare hospice benefit is available, Medicare or Medicaid is not a requirement nor are the other incorrect answers. The prognosis requirement is a barrier for those with uncertain prognoses, such as with Alzheimer's disease.

Blazer DG, Steffens DC (eds): The American Psychiatric Publishing Textbook of Geriatric Psychiatry, 4th ed. Arlington, VA, American Psychiatric Publishing, 2009, p 610

337 A 38-year-old patient with schizophrenia is observed holding her arms in bizarre positions for hours at a time. On interview, the patient does not answer any questions but rather repeats everything the psychiatrist says. Which of the following is the most appropriate initial treatment?

A. Lorazepam.
B. Propranolol.
C. Diphenhydramine.
D. Phenobarbital.
E. Botulinum toxin.

The correct response is option A: Lorazepam.

This patient is experiencing catatonia, with posturing and echolalia. Benzodiazepines are recommended for the initial treatment of catatonic reactions.

American Psychiatric Association Practice Guideline for the Treatment of Patients with Schizophrenia, 2nd ed (2004), pp 659–60. http://psychiatryonline.org/guidelines.aspx

338 Procedural justice in the process of civil commitment refers to:

A. Physician decision making that supports a beneficial outcome for patients.
B. A style of communication that alleviates patients' experience of coercion.
C. The inclusion of a patient's family in commitment decisions.
D. Judicial decision making that takes into account patients' therapeutic options.
E. Choosing the least restrictive alternative for patients.

The correct response is option B: A style of communication that alleviates patients' experience of coercion.

Procedural justice is a style of communication that is intended to limit patients' experience of coercion during the processes of civil commitment. Relevant components include listening to patients and validating their concerns, informing patients about the issues at stake, and treating them with dignity and respect. The style of communication that is most important to avoid when committing patients, because it is most closely associated with their experience of coercion, is the use of threats and force. Therapeutic jurisprudence applies to judges choosing options that are "therapeutic" for the patient. Including a patient's family in commitment decisions might be helpful, with the patient's agreement, but is not relevant to the concept. Similarly, the remaining options do not directly relate to patients' experience of coercion.

McKenna BG, Simpson AIF, Laidlaw TM. Patient perception of coercion on admission to acute psychiatric services: the New Zealand experience. International Journal of Law and Psychiatry. 1999; 22:143–153

Simon RI, Shuman DW. Clinical Manual of Psychiatry and Law. Arlington, VA, American Psychiatric Publishing, 2007, p 127

---

339 A review of the current evidence suggests that the BEST explanation for an increase in the rate of autism spectrum disorders is:

A. Exposure to childhood vaccines.
B. Rates of genetic mutations.
C. Exposure to environmental toxins.
D. Screening and diagnosis.
E. Survival of premature infants.

The correct response is option D: Screening and diagnosis.

On the basis of the current evidence, the best explanation for the increased rate of autism spectrum disorders is broader diagnosis, improved screening and diagnosis, and identification at an earlier age. The current evidence does not support the other options.

Westphal A, Volkmar F. An update on autism. FOCUS: Child and Adolescent Psychiatry. Summer 2008; 6(3):286:288–291

Wazana A, Bresnahan M, Kline J. The autism epidemic: fact or artifact? J Am Acad Child Adolesc Psychiatry. 2007; 46:723–30

Naqvi S. Review of Child and Adolescent Psychiatry. FOCUS: Child and Adolescent Psychiatry. Fall 2004; 2(4):536

---

340 A 22-year-old male college student has a positive HIV test. History reveals he had unprotected sex with multiple partners. His complete blood count is consistent with anemia. Which of the following factors places him at highest risk for eventually developing an HIV dementia?

A. Age.
B. Anemia.
C. Educational level.
D. Gender.
E. Multiple sexual partners.

The correct response is option B: Anemia.

HIV-associated dementias are reported in up to two-thirds of AIDS patients. Risk factors associated with eventual development of HIV dementia include lower educational level, older age, anemia, illicit drug use, and female gender.

Levenson JL (ed): Essentials of Psychosomatic Medicine, American Psychiatric Publishing, Washington, DC, 2007, p 209

341 The symptom that is most suggestive that an individual has generalized anxiety disorder (GAD) is worrying about:

A. Specific behaviors.
B. Physical symptoms.
C. Embarrassment.
D. All experiences.
E. Past events.

The correct response is option D: All experiences.

Worry is a relatively generic feature of anxiety disorders. The primary distinction between GAD and other anxiety disorders is the focus of the patient's concern. Worrying about physical symptoms occurs in panic disorder. Concern about being embarrassed is usually the focus of individuals with social phobia. Patients with GAD experience uncontrollable worry about a number of different areas and often worry about their worrying (metaworrying). Ruminating about past events tends to be associated with depression.

Huppert JD, Rynn M. Generalized anxiety disorder in Clinical Manual of Anxiety Disorders. Edited by Stein DJ. American Psychiatric Publishing, Washington DC, 2004; pp 150–151
Hoge EA, Oppenheimer JE, Simon NM: Generalized anxiety disorder. FOCUS: Anxiety Disorders, Summer 2004; 3:346–347

342 A 7-year-old boy with an anxiety disorder is in cognitive-behavior therapy. The parents ask how they should approach getting the child to do activities that he is fearful about, such as socializing with peers and participating in competitive situations. Which of the following is the MOST appropriate response?

A. Wait until the anxiety and fearfulness have been resolved.
B. Start when the child understands his anxieties.
C. Gradually approach with reinforcement for trying.
D. Find appropriate non-anxiety-producing substitutes.
E. Make fun activities contingent on doing anxiety-provoking things.

The correct response is option C: Gradually approach with reinforcement for trying.

Cognitive and behavioral therapies for anxiety have demonstrated effectiveness for a variety of anxiety disorders. Although there is some variation in approaches, the focus is on helping children and adolescents identify and manage their anxiety as well as reinforcing ongoing attempts to deal with anxiety-provoking situations successfully.

Naqvi S. Review of Child and Adolescent Psychiatry. FOCUS: Child and Adolescent Psychiatry. Fall 2004; 2(4):536–7
AACAP practice parameter for the assessment and treatment of children and adolescents with anxiety disorders. J Am Acad Child Adolesc Psychiatry. 2007; 46:273–274

343 A patient presents with a well-defined history of recurrent hypomanic episodes but denies ever having had depressive symptoms or full manic episodes. According to DSM-5 criteria, the most appropriate diagnosis would be:

A. Cyclothymic disorder.
B. Schizoaffective disorder.
C. Bipolar I disorder.
D. Bipolar II disorder.
E. Other specified bipolar and related disorder.

The correct response is option E: Other specified bipolar and related disorder.

DSM-5 allows the specification of particular conditions for other specified bipolar and related disorder. A diagnosis of bipolar II disorder is defined by one or more major depressive episodes accompanied by at least one hypomanic episode; cyclothymic disorder is characterized by numerous periods with hypomanic symptoms and numerous periods with depressive symptoms; and criteria for schizoaffective disorder include at least one manic, mixed, or major depressive episode. Unless additional history is obtained to the contrary, the patient's diagnosis would be other specified bipolar and related disorder.

American Psychiatric Association: Diagnostic and Statistical Manual of Mental Disorders, 5th Edition. Arlington, VA, American Psychiatric Association, 2013, p 148

344 Which of the following is a required criterion for the diagnosis of depression with melancholic features?

A. Mood worse in the late afternoon.
B. Middle or late insomnia.
C. Significant hyperphagia or weight gain.
D. Mood changes similar to those found in bereavement.
E. Loss of pleasure in all, or almost all, activities.

The correct response is option E: Loss of pleasure in all, or almost all, activities.

To diagnose depression with melancholic features, a person must have either a loss of pleasure in all or almost all activities OR a lack of reactivity to usually pleasurable stimuli (criteria A). They also must have three of six additional criteria, including depression worse in the morning, early morning awakening, significant anorexia or weight loss, a distinct quality of depressed mood characterized by despondency, psychomotor agitation, and excessive guilt.

American Psychiatric Association: Diagnostic and Statistical Manual of Mental Disorders, 5th Edition. Arlington, VA, American Psychiatric Association, 2013, p 185

345 A 10-year-old boy is referred for psychiatric assessment after setting his family's home on fire. His mother smoked cigarettes during the pregnancy. The patient grew up in an extremely impoverished neighborhood with his mother as his sole caregiver. His mother describes the boy as being extremely oppositional and defiant as a preschooler. She has primarily used corporal punishment including beating him with a belt and electric cords. Since starting school, he has had multiple suspensions for fighting with peers and teachers. Intelligence testing is consistent with borderline intellectual functioning. Which of these factors from the patient's history is MOST predictive of a poor outcome in this patient's conduct disorder?

A. Early age at onset of symptoms.
B. Exposure to toxins in utero.
C. Lack of a father figure in his life.
D. Impaired intellectual functioning.

The correct response is option A: Early age at onset of symptoms.

Early age at onset is the factor most consistently found to be associated with poor outcome in conduct disorder. A combination of demographic, individual, school, and family variables predicts age at onset. However, each variable individually does not predict the persistence of symptoms as well as the development of symptoms at an early age.

AACAP practice parameter for the assessment and treatment of children and adolescents with depressive disorders. J Am Acad Child Adolesc Psychiatry. 2007. FOCUS. 2008; 6(3):380–381

Dulcan MK, Weiner JM. Essentials of Child and Adolescent Psychiatry. Arlington (VA): American Psychiatric Publishing, 2006, p 374

Hales RE, Yudofsky SC, Gabbard GO (eds): The American Psychiatric Publishing Textbook of Psychiatry, 5th ed. Arlington, VA, American Psychiatric Publishing, 2008. p 895

346 During the assessment of a 3½-year-old boy who has been referred for biting other children at preschool, the mother discloses that the boy's stepfather has been physically abusive toward her. The child may have witnessed some of the abusive episodes. Which of the following MUST be done prior to the end of the session?

A. Explain that the child is at risk for PTSD.
B. Refer the mother for her own treatment.
C. Find contact information for shelters.
D. Explore whether the child has been abused.
E. Explore mother's reasons for staying with the stepfather.

The correct response is option D: Explore whether the child has been abused.

In terms of safety, it is essential to determine whether the child is being abused. A significant risk factor for child maltreatment is living in a household with domestic violence. The other options are important but not necessarily immediate.

Kaufman J. Child abuse and neglect, in Martin A, Volkmar FR (eds) Lewis' Comprehensive Textbook of Child and Adolescent Psychiatry 4th ed. Philadelphia, Lippincott Williams & Wilkins; 2007, pp 692–701

347 Which of the following signs differentiates patients with cognitive symptoms of depression from patients who are severely demented?

A. Less attention to self-care.
B. Cognitive impairment.
C. Complaints of memory loss.
D. Less attention to environment.
E. Memory storage and retrieval.

The correct response is option C: Complaints of memory loss.

Unlike patients with cognitive symptoms of depression, demented patients with impaired insight are not aware of their cognitive losses and therefore do not complain about them. In addition, depressed patients lack signs of cortical dysfunction such as apraxia, aphasia, and agnosia. Diagnosing patients who have cognitive symptoms of depression is critical so they can be treated. Distinguishing dementia from depression-related cognitive dysfunction can be difficult, particularly as the two may coexist.

American Psychiatric Association Practice Guideline for the Treatment of Patients With Major Depressive Disorder, 3rd ed. (2010). http://psychiatryonline.org/guidelines.aspx

348 A 32-year-old woman who does not want to take medication complains about shortness of breath, chest pain, and diaphoresis. She has had multiple attacks in the past 3 weeks. Her medical workup is negative. Which of the following treatments has the strongest evidence supporting it as first choice for this patient?

A. Dialectical behavioral therapy.
B. Family therapy.
C. Group therapy.
D. Patient support groups.
E. Cognitive-behavioral therapy.

The correct response is option E: Cognitive-behavioral therapy.

Cognitive-behavioral therapy has the most robust evidence of all the psychosocial treatments listed for the treatment of panic disorder. Family therapy, group therapy, and patient support groups may be useful as supplementary approaches depending on the patient's profile and needs. Dialectical behavioral therapy is currently used as a treatment for borderline personality disorder.

American Psychiatric Association Practice Guideline for the Treatment of Patients With Panic Disorder, 2nd ed (2008). http://psychiatryonline.org/guidelines.aspx

349 A 74-year-old man with known dementia is admitted to the hospital for workup and treatment of a presumed delirium. He scores a 21 on the Mini-Mental State Examination (MMSE) on admission and a 15 two days later. Nursing notes from his hospitalization indicate that there are times when he is completely alert and other times when he is nearly stuporous. Without appearing bothered, he has occasionally described seeing brightly colored birds perching on the windowsill of his room. A thorough delirium workup reveals no cause for his waxing and waning mental status findings. This description is most consistent with which dementing process?

A. Vascular dementia.
B. Alzheimer's dementia.
C. Frontotemporal dementia.
D. Lewy body dementia.
E. Korsakoff dementia.

The correct response is option D: Lewy body dementia.

Lewy body dementia is distinguished from other neurocognitive disorders by marked day-to-day fluctuations in cognitive performance. Spontaneous vivid visual hallucinations, with detailed evocations of humans and animals, are common. Also characteristic are relatively preserved memory function, prominent attentional and visuospatial dysfunction, and extrapyramidal motor signs. Systematic clinical evaluations, such as the National Institute of Neurological and Communicative Disorders and Stroke–AD and Related Disorders Association criteria, are generally accurate for diagnosing Alzheimer's disease, with a positive predictive value of as much as 88% when compared with neuropathological diagnosis. Although these criteria are accurate at distinguishing Alzheimer's disease from most other forms of neurocognitive disorders, differentiating Lewy body disease from Alzheimer's disease appears to be most difficult in clinical diagnosis. This is likely because, at least early on, patients often do not develop the extrapyramidal symptoms and hallucinations that help to distinguish this disorder from Alzheimer's disease.

Ranginwala NA, Hynan LS, Weiner MF, White CL, III Clinical criteria for the diagnosis of Alzheimer disease: still good after all these years. Am J Geriatr Psychiatry. 2008; 16(5):384–388

Geser F, Wenning GK, Poewe W, McKeith I. How to diagnose dementia with Lewy bodies: state of the art. Mov Disord. 2005; 20 Suppl 12: S11–S20

---

350 In DSM-5, which of the following disorder(s) of children and adolescents is NOT classified among the neurodevelopmental disorders?

A. Tic disorders.
B. Attention-deficit/hyperactivity disorder.
C. Disruptive mood dysregulation disorder.
D. Learning disorders.
E. Social (pragmatic) communication disorder.

The correct response is option C: Disruptive mood dysregulation disorder.

In DSM-5, disruptive mood dysregulation disorder is classified with depressive disorders. This is a diagnosis for children up to 18 years of age who exhibit persistent irritability and frequent episodes of severe behavioral dyscontrol.

American Psychiatric Association: Diagnostic and Statistical Manual of Mental Disorders, 5th Edition. Arlington, VA, American Psychiatric Association, 2013. pp 49, 156–157, Highlights of changes from DSM-IV to DSM-5, p 810

---

351 Which of the following psychosocial treatments for depression has the most robust data supporting its use?

A. Cognitive-behavioral therapy.
B. Dialectical behavioral therapy.
C. Group therapy.
D. Psychodynamic psychotherapy.
E. Supportive therapy.

The correct response is option A: Cognitive-behavioral therapy.

Cognitive-behavioral therapy, interpersonal psychotherapy, and behavioral psychotherapies (e.g., behavioral activation) have demonstrated acute efficacy in treating major depressive disorder. There is less evidence for other psychotherapies.

American Psychiatric Association: Practice Guideline for the Treatment of Patients With Major Depressive Disorder, 3rd ed (2010), p 47. http://psychiatryonline.org/guidelines.aspx

352 A 25-year-old patient with schizophrenia is admitted to the hospital with auditory hallucinations and persecutory delusions. The psychiatrist initiates haloperidol 5 mg orally twice per day. After 48 hours of receiving medication, the patient becomes increasingly irritable and agitated and is noted to be restless and pacing. The patient's blood pressure is 130/85 with a pulse of 88. The next step in management of this patient's symptoms should be to:

A. Increase the haloperidol to 10 mg orally twice per day.
B. Administer benztropine 1 mg orally twice per day.
C. Administer a one-time dose of haloperidol 5 mg intramuscularly.
D. Administer a one-time dose of diphenhydramine 25 mg intramuscularly.
E. Initiate propranolol 20 mg orally three times per day.

The correct response is option E: Initiate propranolol 20 mg orally three times per day.

Akathisia is a common reaction to treatment with typical neuroleptic agents. Because akathisia may be mistaken for an increase in psychosis or anxiety, it is sometimes inappropriately addressed by increasing the antipsychotic dosage, which results in a worsening of symptoms. The treatment of choice is either to change to an atypical neuroleptic agent or to add a beta-blocking agent, such as propranolol. Anticholinergic agents have not been found to be effective.

Haddad PM, Dursun SM. Neurological complications of psychiatric drugs: clinical features and management. Hum Psychopharmacol. 2008 Jan: 23 Suppl 1:15–26

Rathbone J, Soares-Weiser K. Anticholinergics for neuroleptic-induced acute akathisia. Cochrane Database Syst Rev. 2006 Oct 18; (4): D003727

Hales RE, Yudofsky SC, Gabbard GO (eds): The American Psychiatric Publishing Textbook of Psychiatry, 5th ed. Arlington, VA, American Psychiatric Publishing, 2008. pp 1089–1090

353 Which of the following doses of haloperidol decanoate has been shown to have the lowest rate of symptomatic exacerbation yet minimal increased risk of adverse effect or subjective discomfort?

A. 25 mg/month.
B. 50 mg/month.
C. 100 mg/month.
D. 200 mg/month.

The correct response is option D: 200 mg/month.

In a multidose study of haloperidol decanoate in the maintenance treatment of schizophrenia, 200 mg/month was associated with the lowest rate of symptomatic exacerbation combined with a minimal increased risk of adverse effect of subjective discomfort when compared with doses of 25, 50, and 100 mg/month.

Kane JM, Davis JM, Schooler N, Marder S, Casey D, Brauzer B, Mintz J, Conley R A multidose study of haloperidol decanoate in the maintenance treatment of schizophrenia. Am J Psychiatry. 2002; 159:554–60

354 Which of the following medications has the potential for a significantly increased risk of hemorrhagic pancreatitis?

A. Clozapine.
B. Divalproex.
C. Nefazodone.
D. Pemoline.
E. Thioridazine.

The correct response is option B: Divalproex.

Divalproex is associated with hemorrhagic pancreatitis and hepatic failure. All of the above medications have the potential for serious side effects: clozapine for agranulocytosis and myocarditis; nefazodone for acute liver failure; pemoline for acute liver failure; and thioridazine for torsades de pointes or QT and QTc prolongation.

Sadock BJ, Sadock VA (eds): Kaplan and Sadock's Comprehensive Textbook of Psychiatry, 9th ed. Philadelphia, Lippincott Williams & Wilkins, 2009, p 2972

355 Which of the following situations is the individual with social phobia likely to avoid?

A. Crossing bridges.
B. Eating in public.
C. Being in closed spaces.
D. Proximity to spiders.
E. Sitting in movie theaters.

The correct response is option B: Eating in public.

Anxiety that characterizes social phobia occurs when the individual is expected to perform or interact in social situations in which he or she could be embarrassed, especially with strangers or people that he or she feels might judge him or her. Eating in public for some patients becomes impossible because of the fear that others are judging the way they consume food. Others with this disorder may not be able to write in public, use public urinals, or speak in public—the latter is the most common phobia. Marked fear or anxiety of two or more situations such as crossing bridges and attending movie theaters can be a feature of agoraphobia. Avoidance of a specific closed space such as an elevator or fear of spiders is associated with specific phobia. Panic attacks can occur in the presence of any anxiety disorder.

American Psychiatric Association: Diagnostic and Statistical Manual of Mental Disorders, 5th Edition. Arlington, VA, American Psychiatric Association, 2013, pp 202–203

356 A 32-year-old woman with a history of early-childhood abuse and abandonment begins dynamic psychotherapy. Although the initial stages of treatment proceed well, after 3 months her psychiatrist notices that she is becoming more critical of the therapy and frequently questions the value of it. In addition, she is dismissive of the psychiatrist and begins to question whether the psychiatrist is adequately trained. As a result, the psychiatrist begins to dread the sessions and occasionally begins the sessions late. This mode of interaction is best described as a type of:

A. Projective identification.
B. Displacement.
C. Sublimation.
D. Paranoid-schizoid position.
E. Ambivalent/resistant pattern.

The correct response is option A: Projective identification.

A core psychoanalytic concept derived from object relations theory is that patients reenact early internalized relationship patterns through the externalization of these patterns. The recapitulating of old relationships into the present is called *projective identification*, in which the patient exerts pressure on the therapist to conform to the pattern of interaction that he or she is generating. In this case, the patient, fearful of attachment (with its risk of subsequent abandonment) resorts to earlier modes of interaction in which she behaves in a way that irritates the psychiatrist to the point where the professional begins to behave in a way reminiscent of earlier abusive figures in the patient's life.

Displacement refers to the shifting of uncomfortable impulses to a more acceptable or less threatening target (e.g., yelling at one's spouse when angry at an employer). *Sublimation* is the transformation of negative impulses into positive or productive actions or emotions (e.g., frustrated by a failing relationship, one turns to painting). The *paranoid-schizoid position* is another concept from object relations theory in which one can only form partial object relationships. The result is the defense mechanism referred to as *splitting*. The *ambivalent/resistant pattern* is a reference to attachment theory and refers to a child's reaction to a neglectful or inconsistent caregiver by both seeking closeness with the person but then resisting it when offered.

Gabbard GO: Psychodynamic approaches to personality disorders. FOCUS 2005; 3:363–367

357 The parents of a 16-year-old-year boy ask if he can be treated to prevent the development of schizophrenia. For the last year, the boy has been more irritable, staying in his room most of the time playing music. His grades have declined. His uncle was diagnosed with schizophrenia at the age of 17. Which of the following statements BEST describes the current knowledge about the early identification and treatment of individuals who will become schizophrenic?

A. Many adolescents with these symptoms will not become schizophrenic.
B. Treatment with low-dose atypical antipsychotics will prevent schizophrenia.
C. Long-term use of atypical antipsychotics does not have major adverse effects.
D. Psychosocial interventions are more effective than medication treatment.

The correct response is option A: Many adolescents with these symptoms will not become schizophrenic.

There is increased interest in early identification of adolescents who are at high risk to become schizophrenic and in early interventions to either prevent the development of the disorder or ameliorate its course. Current problems include the following: many adolescents have prodromal symptoms but do not develop schizophrenia, the adverse effects of long-term use of atypical antipsychotics, unnecessary treatment of individuals, and the unclear benefits of early treatment with atypical antipsychotics. There have been no identified psychosocial treatments that prevent the onset of schizophrenia. At this point, further evaluation would be helpful to determine what is going on and whether the adolescent has a condition that would warrant treatment (e.g., psychosis, depression, substance use disorder).

AACAP practice parameters for the assessment and treatment of children and adolescents with schizophrenia. J Am Acad Child Adolesc Psychiatry. 2001; 40(7) Supplement:4S–23S

358 Which of the following is a common adverse effect of monoamine oxidase inhibitors therapy?

A. Serotonin syndrome.
B. Hypertensive crisis.
C. Priapism.
D. Orthostatic hypotension.
E. Weight loss.

The correct response is option D: Orthostatic hypotension.

Hypotension is a frequent adverse effect of MAOIs. Other common side effects include insomnia, dry mouth, weight gain, edema, sexual dysfunction, headache, and afternoon somnolence. Orthostatic hypotension can lead to dizziness and falls. Therefore, cautious upward titration of MAOI dosage should be used. Treatment for orthostatic hypotension includes avoidance of caffeine, intake of 2 L of fluid per day, addition of dietary salt, adjustment of antihypertensive drugs, support stockings, and, in severe cases, treatment with fludrocortisones. Hypertensive crises and serotonin syndrome are rare but life-threatening events.

Sadock BJ, Sadock VA (eds): Kaplan and Sadock's Synopsis of Psychiatry: Behavioral Sciences/Clinical Psychiatry. Philadelphia, Lippincott Williams & Wilkins, 10th edition, 2007, p1067
Yudofsky SC, Hales RE (eds): The American Psychiatric Publishing Textbook of Neuropsychiatry and Behavioral Sciences, 5th ed. Arlington, VA, American Psychiatric Publishing, 2008, pp 1061, 1071–1074

359 A patient who was recently diagnosed with panic disorder complains 2 days after starting citalopram that she continues to be very anxious about having another panic attack. Even her sleep has been disrupted. Which of the following would treat her anxiety best?

A. Increase the citalopram.
B. Add lithium.
C. Lower citalopram.
D. Add clonazepam.
E. Add trazodone.

The correct response is option D: Add clonazepam.

The patient's complaint is likely due to anticipatory anxiety. Clonazepam or another benzodiazepine would lower her anxiety until the citalopram can both treat anxiety and reassure her that a panic attack is unlikely in the future. If she complained about jitteriness in general, lowering the citalopram dose would be indicated. The addition of trazodone would address the sleep problem, but that is not her primary problem. Currently, there is no indication for increasing the citalopram or adding lithium.

American Psychiatric Association Practice Guideline for the Treatment of Patients With Panic Disorder, 2nd ed (2008). http://psychiatryonline.org/guidelines.aspx

---

360 A 32-year-old woman presents to the emergency department after being raped. She appears confused and extremely frightened. She mentions a history of prior rapes. Which of the following psychotherapies, if administered soon after the event, has the best body of evidence in preventing the patient from progressing to PTSD?

A. Supportive psychotherapy.
B. Psychological debriefing.
C. Hypnosis.
D. Cognitive-behavioral therapy.
E. Single-session exposure therapy.

The correct response is option D: Cognitive-behavioral therapy.

Victims of multiple traumas are at particular risk for developing PTSD. A number of psychotherapeutic techniques have been attempted to prevent the onset of PTSD. By desensitizing individuals to trauma-related triggers, cognitive-behavioral therapies have been shown to speed recovery and prevent PTSD in rape and accident victims. In patients who have experienced multiple recurrent traumas, there is little evidence that supportive therapy or psychoeducation will, in and of themselves, result in lasting reductions in symptoms, although they are unlikely to do harm. In contrast, single-session techniques such as psychological debriefing and single-session exposure therapies may exacerbate symptoms in some patients. Hypnosis has been used for PTSD patients, generally not as a preventive treatment, nor has it been used in the acute setting.

American Psychiatric Association Practice Guideline for the Treatment of Patients with Acute Stress Disorder and Posttraumatic Stress Disorder. 2004. p 13. http://psychiatryonline.org/guidelines.aspx

---

361 A 28-year-old patient with schizophrenia is prescribed an atypical antipsychotic medication. A baseline fasting plasma glucose level is obtained and is within normal limits. After what period of time should this test be repeated?

A. 2 weeks, and then quarterly.
B. 3 months, and then annually.
C. 6 months, and then annually.
D. Every 6 months.
E. Annually.

The correct response is option B: 3 months, and then annually.

According to the Consensus Development Conference on Antipsychotic Drugs and Obesity and Diabetes, individuals prescribed an antipsychotic medication should have a fasting plasma glucose level performed at baseline, then again in 3 months, and then annually thereafter. The APA Practice Guideline on Schizophrenia (2004) mentions "Fasting blood glucose or hemoglobin A1c at 4 months after initiating a new treatment and annually thereafter."

American Psychiatric Association Practice Guideline for the Treatment of Patients with Schizophrenia, 2nd ed (2004) pp 272–273. http://psychiatryonline.org/guidelines.aspx

Consensus Development Conference on Antipsychotic Drugs and Obesity and Diabetes. (Reviews/Commentaries/Position Statements). Diabetes Care. 2004; 27:596–601

---

362 Which of the following reflects the APA's position on psychiatrists' participation in legally authorized executions?

A. Sanctioning of participation is determined by state associations.
B. Psychiatrists should not participate in executions.
C. Participation is left up to the discretion of the psychiatrist.
D. Psychiatrists may only perform a mental status exam prior to execution.
E. Psychiatrists may participate if they are only in a supervisory role.

The correct response is option B: Psychiatrists should not participate in executions.

A physician shall be dedicated to providing competent medical care with compassion and respect for human dignity and rights. APA ethical guidelines state a psychiatrist should not be a participant in a legally authorized execution.

Opinions of the Ethics Committee on The Principles of Medical Ethics With Annotations Especially Applicable to Psychiatry 2014. American Psychiatric Association, Arlington, VA. http://www.psychiatry.org/practice/ethics/resources-standards

---

363 A 20-year-old college student presents to the mental health clinic because for the past 6 months he worries constantly about things going on at his part-time job and about exams that he must take in his classes. He has chronic problems with concentration and sleep and complains that he is easily fatigued. He states that he is tired of the pressure he always feels. He adds that he has also been to the medical clinic because he feared that his frequent muscle tension meant he had a neurological disease. Which of the following is the most likely diagnosis?

A. Major depression.
B. Illness anxiety disorder.
C. Generalized anxiety disorder (GAD).
D. Adjustment disorder.
E. Somatic symptom disorder.

The correct response is option C: Generalized anxiety disorder (GAD).

The patient's history includes virtually all the criteria for GAD. Excessive worry more days than not for at least 6 months, the worry is about a number of events or activities, and at least three additional specific symptoms of anxiety such as fatigue, concentration difficulties, and muscle tension. The disorder can be comorbid with depression, but this history does not provide much evidence for that diagnosis. Options B and E refer to disorders where the chief complaints are focused on the body. Adjustment disorder requires a known precipitant and would have less extensive and intensive symptomatology.

American Psychiatric Association: Diagnostic and Statistical Manual of Mental Disorders, 5th Edition. Arlington, VA, American Psychiatric Association, 2013, p 222

---

364 Which medication has the most evidence supporting its use as an augmenting agent for treatment-resistant major depression?

A. Divalproex sodium.
B. Lamotrigine.
C. Lithium.
D. Lorazepam.
E. Phenelzine.

The correct response is option C: Lithium.

Accepted augmentation agents for treatment-resistant major depression include lithium, thyroid hormone, buspirone, and atypical antipsychotics. Augmentation of antidepressant medications can utilize another non-MAOI antidepressant, generally from a different pharmacological class, or a non-antidepressant medication such as lithium. Lithium has been found to be effective in augmenting antidepressants when treating depressive disorders and has the most evidence for its use. Lorazepam can be used to reduce associated anxiety, which may indirectly relieve depressive symptoms. Several anticonvulsants have been studied as augmentation agents, but the evidence for agents like lamotrigine or divalproex sodium is not as strong as it is for lithium. Phenelzine is a monoamine oxidase inhibitor (MAOI) that should not be given with a selective serotonin reuptake inhibitor (SSRI, e.g., fluoxetine) because it can result in serious life-threatening reactions. Aripiprazole and quetiapine have received approval, but adverse effects must be considered.

Crossley NA, Bauer M. Acceleration and augmentation of antidepressants with lithium for depressive disorders: two metaanalyses of randomized, placebo-controlled trials. J Clin Psychiatry. 2007 Jun; 68(6):935–40

American Psychiatric Association Practice Guideline for the Treatment of Patients With Major Depressive Disorder, 3rd ed. (2010). http://psychiatryonline.org/guidelines.aspx

---

365 Eye movement desensitization and reprocessing (EMDR) has several features that distinguish it from the other cognitive-behavioral treatments for PTSD. In addition to the directed eye movements, which of the following also distinguishes EMDR?

A. Having patients think about the trauma rather than verbalize it.
B. Encouraging patients to learn to identify cognitive distortions.
C. Utilizing and emphasizing exposures to the traumatic material.
D. Teaching relaxation and imaging techniques to manage anxiety.
E. Employing homework assignments to reinforce session work.

The correct response is option A: Having patients think about the trauma rather than verbalize it.

EMDR is a form of psychotherapy that includes an exposure-based therapy (with multiple brief, interrupted exposures to traumatic material), eye movement, and recall of traumatic memories of an event or events. It combines multiple perspectives and techniques, including cognitive-behavior therapy. The use of directed eye movements as a feature distinguishes this form of therapy from other cognitive-behavior approaches. Additionally, the traumatic material need not be verbalized; instead, patients are directed to think about their traumatic experiences without having to discuss them.

American Psychiatric Association Practice Guideline for the Treatment of Patients with Acute Stress Disorder and Posttraumatic Stress Disorder. Am J Psychiatry. 2004; 161(11):18. http://psychiatryonline.org/guidelines.aspx

---

366 A 28-year-old woman with bipolar II disorder has been using an oral contraceptive for birth control. She currently presents with a hypomanic episode. Which of the following medications would be best to treat her hypomania without impairing the efficacy of the oral contraceptive?

A. Carbamazepine.
B. Lithium.
C. Oxcarbamazepine.
D. Topirimate.

The correct response is option B: Lithium.

Carbamazepine, oxcarbamazepine, and topiramate increase the metabolism of oral contraceptives. As a result, women taking these medications should not rely on oral contraceptives for birth control. This effect does not occur with other medications used to treat bipolar disorder.

American Psychiatric Association Practice Guideline for the Treatment of Patients with Bipolar Disorder, 2nd Edition (2002). Reprinted in FOCUS: Bipolar Disorder 2003; 1:74. http://psychiatryonline.org/guidelines.aspx

Altshuler LL, Hendrick V, Cohen LS: Course of mood and anxiety disorders during pregnancy and the postpartum period. J Clin Psychiatry 1998; 59(suppl 2):29–33 87

Spina E, Pisani F, Perucca E: Clinically significant pharmacokinetic drug interactions with carbamazepine: an update. Clin Pharmacokinet 1996; 31:198–214

---

367 Which psychotherapeutic modality involves teaching patients to tolerate distress, regulate their emotions, reduce vulnerability to cues, and avoid or distract without problem behavior, while concomitantly reducing reinforcement of maladaptive behavior?

A. Psychoanalytic psychotherapy.
B. Cognitive-behavioral therapy.
C. Interpersonal psychotherapy.
D. Dialectical behavior therapy.
E. Supportive therapy.

The correct response is option D: Dialectical behavior therapy.

Dialectical behavior therapy focuses on expanding the patient's repertoire of coping skills, reducing reinforcement of maladaptive behavior, increasing reinforcement of adaptive behaviors, generalizing new behaviors from the therapeutic environment to the natural environment, and supporting the motivation and capability of the therapist.

Sadock BJ, Sadock VA: Kaplan and Sadock's Synopsis of Psychiatry, 10th ed. Philadelphia, Lippincott Williams & Wilkins, 2007, pp 944–5

Textbook of Psychotherapeutic Treatments. Gabbard GO (ed). Arlington VA, American Psychiatric Publishing, 2009, pp 727–731

---

368 Which of the following drug classes is the preferred initial pharmacotherapy for social anxiety disorder?

A. Tricyclic antidepressant (TCA).
B. Monoamine oxidase inhibitor (MAOI).
C. Benzodiazepine (BDZ).
D. Selective serotonin reuptake inhibitor (SSRI).
E. Beta-blockers.

The correct response is option D: Selective serotonin reuptake inhibitor (SSRI).

Both paroxetine and sertraline are SSRIs that are FDA-approved for treating social anxiety disorder (social phobia). Research studies have also supported the efficacy of other SSRIs. Venlafaxine XR (serotonin-norepinephrine reuptake inhibitor [SNRI]) is also FDA-approved for anxiety disorders. Research evidence does support efficacy for both MAOIs and benzodiazepines; however, neither is FDA-approved, and they have disadvantages that prevent them from being first-line medications for social anxiety. Beta-blockers may have some value for treatment of performance anxiety, but their effectiveness for generalized social phobia is marginal. There is little evidence that TCAs are useful for treating social anxiety disorder.

Delong H, Pollack M. Update on the assessment, diagnosis, and treatment of individuals with social anxiety disorder. FOCUS: Panic and Social Phobia. Fall 2008; (6)4

Davidson JRT. Pharmacotherapy of social anxiety disorder: what does the evidence tell us? J Clin Psychiatry. 2006; 67(suppl 12):20–26

Muller JE, Koen L, Seedat S, Stein DJ. Social anxiety disorder: current treatment recommendations. CNS Drugs 2005; 19:377–391

Hales RE, Yudofsky SC and Gabbard GO (eds): The American Psychiatric Publishing Textbook of Psychiatry, 5th ed. Arlington, VA, American Psychiatric Publishing, 2008. p 542

369 Which of the following factors is most likely to be associated with bacterial soft-tissue infections in drug users?

A. Cleaning the skin before injection.
B. Being HIV negative.
C. Being an experienced injector.
D. Intravenous injection.
E. Subcutaneous injection.

The correct response is option E: Subcutaneous injection.

Subcutaneous injection or intramuscular injection ("skin popping"), repeatedly flushing and pulling back during an injection ("booting"), being human immunodeficiency virus positive, and failing to clean the skin before injection all increase the risk of bacterial soft-tissue infections. Intravenous injection, particularly by an experienced injector with a single drug does not increase the risk as much as these other factors. Being an inexperienced injector and combining heroin and cocaine ("speed balls") may increase the risk of infection. *Staphylococcus aureus* and *streptococcus* species are the most common sources of infection.

Gordon RJ, Lowy FD: Bacterial infections in drug users. N Engl J Med 2005; 353:1945–54

370 A 40-year-old patient complains of episodes of intense fear with associated somatic symptoms that have a sudden onset and peak within minutes. Which of the following is the essential feature required for a diagnosis of panic disorder?

A. Anticipatory anxiety and avoidance of public speaking.
B. Unexpected, "out-of-the-blue" nature of the episodes.
C. Presence of four or more characteristic symptoms during episodes.
D. Episodes precipitated by memories of a past trauma.
E. Episodes triggered by contact with "contaminated" objects.

The correct response is option B: Unexpected, "out-of-the-blue" nature of the episodes.

According to DSM-5, key to a diagnosis of panic disorder is the occurrence of unexpected, recurrent panic attacks. Panic attacks can occur in association with many other conditions such as social anxiety (e.g., public speaking), posttraumatic stress disorder (e.g., when recalling the stressor), and obsessive-compulsive disorder. At least 4 of 13 characteristic symptoms are necessary to diagnose both a panic attack and panic disorder.

American Psychiatric Association: Diagnostic and Statistical Manual of Mental Disorders, 5th Edition. Arlington, VA, American Psychiatric Association, 2013, pp 208, 214

371 A 53-year-old man with a history of alcohol dependence has been abstinent from alcohol for 3 months. Although he continues to attend peer support groups, he reports that he has recently begun drinking one to two drinks approximately every other day and is fearful that his relapse will worsen. Which of the following medications would be the most appropriate first-line pharmacological intervention for this patient?

A. Naltrexone.
B. Acamprosate.
C. Bupropion.
D. Fluoxetine.
E. Disulfiram.

The correct response is option B: Acamprosate.

Of medications used for the treatment or prevention of alcohol disorder, naltrexone and acamprosate have the best support in the literature. Naltrexone, an opioid antagonist, appears to be most effective at reducing heavy drinking. Acamprosate, which is thought to work through an effect on NMDA-mediated glutamatergic transmission, appears to have a unique role in supporting abstinence in individuals who are abstinent or only recently relapsed. Disulfiram, which has had mixed results, should not be used in patients who are actively drinking even small amounts. Antidepressants have only equivocal results for treating alcohol use disorder.

Mason BJ: Acamprosate for alcohol dependence: An update for the clinician. FOCUS 2006; 4:505–511

Yudofsky SC, Hales RE (eds): The American Psychiatric Publishing Textbook of Neuropsychiatry and Behavioral Sciences, 5th ed. Arlington, VA, American Psychiatric Publishing, 2008, p 380

---

372 A 20-year-old patient with schizophrenia receiving antipsychotic treatment complains of breast tenderness, galactorrhea, and amenorrhea. Which of the following medications is the patient most likely taking?

A. Aripiprazole.
B. Risperidone.
C. Quetiapine.
D. Clozapine.
E. Ziprasidone.

The correct response is option B: Risperidone.

This patient is experiencing the effects of hyperprolactinemia. Of the atypical antipsychotic agents, risperidone is most likely to cause increased prolactin levels.

Schatzberg AF, Nemeroff CB (eds): Essentials of Clinical Psychopharmacology, 2nd ed. Washington, DC, American Psychiatric Publishing, 2006, p 291–2

---

373 Which of the following statements most accurately reflects the position of the *APA's Principles of Medical Ethics* on faculty psychiatrists having sex with trainees?

A. There is no established APA position on sexual relationships with trainees.
B. Sexual relationships with trainees are absolutely unethical.
C. Sexual relationships are permissible when both parties are consenting adults.
D. Sexual behavior in faculty-trainee relationships may negatively impact patient care.

The correct response is option D: Sexual behavior in faculty-trainee relationships may negatively impact patient care.

APA ethical guidelines state that sexual involvement between supervisors and trainees may be unethical because the patient whose treatment is being supervised may be negatively affected, trust between the student and teacher may be damaged, and teachers are important role models for trainees and affect their trainees' future professional behavior.

American Psychiatric Association. The Principles of Medical Ethics With Annotations Especially Applicable to Psychiatry, 2013, http://www.psychiatry.org/practice/ethics

---

374 In which of the following situations would a high-potency benzodiazepine be the preferred initial pharmacotherapy for panic disorder?

A. Comorbid major depression.
B. Need for rapid onset of action.
C. Anticipation of long-term treatment.
D. Associated agoraphobia.
E. Comorbid cardiovascular disease.

The correct response is option B: Need for rapid onset of action.

Although SSRIs are usually the preferred treatment for panic disorder, their onset of action is slow compared with that of benzodiazepines. On the other hand, benzodiazepines are not effective antidepressants, and they carry risks of dependence and abuse with long-term treatment. Both classes of drugs can benefit associated agoraphobia and are well tolerated in the presence of cardiovascular disease.

Bakker A, van Balkom AJ, Stein DJ. Evidence-based pharmacotherapy of panic disorder. Int J Neuropsychopharmacol 2005; 8:473–482

Pollack MH, Allgulander C, Bandelow B, Cassano GB, et al: WCA recommendations for the long-term treatment of panic disorder. CNS Spectrums 2003; 8(suppl 1):17–30

Roy-Byrne PP, Craske MG, Stein MG. Panic disorder. Lancet 2006; 368:1023–1032 American Psychiatric Association Practice Guideline for the Treatment of Patients With Panic Disorder, 2nd ed (2008). http://psychiatryonline.org/guidelines.aspx

---

375 Which of the following substance abuse therapist attributes has the greatest and most consistent impact on patient retention and reduced substance use?

A. Therapists skilled at limit setting.
B. Therapists who were successfully treated for substance dependence.
C. Therapists who have a first-degree relative who was substance dependent.
D. Therapists with strong interpersonal skills.
E. Therapists who are knowledgeable about both biological and psychosocial interventions.

The correct response is option D: Therapists with strong interpersonal skills.

Limit setting has an important role in treatment of substance use disorders and may be particularly important for individuals with co-occurring personality disorders. However, a review of the literature on effective characteristics of therapists concluded that the characteristic most associated with patient retention and reduced substance use was strong interpersonal skills.

American Psychiatric Association Practice Guideline for the Treatment of Patients with Substance Use Disorders, Second Edition, 2nd Edition (2006), pp 316–317. http://psychiatryonline.org/guidelines.aspx

---

376 The daughter of an 89-year-old man with severe dementia requests that her father be deemed incompetent. The ultimate decision to determine competence is made by the:

A. Daughter.
B. Court
C. Psychiatrist.
D. Treating physician.
E. Health care power of attorney.

The correct response is option B: Court.

Although anyone can offer an opinion as to whether or not someone should be deemed incompetent, the final decision is made by the court.

Blazer DG, Steffens DC (eds): The American Psychiatric Publishing Textbook of Geriatric Psychiatry, 4th ed. Arlington, VA, American Psychiatric Publishing, 2009, pp 612–13

---

377 Anger is most closely associated with which of the following temperament traits?

A. Harm avoidance.
B. Novelty seeking.
C. Reward dependence.
D. Persistence.

The correct response is option B: Novelty seeking.

Temperament, a heritable factor in personality development, has been divided into four dimensions: harm avoidance, novelty seeking, reward dependence, and persistence. These are associated with the four basic emotions of fear, anger, attachment, and ambition, respectively.

Sadock BJ, Sadock VA: Kaplan & Sadock's Comprehensive Textbook of Psychiatry. 9th Ed, 2009 pp 2199–2204

Angres DH. The Temperament and Character Inventory in addiction treatment. Focus 2010 8: 192

378 An 80-year-old man is brought to the emergency room after suffering a grand mal seizure. His serum sodium concentration is 107 mmol/L. Which of the following medications is most likely to have caused the hyponatremia?

A. Topiramate.
B. Lamotrigine.
C. Gabapentin.
D. Oxcarbazepine.
E. Valproate.

The correct response is option D: Oxcarbazepine.

Of the options given, only oxcarbazepine use has been associated with hyponatremia. The mechanism has not been resolved fully, but considerations include increased antidiuretic hormone (ADH) release, increased renal vasopressin receptor sensitivity, and vasopressinase inhibition. Risk factors include increased age, low baseline sodium concentration, smoking, and diuretic use.

Dong X, Leppik IE, White J, Rarick J: Hyponatremia from oxcarbazepine and carbamazepine. Neurology 2005; 65:1976–1978

Van Amelsvoort T, Bakshi R., Devaux CB, Schwabe S: Hyponatremia associated with carbamazepine and oxcarbazepine therapy: a review. Epilepsia 1994; 35:181–188

379 In children with major depressive disorder, which of the following is MORE likely to occur in boys than girls?

A. Feelings of anxiety.
B. Acting-out behaviors.
C. Poorer self-esteem.
D. Severe symptoms of depression.
E. Shorter period of recovery.

The correct response is option B: Acting-out behaviors.

Epidemiological studies have demonstrated gender differences in children and adolescents with depressive disorders. Gender is not believed to affect recovery from depression. Girls tend to report higher levels of depressive symptoms than boys and have more inwardly directed symptoms related to feeling anxious. Girls have lower self-worth and poorer self-esteem than boys. Boys have higher rates of irritability and acting-out behaviors such as running away, theft, or substance abuse.

Dulcan MK, Weiner JM. Essentials of Child and Adolescent Psychiatry. Arlington (VA); 2006, p 270

380 A 21-year-old patient dropped out of college and has been unable to attend social gatherings as a result of extreme fear of embarrassing herself. She has failed to respond to therapeutic trials of paroxetine, fluvoxamine, sertraline, clonazepam, and buspirone. Which of the following medications would be most appropriate to prescribe next?

A. Fluoxetine.
B. Propranolol.
C. Phenelzine.
D. Lithium.
E. Risperidone.

The correct response is option C: Phenelzine.

MAOIs such as phenelzine are very effective in the treatment of social anxiety, but because of side effects and the requirement of extensive medication and dietary restrictions, they are not first-line treatments. However, in individuals who have failed to respond to therapeutic trials of several other agents with better side-effect profiles, such as the patient described in this case, MAOIs are another option. Fluoxetine would not be a good choice, given failed trials of more than two other SSRIs. Propranolol is typically useful on an as-needed basis for performance anxiety and is not likely to be helpful in treatment-refractory social anxiety. Lithium and risperidone have not been proven to be effective in the treatment of social anxiety.

Hales RE, Yudofsky SC, Gabbard GO (eds): The American Psychiatric Publishing Textbook of Psychiatry, 5th ed. Arlington, VA, American Psychiatric Publishing, 2008, pp 542–44

Blanco C, Raza MS, Schneier FR, et al. The evidence-based pharmacological treatment of social anxiety disorder. Int J Neuropsychopharmacol 2003; 6:427–442

---

381 Which of the following psychotropic medications has been associated with polycystic ovarian syndrome?

A. Lithium.
B. Divalproex.
C. Methylphenidate.
D. Citalopram.
E. Aripiprazole.

The correct response is option B: Divalproex.

Divalproex has been associated with the polycystic ovarian syndrome. Patients taking valproic acid medications should be counseled to avoid weight gain. If they have oligomenorrhea or hirsutism, then a referral may be appropriate for initiation of treatment with either a combination oral contraceptive or progestin and treatments for hirsutism. The mood stabilizers (e.g., lithium, lamotrigine) do not appear to be associated with polycystic ovarian syndrome and may be substituted for divalproex if needed.

Correll CU, Carlson HE: Endocrine and metabolic adverse effects of psychotropic medications in children and adolescents. J Am Acad Child Adolesc Psychiatry. 2006; 45:771–91

---

382 A 58-year-old patient with diabetic peripheral neuropathic pain presents with major depressive disorder. Which of the following antidepressants is most likely to have beneficial effects on both conditions?

A. Bupropion.
B. Duloxetine.
C. Escitalopram.
D. Nefazodone.
E. Mirtazapine.

The correct response is option B: Duloxetine.

Although all of the options are FDA-approved for the treatment of major depressive disorder, only duloxetine is also approved for the treatment of diabetic peripheral neuropathic pain. Hepatotoxicity can be caused by nefazadone and should be avoided in patients with liver disease, persons with alcohol misuse, or those consuming high doses of acetaminophen.

Sedky K, Nazir R, Joshi A, Kaur G, Lippmann S. Which psychotropic medications induce hepatotoxicity? Gen Hosp Psychiatry. 2012 Jan-Feb; 34(1):53–61

Smith TR. Duloxetine in diabetic neuropathy. Expert Opin Pharmacother 2006; 7:215–223

---

383 When initiating treatment with risperidone long-acting injection, oral risperidone should be concomitantly prescribed for what length of time?

A. 1 week.
B. 3 weeks.
C. 6 weeks.
D. 8 weeks.
E. 12 weeks.

The correct response is option B: 3 weeks.

According to the package insert, oral risperidone (or another oral antipsychotic medication) should be prescribed for 3 weeks following the first injection (and then discontinued) to maintain therapeutic plasma concentrations.

Lasser RA, Bossie CA, Zhu Y, Locklear JC, Kane JM. Long-acting risperidone in young adults with early schizophrenia or schizoaffective illness. Ann Clin Psychiatry. 2007 Apr-Jun; 19(2):65–71

Risperdal® Consta® package insert, Janssen LP, Titusville, NJ, 2007

---

384 Which of the following personality disorders most closely resembles social anxiety disorder?

A. Schizoid.
B. Borderline.
C. Avoidant.
D. Dependent.
E. Histrionic.

The correct response is option C: Avoidant.

According to DSM-5, avoidant personality disorder may be a more severe variant of social phobia that is not qualitatively distinct. Schizoid personality is characterized by odd behavior and beliefs. Borderline personality disorder is characterized by problems with boundaries and others. Histrionic individuals tend to call attention to themselves by their actions, whereas dependent individuals are seeking means to cling to others.

American Psychiatric Association: Diagnostic and Statistical Manual of Mental Disorders, 5th Edition. Arlington, VA, American Psychiatric Association, 2013, pp 672–675

---

385 Which antidepressant has been shown to be most efficacious in the treatment of depression in patients with HIV/AIDS with chronic diarrhea?

A. Fluoxetine.
B. Mirtazapine.
C. Paroxetine.
D. Sertraline.
E. Venlafaxine.

The correct response is option B: Mirtazapine.

Several studies reported efficacy of various antidepressants in HIV-infected patients, but no single antidepressant has been found superior in treating HIV-infected patients as a group. The side effects of certain antidepressants can render them advantageous or disadvantageous in particular patients with HIV. For example, SSRIs are best avoided in patients with chronic diarrhea. SNRIs should also be avoided in patients with chronic diarrhea.

Levenson JL (editor): Essentials of Psychosomatic Medicine. Arlington, VA, American Psychiatric Publishing, 2007, pp 213–14

---

386 Which of the following is the best predictor of a recurrence of depression in someone with major depressive disorder?

A. Family history of depression.
B. Prior episodes of depression.
C. Prior suicidal attempt.
D. Comorbid psychiatric disorder.
E. Comorbid medical condition.

The correct response is option B: Prior episodes of depression.

The number of lifetime major depressive episodes is significantly associated with the probability of recurrence. Risk is higher in individuals whose preceding episode was severe, in younger individuals, and in individuals who have experienced multiple episodes.

American Psychiatric Association Practice Guideline for the Treatment of Patients With Major Depressive Disorder, 3rd ed (2010), p 57. http://psychiatryonline.org/guidelines.aspx
American Psychiatric Association: Diagnostic and Statistical Manual of Mental Disorders, 5th Edition. Arlington, VA, American Psychiatric Association, 2013, p 165

---

387 A patient has been successfully treated with an SSRI for acute panic episodes. What is the minimum length of time recommended for maintenance pharmacotherapy for this patient?

A. 2–4 months.
B. 6–12 months.
C. 18 months.
D. Over 24 months.

The correct response is option B: 6–12 months.

The American Psychiatric Association Guideline for the Treatment of Patients With Panic Disorder (2008) recommends maintenance pharmacotherapy for at least 6–12 months following acute treatment. Studies of fluoxetine, paroxetine, sertraline, imipramine, and clomipramine have demonstrated a benefit of continuing medication for 6–12 months. Maintenance pharmacotherapy should be considered for most patients as a means of preventing recurrence of panic disorder symptoms and promoting continued symptom relief and better functioning.

American Psychiatric Association Practice Guideline for the Treatment of Patients with Panic Disorder (2009). http://psychiatryonline.org/guidelines.aspx

388 Which of the following is a required gateway symptom for major depressive disorder?

A. Insomnia or hypersomnia.
B. Recurrent thoughts of death.
C. Feelings of worthlessness.
D. Psychomotor agitation or retardation.
E. Loss of interest or pleasure.

The correct response is option E: Loss of interest or pleasure.

According to DSM-5, the diagnosis of either a major depressive episode or major depressive disorder requires the presence of either a depressed mood (a change from previous functioning) or a loss of interest or pleasure as one of five required symptoms from nine symptom categories. Symptoms must have been evident for at least 2 weeks.

American Psychiatric Association: Diagnostic and Statistical Manual of Mental Disorders, 5th Edition. Arlington, VA, American Psychiatric Association, 2013, pp 160–161

389 In contrast to delusional disorder, schizophrenia is characterized by which of the following?

A. Disorganized speech.
B. Grandiosity.
C. Mood episodes.
D. Paranoid beliefs.
E. Physiological effects of a general medical condition.

The correct response is option A: Disorganized speech.

The differential diagnosis between schizophrenia and delusional disorder rests on the presence of other characteristic symptoms of schizophrenia (hallucinations, disorganized speech or behavior, prominent negative symptoms). Both paranoid beliefs and grandiosity may be common to schizophrenia and delusional disorder. General medical conditions must be ruled out prior to making a diagnosis of schizophrenia.

American Psychiatric Association: Diagnostic and Statistical Manual of Mental Disorders, 5th Edition. Arlington, VA, American Psychiatric Association, 2013, pp 90–93, 99–104

390 In DSM-5, which of the following symptoms of PTSD is classified as a criterion D symptom of negative alteration in cognition or mood?

A. Difficulty falling asleep.
B. Recurrent nightmares.
C. Exaggerated startle response.
D. Inability to recall important aspects of the trauma.
E. Difficulty concentrating.

The correct response is option D: Inability to recall important aspects of the trauma.

Inability to recall important aspects of the trauma is a criterion D symptom of PTSD (negative alteration in cognition or mood). In DSM-5, the DSM-IV avoidance/numbing cluster is divided into criterion C avoidance and criterion D persistent negative alterations in cognitions and mood. This latter category retains most of the DSM-IV numbing symptoms and also includes new or reconceptualized symptoms, such as persistent negative emotional states. Criterion E—alterations in arousal and reactivity—retains most of the DSM-IV arousal symptoms. It also includes irritable or aggressive behavior and reckless or self-destructive behavior. Criterion C avoidance symptoms include efforts to avoid thoughts, feelings, conversations, activities, places, or people that arouse recollection of the event. Options A, C, and E are symptoms of increased arousal and reactivity, whereas B is a symptom of intrusion.

American Psychiatric Association: Diagnostic and Statistical Manual of Mental Disorders, 5th Edition. Arlington, VA, American Psychiatric Association, 2013, pp 271–272

391 The personality disorder most closely associated with social anxiety disorder is which of the following?

A. Schizoid.
B. Obsessive-compulsive.
C. Histrionic.
D. Avoidant.
E. Borderline.

The correct response is option D: Avoidant.

DSM-5 lists the essential features of avoidant personality disorder (APD) as "a pervasive pattern of social inhibition, feelings of inadequacy, and hypersensitivity to negative evaluation that begins by early adulthood...." There is considerable overlap between the features of generalized social anxiety disorder and those of APD, and there is a stronger association with social anxiety disorder and APD than with other personality disorders, "so much so they may be viewed as alternative conceptualizations of the same or similar conditions."

American Psychiatric Association: Diagnostic and Statistical Manual of Mental Disorders, 5th Edition. Arlington, VA, American Psychiatric Association, 2013, pp 672–674

Hummelen B, Wilberg T, Pedersen G, Karterud S: The relationship between avoidant personality disorder and social phobia. Compr Psychiatry 2007; 48:348–356

Stein MB, Stein DJ: Social anxiety disorder. Lancet 2008; 371:1115–1125

---

392 In order to make a diagnosis of bulimia nervosa, the symptoms must have duration of at least:

A. 1 month.
B. 3 months.
C. 6 months.
D. 9 months.
E. 12 months.

The correct response is option B: 3 months.

According to the DSM-5, symptoms of bulimia nervosa must be present at least once a week for at least 3 months. Prior to 3 months the patient would be diagnosed with other specified feeding or eating disorder (bulimia nervosa [of low frequency and/or limited duration]).

American Psychiatric Association: Diagnostic and Statistical Manual of Mental Disorders, 5th Edition. Arlington, VA, American Psychiatric Association, 2013, pp 345, 353

---

393 A 65-year-old man whose wife died 3 months ago presents to the clinic, accompanied by his daughter. The daughter states that the couple were married for 40 years and that he now feels utterly worthless without his wife. Since her death, he has stayed in the house, letting the newspapers pile up, and he doesn't answer the phone. He stopped his weekly fishing trips with his neighbor, a pastime of his for 20 years. He denies suicidal ideation but states that he wishes to join his wife. He has lost 30 pounds over the past 3 months and has stopped taking his hypertension medications. What is the most likely diagnosis?

A. Bereavement.
B. Adjustment disorder with depressed mood.
C. Major depressive disorder.
D. Depressive disorder, not otherwise specified.
E. Persistent depressive disorder (dysthymic disorder).

The correct response is option C: Major depressive disorder.

Although the death of his spouse clearly precipitated his current symptoms, their severity places his diagnosis past the point of normal bereavement or an adjustment disorder, which, by definition, cannot be represented by normal bereavement. He has enough symptoms to meet criteria for major depressive disorder. The bereavement exclusion is omitted in DSM-5 to remove the implication that bereavement typically lasts only 2 months; bereavement is recognized as a severe psychosocial stressor that can precipitate a major depressive episode; a detailed footnote has replaced the DSM-IV exclusion to aid clinicians in making the critical distinction between the symptoms characteristic of bereavement and those of a major depressive episode. Dysthymia in DSM-IV now falls under the category of persistent depressive disorder, which includes both chronic major depressive disorder and the previous dysthymic disorder. An inability to find scientifically meaningful differences between these two conditions led to their combination with specifiers included to identify different pathways to the diagnosis and to provide continuity with DSM-IV.

American Psychiatric Association: Diagnostic and Statistical Manual of Mental Disorders, 5th Edition. Arlington, VA, American Psychiatric Association, 2013, pp 160–168

394 In dialectical behavior therapy (DBT), the term *dialectical* refers to which of the following therapeutic principles?

A. Psychic integration of good and bad objects.
B. A simultaneous emphasis on validation and change.
C. Efforts to treat both the manic and depressed phases of bipolar disorder.
D. A simultaneous focus on both thoughts and behaviors.
E. A dual focus on one's feelings and their impact on others.

The correct response is option B: A simultaneous emphasis on validation and change.

DBT was developed by Linehan, in part based on the observation that patients with borderline personality disorder often find an emphasis on behavioral change feels as though it invalidates their painful inner experiences. The "dialectic" of this new therapy would be a dual emphasis on both validation of these painful feelings alongside change strategies, which are also necessary for providing hope and improving functioning. The first option refers to the psychodynamic concept of integrating split objects, most attributable to Melanie Klein but also further developed within object relations theory. Dialectical behavior therapy does not target bipolar disorder. Option D describes cognitive-behavioral therapy, and option E does not refer to any specific type of psychotherapy formally, although it may be a target of many therapeutic treatments.

Shearin EN, Linehan MM: Dialectical behavior therapy for borderline personality disorder: theoretical and empirical foundations. Acta Psychiatr Scand Suppl, 1994; 379:61–8

Textbook of Psychotherapeutic Treatments. Gabbard GO (ed) Arlington VA, American Psychiatric Publishing, 2009, pp 731–732

395 Which of the following approaches to neurotransmitter modulation would be most appropriate in treating a patient with Tourette's disorder?

A. Dopaminergic modulation at the striatum and serotonergic modulation at the orbitofrontal cortex.
B. Dopaminergic modulation at the striatum.
C. Serotonergic modulation at the orbitofrontal cortex.
D. Noradrenergic modulation.

The correct response is option B: Dopaminergic modulation at the striatum.

Body dysmorphic disorder and non-tic-related OCD respond best to serotonergic modulation. Tic-related OCD responds best to a combination of serotonergic and dopaminergic modulation. Tourette's disorder responds to dopaminergic modulation at the level of the striatum but not to serotonergic modulation at the orbitofrontal cortex. Noradrenergic modulation does not seem to be active in the treatment of Tourette's disorder.

Fineberg NA, Gale TM, Sivakumaran T. A review of antipsychotics in the treatment of obsessive compulsive disorder. J Psychopharmacology 2006; 20:97–103. Reprinted in FOCUS: OCD summer 2007; 3:354–360

Dougherty DD, Rauch SL, Greenberg BD. Pathophysiology of Obsessive-Compulsive Disorders, in American Psychiatric Publishing Textbook of Anxiety Disorders. Edited by Stein DJ, Hollander E, Rothbaum BO. Arlington, VA, American Psychiatric Publishing, 2010, pp 291–92

396 Features that support the diagnosis of somatic symptom disorder include distressing somatic symptoms plus abnormal thoughts, persistently high level of anxiety, and

A. State of being symptomatic that is persistent.
B. Distinct, clearly delineated symptoms of limited duration.
C. Symptoms that are different from those of organic disorders.
D. Symptoms that do not cause functional impairment.
E. Signs that are not acknowledged or recognized by the patient.

The correct response is option A: State of being symptomatic is persistent.

Individuals with somatic symptom disorder tend to have ongoing symptoms without physical signs or structural abnormalities. Often the symptoms are vague, multiple, confusing, and persistent and similar to the symptoms of organically based disorders.

Sadock BJ, Sadock VA, Ruiz P (eds): Kaplan & Sadock's Comprehensive Textbook of Psychiatry, 9th ed. Philadelphia, Lippincott Williams & Wilkins, 2009, pp 1928–35

American Psychiatric Association: Diagnostic and Statistical Manual of Mental Disorders, 5th Edition. Arlington, VA, American Psychiatric Association, 2013, p 311

---

397 Demographic and clinical factors associated with suicide in patients with schizophrenia include:

A. Older age.
B. Female gender.
C. Higher cognitive function.
D. Lower socioeconomic status.
E. Good social support.

The correct response is option C: Higher cognitive function.

About 20%–50% of patients with schizophrenia attempt suicide, whereas up to 10% eventually commit suicide. Demographic and clinical factors associated with suicide include young age, male gender, single marital status, depressive symptoms and hopelessness, more severe illness, frequent relapses, recent hospitalization, good insight, higher cognitive functions, higher socioeconomic background, poor social functioning, and lack of social support.

American Psychiatric Association Practice Guideline for the Treatment of Patients with Schizophrenia, 2nd ed (2004), pp 577–78, 607–608. http://psychiatryonline.org/guidelines.aspx

Kirkpatrick B and Tek C. Schizophrenia: Clinical Features and Psychopathology Concepts, in: Sadock BJ, Sadock VA (eds): Kaplan and Sadock's Comprehensive Textbook of Psychiatry, 8th ed. Philadelphia, Lippincott Williams & Wilkins, 2005, pp 1416–36

VanOs J and Allardyce J. The Clinical Epidemiology of Schizophrenia, in Sadock BJ, Sadock VA, Ruiz P (eds): Kaplan & Sadock's Comprehensive Textbook of Psychiatry, 9th ed. Philadelphia, Lippincott Williams & Wilkins, 2009, pp 1475–87

---

398 Which of the following therapeutic strategies for OCD maintains treatment success for the longest period of time after active therapy is discontinued?

A. Psychoeducation.
B. Record keeping.
C. A selective serotonin reuptake inhibitor.
D. Exposure and response prevention.
E. Supportive psychotherapy.

The correct response is option D: Exposure and response prevention.

Exposure and response prevention has the strongest research supporting effectiveness in maintaining long-term gains after active treatment. SSRIs and other agents are as effective while the patient is on the drugs, but relapse may occur when patients discontinue pharmacotherapy. Supportive therapy has not been shown to be efficacious. Psychoeducation and record keeping are useful adjuncts to treatment.

American Psychiatric Association Practice Guideline for the Treatment of Patients with Obsessive-Compulsive Disorder 2007. http://psychiatryonline.org/guidelines.aspx

Greist J, Jefferson J. Obsessive-compulsive disorder. FOCUS: OCD: Summer 2007; 3:283–298

---

399 The highest level of decision-making capacity is required for which of the following actions?

A. Making a will.
B. Appointing a substitute decision maker.
C. Agreeing to participate in a research study.
D. Making a decision about treatment.
E. Consenting to phlebotomy.

The correct response is option C: Agreeing to participate in a research study.

Drane proposed a sliding scale for capacity: the more serious the issue at stake, the higher the threshold for decisional capacity. Agreement to participate in clinical research requires the highest standard because the patient must be able to understand that he or she will not necessarily be in an active treatment arm.

Rosenstein DL, Miller FG. Ethical issues. in: American Psychiatric Publishing Textbook of Psychosomatic Medicine, edited by Levenson JL. Arlington, VA, American Psychiatric Publishing, 2005, p 58

Drane JF. Competency to give an informed consent. A model for making clinical assessments. JAMA. 1984 Aug 17; 252(7):92 5–7

---

400 Which of the following agents has been shown to be effective in the treatment of trauma-related nightmares and sleep disruption?

A. Phenelzine.
B. Prazosin.
C. Bupropion.
D. Cyproheptadine.
E. Diphenhydramine.

The correct response is option B: Prazosin.

A series of controlled studies have shown that the α-adrenergic antagonist prazosin is effective in increasing total sleep time and REM sleep and in reducing nightmares.

Maher MJ, Rego SA, Asnis GM. Sleep disturbances in patients with post-traumatic stress disorder: epidemiology, impact and approaches to management. CNS Drugs. 20(7):567–590

Benedek DM, Friedman MJ, Zatzick D, Ursano RJ. Guideline Watch (March 2009): Practice Guideline for the Treatment of Patients with Acute Stress Disorder and Posttraumatic Stress Disorder. FOCUS. 2009; 2:204–213. http://psychiatryonline.org/guidelines.aspx

Raskind MA, Peterson K, Williams T, et al: A trial of prazosin for combat trauma PTSD with nightmares in active-duty soldiers returned from Iraq and Afghanistan. Am J Psychiatry. 2013 Sep 1; 170(9):1003–10

FOCUS Psychiatry Review (Volume 2, DSM® Revised Edition): Answer Sheet

1. A	51. D	101. D	151. A	201. A	251. C	301. B	351. A
2. B	52. E	102. E	152. E	202. B	252. B	302. A	352. E
3. D	53. D	103. E	153. D	203. A	253. A	303. B	353. D
4. C	54. C	104. C	154. A	204. B	254. E	304. D	354. B
5. B	55. B	105. E	155. C	205. C	255. B	305. B	355. B
6. B	56. C	106. D	156. A	206. C	256. B	306. E	356. A
7. A	57. A	107. A	157. C	207. E	257. A	307. B	357. A
8. C	58. C	108. C	158. C	208. E	258. C	308. C	358. D
9. E	59. A	109. D	159. A	209. C	259. D	309. D	359. D
10. C	60. B	110. D	160. A	210. A	260. D	310. D	360. D
11. B	61. B	111. C	161. E	211. A	261. C	311. D	361. B
12. B	62. C	112. C	162. C	212. A	262. B	312. C	362. B
13. C	63. B	113. D	163. D	213. A	263. D	313. B	363. C
14. E	64. D	114. B	164. E	214. D	264. E	314. B	364. C
15. B	65. D	115. A	165. B	215. D	265. C	315. E	365. A
16. A	66. B	116. C	166. C	216. A	266. D	316. D	366. B
17. C	67. A	117. A	167. A	217. C	267. D	317. B	367. D
18. A	68. A	118. E	168. B	218. A	268. E	318. D	368. D
19. C	69. B	119. C	169. D	219. D	269. E	319. C	369. E
20. B	70. C	120. D	170. C	220. A	270. E	320. B	370. B
21. B	71. B	121. D	171. D	221. C	271. B	321. C	371. B
22. D	72. B	122. E	172. C	222. B	272. E	322. B	372. B
23. A	73. D	123. C	173. A	223. D	273. E	323. C	373. D
24. D	74. C	124. B	174. A	224. C	274. B	324. C	374. B
25. B	75. B	125. B	175. B	225. D	275. A	325. E	375. D
26. E	76. C	126. A	176. C	226. A	276. B	326. E	376. B
27. E	77. C	127. E	177. D	227. D	277. A	327. C	377. B
28. A	78. A	128. B	178. A	228. A	278. B	328. D	378. D
29. E	79. C	129. B	179. E	229. E	279. A	329. D	379. B
30. A	80. A	130. B	180. B	230. D	280. E	330. A	380. C
31. C	81. B	131. A	181. E	231. A	281. B	331. A	381. B
32. D	82. C	132. C	182. E	232. C	282. C	332. B	382. B
33. A	83. A	133. D	183. C	233. E	283. B	333. A	383. B
34. B	84. C	134. B	184. C	234. A	284. A	334. C	384. C
35. D	85. A	135. C	185. C	235. A	285. D	335. E	385. B
36. C	86. B	136. D	186. C	236. D	286. A	336. C	386. B
37. A	87. B	137. C	187. E	237. A	287. A	337. A	387. B
38. C	88. C	138. C	188. B	238. D	288. C	338. B	388. E
39. D	89. E	139. C	189. B	239. A	289. B	339. D	389. A
40. D	90. A	140. B	190. D	240. E	290. D	340. B	390. D
41. A	91. B	141. B	191. B	241. E	291. B	341. D	391. D
42. E	92. B	142. B	192. D	242. B	292. D	342. C	392. B
43. A	93. B	143. D	193. D	243. E	293. D	343. E	393. C
44. B	94. C	144. B	194. A	244. A	294. C	344. E	394. B
45. E	95. D	145. B	195. B	245. C	295. A	345. A	395. B
46. E	96. C	146. D	196. A	246. C	296. B	346. D	396. A
47. D	97. C	147. E	197. B	247. D	297. B	347. C	397. C
48. A	98. E	148. E	198. B	248. E	298. E	348. E	398. D
49. C	99. C	149. B	199. B	249. C	299. A	349. D	399. C
50. E	100. E	150. C	200. D	250. D	300. D	350. C	400. B

1. _____	51. _____	101. _____	151. _____	201. _____	251. _____	301. _____	351. _____
2. _____	52. _____	102. _____	152. _____	202. _____	252. _____	302. _____	352. _____
3. _____	53. _____	103. _____	153. _____	203. _____	253. _____	303. _____	353. _____
4. _____	54. _____	104. _____	154. _____	204. _____	254. _____	304. _____	354. _____
5. _____	55. _____	105. _____	155. _____	205. _____	255. _____	305. _____	355. _____
6. _____	56. _____	106. _____	156. _____	206. _____	256. _____	306. _____	356. _____
7. _____	57. _____	107. _____	157. _____	207. _____	257. _____	307. _____	357. _____
8. _____	58. _____	108. _____	158. _____	208. _____	258. _____	308. _____	358. _____
9. _____	59. _____	109. _____	159. _____	209. _____	259. _____	309. _____	359. _____
10. _____	60. _____	110. _____	160. _____	210. _____	260. _____	310. _____	360. _____
11. _____	61. _____	111. _____	161. _____	211. _____	261. _____	311. _____	361. _____
12. _____	62. _____	112. _____	162. _____	212. _____	262. _____	312. _____	362. _____
13. _____	63. _____	113. _____	163. _____	213. _____	263. _____	313. _____	363. _____
14. _____	64. _____	114. _____	164. _____	214. _____	264. _____	314. _____	364. _____
15. _____	65. _____	115. _____	165. _____	215. _____	265. _____	315. _____	365. _____
16. _____	66. _____	116. _____	166. _____	216. _____	266. _____	316. _____	366. _____
17. _____	67. _____	117. _____	167. _____	217. _____	267. _____	317. _____	367. _____
18. _____	68. _____	118. _____	168. _____	218. _____	268. _____	318. _____	368. _____
19. _____	69. _____	119. _____	169. _____	219. _____	269. _____	319. _____	369. _____
20. _____	70. _____	120. _____	170. _____	220. _____	270. _____	320. _____	370. _____
21. _____	71. _____	121. _____	171. _____	221. _____	271. _____	321. _____	371. _____
22. _____	72. _____	122. _____	172. _____	222. _____	272. _____	322. _____	372. _____
23. _____	73. _____	123. _____	173. _____	223. _____	273. _____	323. _____	373. _____
24. _____	74. _____	124. _____	174. _____	224. _____	274. _____	324. _____	374. _____
25. _____	75. _____	125. _____	175. _____	225. _____	275. _____	325. _____	375. _____
26. _____	76. _____	126. _____	176. _____	226. _____	276. _____	326. _____	376. _____
27. _____	77. _____	127. _____	177. _____	227. _____	277. _____	327. _____	377. _____
28. _____	78. _____	128. _____	178. _____	228. _____	278. _____	328. _____	378. _____
29. _____	79. _____	129. _____	179. _____	229. _____	279. _____	329. _____	379. _____
30. _____	80. _____	130. _____	180. _____	230. _____	280. _____	330. _____	380. _____
31. _____	81. _____	131. _____	181. _____	231. _____	281. _____	331. _____	381. _____
32. _____	82. _____	132. _____	182. _____	232. _____	282. _____	332. _____	382. _____
33. _____	83. _____	133. _____	183. _____	233. _____	283. _____	333. _____	383. _____
34. _____	84. _____	134. _____	184. _____	234. _____	284. _____	334. _____	384. _____
35. _____	85. _____	135. _____	185. _____	235. _____	285. _____	335. _____	385. _____
36. _____	86. _____	136. _____	186. _____	236. _____	286. _____	336. _____	386. _____
37. _____	87. _____	137. _____	187. _____	237. _____	287. _____	337. _____	387. _____
38. _____	88. _____	138. _____	188. _____	238. _____	288. _____	338. _____	388. _____
39. _____	89. _____	139. _____	189. _____	239. _____	289. _____	339. _____	389. _____
40. _____	90. _____	140. _____	190. _____	240. _____	290. _____	340. _____	390. _____
41. _____	91. _____	141. _____	191. _____	241. _____	291. _____	341. _____	391. _____
42. _____	92. _____	142. _____	192. _____	242. _____	292. _____	342. _____	392. _____
43. _____	93. _____	143. _____	193. _____	243. _____	293. _____	343. _____	393. _____
44. _____	94. _____	144. _____	194. _____	244. _____	294. _____	344. _____	394. _____
45. _____	95. _____	145. _____	195. _____	245. _____	295. _____	345. _____	395. _____
46. _____	96. _____	146. _____	196. _____	246. _____	296. _____	346. _____	396. _____
47. _____	97. _____	147. _____	197. _____	247. _____	297. _____	347. _____	397. _____
48. _____	98. _____	148. _____	198. _____	248. _____	298. _____	348. _____	398. _____
49. _____	99. _____	149. _____	199. _____	249. _____	299. _____	349. _____	399. _____
50. _____	100. _____	150. _____	200. _____	250. _____	300. _____	350. _____	400. _____

Index of Questions by Topic

This index provides a guide for review of questions by topic area. Many questions apply to more than one topic area but are indexed by one or two topics only.

CPSIA information can be obtained
at www.ICGtesting.com
Printed in the USA
LVOW05s0718210417
531605LV00002B/2/P

9 780890 424629